PROTEIN BLOOD GROUP ANTIGENS OF THE HUMAN RED CELL

THE JOHNS HOPKINS SERIES IN HEMATOLOGY/ONCOLOGY

CONSULTING EDITORS

Jerry L. Spivak, M.D.
Martin D. Abeloff, M.D.

PROTEIN BLOOD GROUP ANTIGENS OF THE HUMAN RED CELL

STRUCTURE, FUNCTION, AND CLINICAL SIGNIFICANCE

Edited by

PETER C. AGRE, M.D.
Departments of Medicine and Cell Biology/Anatomy
Johns Hopkins University School of Medicine
Baltimore, Maryland

and

JEAN-PIERRE CARTRON, Ph.D.
Institut National de la Santé et de la Recherche Médicàle (INSERM)
Institut National de Transfusion Sanguine
Paris, France

THE JOHNS HOPKINS UNIVERSITY PRESS
Baltimore and London

Printed in the United States of America on acid-free paper

The Johns Hopkins University Press
701 West 40th Street
Baltimore, Maryland 21211-2190
The Johns Hopkins Press Ltd., London

Library of Congress Cataloging-in-Publication Data

Protein blood group antigens of the human red cell : structure, function, and clinical significance / edited by Peter C. Agre and Jean-Pierre Cartron.
p. cm. — (The Johns Hopkins series in hematology/oncology)
Includes bibliographical references and index.
ISBN 0-8018-4493-2 (hc)
1. Blood group antigens. 2. Erythrocyte membranes. 3. Membrane proteins. 4. Anemia—Pathophysiology. I. Agre, Peter, 1949– . II. Cartron, Jean-Pierre. III. Series.
[DNLM: 1. Antigens. 2. Blood Groups—immunology. 3. Erythrocytes—physiology. 4. Hematologic Diseases—physiopathology. WH 150 P9665]
QP98.P75 1992
616.07′92—dc20
DNLM/DLC
for Library of Congress 92-49755
CIP

To our children:
Sara, Claire, Clarke, and Anne Carlyle Agre
Valerie and Cecile Cartron

CONTENTS

FOREWORD

Human blood groups constitute an increasing list of symbols, each denoting a red cell polymorphism. Until recently, little biochemical information existed for many of these antigens. Nevertheless, the serologic recognition of them has made possible much clinical research and the treatment of diseases such as hemolytic disease of the newborn.

At present, the fields of immunology, genetics, and biochemistry have merged to advance our understanding of the human blood group antigens. Serologists make immunologic observations on inherited antigenic structures, and biochemists identify the molecular basis of the structures using methods of protein chemistry and molecular genetics. This was the case, for example, for the M^c variant of the MNSs system. Confusing serologic reactions with M and N reagents were explained when the amino acid sequence of the M^c protein was found to contain serine at position 1 and glutamate at position 5, which is intermediate between the sequences of the M and N proteins. Thus the molecular explanation of the "epitope" was revealed. It is likely that similar efforts will be needed to elucidate the molecular basis of the many blood group antigens that still await explanation.

This book describes many new biochemical aspects of human blood group antigens carried by proteins in the red cell membrane. This membrane is ideal for biologic research, since it is readily available and may be purified in large amounts. These properties have made possible recent work that has led to the molecular understanding of the enigmatic Rh antigens. Human monoclonal Rh-specific antibodies permitted immunologic isolation of the core structural protein, which was analyzed by flow cytometry, radioimmunoassay, and iodopeptide map and demonstrated to be the site of the Rh polymorphism. Molecular genetic studies permitted the isolation of the complementary DNA encoding a 416–amino acid Rh protein. Subsequent molecular genetic research demonstrated a gene duplication and other findings that together provide insight into this highly polymorphic antigen group. It is to be hoped that the physiologic role of Rh may also be defined.

Besides Rh, many other examples of blood group research are contained in this book. Molecular research of several blood group antigens has provided a highly refined understanding of the antigen structures, thereby providing the molecular perspective from which to view their involvement in blood transfusion, hemolytic disease of the newborn, and autoimmunity. Red cell diseases and abnormalities may be associated with blood groups or antigenic markers such as Rh_{null}, Leach, McLeod, HEMPAS, and others.

The reader will find extensive recent data in this book. The contributors are to be congratulated for giving us the opportunity to absorb these new approaches to studying the blood group antigens. The message of the book is to challenge the next generation to continue this type of study, which may eventually unveil the molecular basis of most blood group antigens and may provide tools for the elucidation of many topics that are still speculative. I encourage you to read this book, to know the current state of this field and to understand future discoveries.

Charles Salmon, M.D., D.Sc.
Emeritus Director, Institut National de Transfusion Sanguine, Paris
Karl Landsteiner Award, 1988

PREFACE

In addition to the ABH antigens and a few other well-understood oligosaccharide structures, red cells are known to contain over 400 other antigens, many being membrane proteins that fit into several families known as the "blood groups." Despite long-recognized clinical importance, the molecular basis of most protein blood group antigens is still obscure.

It was a pleasant surprise when the two of us met at the 1987 Red Cell Gordon Conference in Plymouth, New Hampshire. Without knowing of each other's work, our laboratories had both set about isolating and characterizing the core structural proteins of the Rh blood group antigens. From our conversations during those summer afternoons, we recognized that each of us had independently arrived at the same tenet—that most serologically described blood group antigens probably represent polymorphisms within functionally important but yet unidentified membrane proteins. We also knew of several other investigators who were studying different protein blood group antigens.

Our laboratories have pursued a few common studies since that time, and we have maintained our discussions of blood group antigens. Indeed, several of our early speculations have proven to be correct. When the Johns Hopkins University Press presented us with the opportunity of assembling a volume on red cell blood group antigens, it was quickly apparent that this area of research was ripe for presentation.

It was not our goal to provide an encyclopedic collection of all relevant materials. We planned a series of reviews written by investigators who are leading authorities on each of the respective antigens. We hope that this volume is of interest to a wide scientific audience, including laboratory investigators, blood bank technologists, physicians, and students. Because of constraints on size and cost, we decided to restrict our scope to the protein blood group antigens.

The contents of this book are empirically split into two parts: Part I (structure and function) and Part II (diseases), but there is considerable overlap. All chapters illustrate the concept that blood group antigens are of functional importance to normal red cell membrane physiology and are of primary pathologic significance in certain diseases.

Each of the major protein blood groups is presented in this volume. The discovery of several proteins carrying blood group antigens is told in Chapter 1 by an investigator who had a pioneering role in that work. Full accounts of the molecular structure of the Rh antigens, their involvement in hemolytic disease of the newborn, and the structure of the immunoglobulins are presented in Chapters 2, 9, and 10. The molecular structure of the enigmatic Kell antigens was recently solved, and it revealed an unforeseen homology with a class of membrane proteases that may be involved in degradation of peptide hormones, the subject of Chapter 3. The complex biology of Lutheran antigen expression is presented in Chapter 4, which describes how a distinct gene product essential for the expression of Lutheran antigens also controls the expression of a large class of membrane immunoregulatory structures. Although still incompletely defined, provocative studies linking Kidd antigens and the urea transporter are discussed in Chapter 5. Chapters 6 and 7 present the detailed molecular structure of the glycophorins and full accounts of their evolution and functional significance to membrane integrity. The distribution of these antigens is not entirely specific for red cells, and new primary data are presented in Chapter 8. The existence of phosphatidylinositol-glycan–linked membrane antigens represents a very new revelation in blood group antigen biology, and explains paroxysmal hemoglobinuria, a longstanding clinical puzzle, discussed in Chapter 11. Malaria is the red cell disease of largest worldwide importance, and the molecular involvement of Duffy antigens and glycophorins in the invasion of red cells is presented in Chapter 12. Red cell membrane proteins are known to be pathologically involved in congenital dyserythropoietic anemias; this is discussed in Chapter 13.

The members of our research staff at Johns Hopkins and at INTS-Paris are acknowledged for their excellent suggestions and encouragement. Special thanks go to our colleagues whose work appears in this book and who generously spent many hours composing the chapters. We look forward to continued scientific progress in this exciting area of biomedical research.

Support for this volume was provided by NATO grant 0556/88 and by grants from NIH and INSERM.

LIST OF CONTRIBUTORS

David J. Anstee, Ph.D., Director, International Blood Group Reference Laboratory, South Western Regional Blood Transfusion Centre, Bristol, United Kingdom

Joel Anne Chasis, M.D., Staff Scientist, Division of Cell and Molecular Biology, Lawrence Berkeley Laboratory, University of California, Berkeley, California

Otto Fröhlich, Ph.D., Associate Professor, Department of Physiology, Emory University School of Medicine, Atlanta, Georgia

Michiko N. Fukuda, Ph.D., Staff Scientist, La Jolla Cancer Research Foundation, La Jolla, California

Carl G. Gahmberg, M.D., Professor, Department of Biochemistry, University of Helsinki, Helsinki, Finland

J. Jay Gargus, M.D., Ph.D., Associate Professor, Department of Physiology, Emory University School of Medicine, Atlanta, Georgia

Robert B. Gunn, M.D., Professor and Chairman, Department of Physiology, Emory University School of Medicine, Atlanta, Georgia

Terence J. Hadley, M.D., Associate Professor, Division of Hematology/ Oncology, Department of Medicine, James Graham Brown Cancer Center, University of Louisville, Louisville, Kentucky

Christopher H. Holmes, Ph.D., Research Fellow, University Department of Obstetrics and Gynaecology, St. Michael's Hospital, Bristol, United Kingdom

Nevin C. Hughes-Jones, M.D., Ph.D., Senior Investigator, Division of Transfusion Medicine, Blood Transfusion Centre, Cambridge, United Kingdom

Philip A. Judson, Ph.D. Clinical Scientist, Department of Immunochemistry, South Western Regional Blood Transfusion Centre, Bristol, United Kingdom

Jacqueline London, Ph.D., Professor, University of Paris VII; and Senior Investigator, Unité INSERM U76, Institut National de Transfusion Sanguine, Paris, France

W. Laurence Marsh, Ph.D., Senior Investigator and Vice President for Research Emeritus, Lindsley F. Kimball Research Institute, New York Blood Center, New York, New York

Louis H. Miller, M.D., Chief, Laboratory of Malaria Research, National Institute of Allergy and Infectious Diseases, Bethesda, Maryland

Narla Mohandas, D.Sc., Senior Staff Scientist and Director, Division of Cell and Molecular Biology, Lawrence Berkeley Laboratory, University of California, Berkeley, California

Colvin M. Redman, Ph.D., Senior Investigator, Lindsley F. Kimball Research Institute, New York Blood Center, New York, New York

Wendell F. Rosse, M.D., Florence McAlister Professor of Medicine, Division of Hematology/Oncology, Department of Medicine, Duke University Medical Center, Durham, North Carolina

Don L. Siegel, Ph.D., M.D., Assistant Professor, Blood Bank and Transfusion Medicine Section, Department of Pathology and Laboratory Medicine, Hospital of the University of Pennsylvania, Philadelphia, Pennsylvania

Leslie E. Silberstein, M.D., Associate Professor and Director, Blood Bank and Transfusion Medicine Section, Department of Pathology and Laboratory Medicine, Hospital of the University of Pennsylvania, Philadelphia, Pennsylvania

Michael J. A. Tanner, Ph.D., Reader, Department of Biochemistry, School of Medical Sciences, University of Bristol, Bristol, United Kingdom

Marilyn J. Telen, M.D., Associate Professor, Division of Hematology/Oncology, Department of Medicine; and Associate Medical Director, Transfusion Service, Duke University Medical Center, Durham, North Carolina

I

THE STRUCTURE AND FUNCTION OF PROTEIN BLOOD GROUP ANTIGENS

1

RED CELL MEMBRANE PROTEINS CARRYING THE MN, ABH, AND RH ANTIGEN ACTIVITIES

Carl G. Gahmberg, M.D.

Early in this century, Landsteiner, Levine, and others showed that blood transfusion reactions are due to a reaction between red cell membrane surface antigens and specific antibodies in plasma. The development of blood group typing reagents made it possible to define these antigens serologically, an advance that had a major clinical impact. Furthermore, the discovery by Clarke and others that Rh(D) isoimmunization could be prevented by the passive transfer of anti-D immunoglobulin to pregnant Rh(D)-negative women carrying an Rh(D)-positive fetus greatly improved the prognosis of Rh(D)-incompatible pregnancies.

Despite the advances in blood group serology and clinical medicine, the molecular nature of the major human blood group antigens remained poorly understood. Only with the more recent developments in membrane biochemistry has it become possible to reveal the molecular complexity of these structures.

Another major factor leading to our increased understanding of red cell blood group molecules is the fortunate fact that the human red cell membrane proved to be an excellent model of mammalian cell membranes in general. There are several reasons for this: the membrane is easy to isolate in large quantities in pure form, it contains some proteins that are relatively simple to purify, and several interesting mutations affecting the membrane are known. Therefore, much of what we now know about cell membranes derives from studies of the red cell membrane. Several reviews on the structure of the human red cell membrane have been written, and the reader is referred to these for details on non–blood group aspects (Steck 1974; Marchesi et al. 1976; Furthmayr 1978).

Early studies of the ABO blood group system and the MN blood groups showed that sugars are involved in the activity and specificity of blood groups. Using substances purified from ovarian cyst fluids, investigators found fucose to be important for H activity, and α-N-acetyl-D-galactosamine and α-D-galactose for A and B specificities, respectively.

Subsequently, Hakomori and others isolated ABO-active glycolipids from human red cells, determined their structures, and thus firmly established the carbohydrate nature of these red cell antigens (Hakomori and Kobata 1975). Some aspects of the biochemistry of blood groups have been reviewed previously (Gahmberg and Karhi 1986; Anstee 1990).

These results implied to many that blood group antigens in general consist of carbohydrates. Only relatively recently has it become obvious that cell surface proteins act as the major blood group carriers in red cells, whether carbohydrate is involved in the antigenic determinant or not.

The mature mammalian red cell is in many respects inactive: it does not synthesize proteins or actively move. However, red cell precursors have these functions, and also contain many of the plasma membrane proteins of mature red cells. The information available on the proteins of the mature red cell membrane (their structure, localization, interaction with neighboring molecules) has been of utmost value when studying immature, differentiating precursor cells. By combining the structural information with the results of experiments on the more complicated nucleated cells, investigators obtained a most detailed understanding of the mammalian cell plasma membrane.

This chapter deals with the elucidation of the molecular characteristics of the three most important and best understood blood group antigen systems: MN, ABH, and Rh. These blood group antigens are confined to proteins of more general interest.

GLYCOPHORIN A: THE MN BLOOD GROUP GLYCOPROTEIN

Early work using influenza virus neuraminidase (a receptor-destroying enzyme!) showed that MN antigens need sialic acid for activity (Mäkelä and Cantell 1958; Springer and Ansell 1958). The protein carrying the MN blood group activities was purified and identified as a major red cell sialoglycoprotein, subsequently named *glycophorin A* (Tomita and Marchesi 1975). This protein is a major component of the red cell membrane. Mature red cells contain about 10^6 copies per cell (Gahmberg et al. 1979). In several aspects it is a classic model of membrane proteins. It was the first membrane protein shown to span a cell plasma membrane (Bretscher 1971), which is a common property of integral membrane proteins. It was among the first mammalian membrane glycoproteins studied biosynthetically in any detail (Jokinen et al. 1979). Its interaction with the cytoskeleton has been shown to be highly specific (Anderson and Marchesi 1985). It probably exists as a dimer in the membrane, and, interestingly, the polypeptides seem to be held together by noncovalent bonds within the lipid bilayer (Bormann et al. 1989).

Figure 1.1 is a schematic drawing of the structure of glycophorin A. It consists of 131 amino acids, and is a typical class 1 membrane protein.

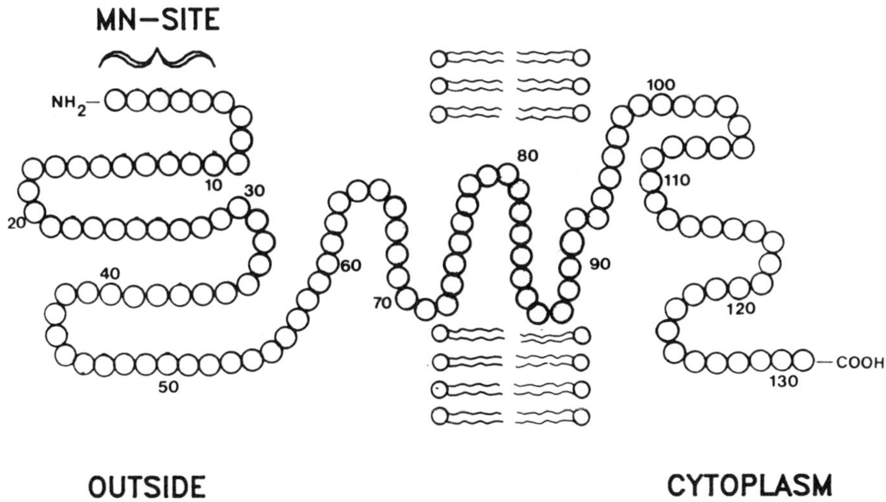

Figure 1.1. The structure of glycophorin A.
Source: Gahmberg, 1988.

Thus, the NH_2-terminal end is external to the lipid bilayer and the polypeptide contains a hydrophobic membrane-spanning sequence and a cytoplasmic COOH-terminal region, which is about 30 amino acids long. Some of the molecules are phosphorylated at serine-102. The sequence has been confirmed and slightly revised by cDNA sequencing (Siebert and Fukuda 1986). Glycophorin A is extensively glycosylated. A single N-glycosidic oligosaccharide is located at asparagine-26, but in addition the protein from mature red cells contains about 15 O-glycosidic oligosaccharides. Figure 1.2 shows the structure of the major O-glycosidic carbohydrate chain.

It was soon realized that the NH_2-terminal sequence was different when obtained from glycophorin A of MM or NN cells. In MM cells glycophorin A has the NH_2-terminal sequence Ser-Ser-Thr-Thr-Gly-, whereas the molecule isolated from NN cells has the sequence Leu-Ser-Thr-Thr-Glu- (Wasniowska et al. 1977; Furthmayr 1978). MN cells have a mixture of both. It now seems obvious that the MN specificity is due to the allelic diversity in the aminoterminal amino acid sequence. However, sialic acids in the NH_2-terminal O-glycosidic oligosaccharides are needed for the MN activity.

NANA-α2-6
|
NANA-α2-3-Gal-β1-3-GalNAc-α1-O-Ser/Thr

Figure 1.2. The structure of the major O-glycosidic carbohydrate chain of glycophorin A.

The gene structure of glycophorin A has been studied in detail (Cartron et al. 1990). It contains seven exons. The first exon codes for the signal sequence, whereas the second specifies the *MN*-specific sequence. As expected, the first and fifth codons in the second exon are different in *M* and *N* genes. The polypeptide is coded for by a gene on chromosome 4.

Glycophorin A is specific for the erythroid lineage of cells in human bone marrow (Gahmberg et al. 1978), but no specific physiologic functions for glycophorin A have been found. In fact, rare individuals are known to lack either glycophorin A [En(a−) red cells], glycophorin B, or both (Gahmberg et al. 1976; Tanner and Anstee 1976). Surprisingly, their red cells seem to function normally, and individuals with these abnormalities appear healthy. It should be pointed out, however, that the anion transport protein band 3, which contains one complex polylactosamine type of oligosaccharide, is overglycosylated in cells lacking or containing reduced levels of glycophorin A (Gahmberg et al. 1976). The oligosaccharide from mutant cells has a larger-than-normal molecular weight, which may partially compensate for the absence of glycophorin A. On the other hand, band 3 seems to be less than normally glycosylated in red cell variants containing abnormal glycophorins. Rare individuals are known to have hybrid glycophorin molecules comprising the NH_2-terminal portion of glycophorin B and the COOH-terminal portion of glycophorin A (Anstee 1990). Red cells homozygous for this defect have a band 3 molecule with an apparent molecular weight about 5 kDa less than the normal value. This correlation between the presence/absence/variability in glycophorin A and the size of the band 3 oligosaccharide could be due to the fact that these glycoproteins are synthesized together and compete for glycosylation. The types of glycosylation of O-glycosidic glycophorin A oligosaccharides and the complex N-linked band 3 oligosaccharide (see below) are very different. These findings reflect our ignorance of how cellular glycosylation is regulated in general.

When red blood cells lacking glycophorin A were found, the absence did not seem to have adverse effects. Therefore it was speculated that glycophorin A could be present and important for red cell precursors in bone marrow (Ekblom et al. 1985). Recent work, however, has established that En(a−) individuals have large deletions in their glycophorin A genes (Cartron et al. 1990), strongly indicating the absence of the protein in precursor cells.

Although the possible importance of glycophorin A for the normal function of red cells remains unclear, it is firmly established that a number of microbes use the protein as a receptor. In this context it is interesting that the *Escherichia coli* strain IH 11165 binds to glycophorin A, but only to molecules of the M type (Jokinen et al. 1985a). Detailed studies have shown that both the O-glycosidic NH_2-terminal carbohydrate and the M-specific peptide sequence are needed for the receptor to function properly.

The human erythroleukemic cell lines K562 (Andersson et al. 1979) and HEL (Martin and Papayannopoulou 1982) contain glycophorin A with the same amino acid sequence as that of mature red cells. Rabbit antiglycophorin A antisera reacted strongly with glycophorin from K562 cells. However, many monoclonal antibodies raised against glycophorin A from red cells fail to react or react weakly with glycophorin A from K562 cells or with the protein from early bone marrow erythroid precursor cells. In addition, such cells show very low MN blood group activity. During the differentiation of bone marrow erythroid cells, a substantial increase in MN activity was seen (Ekblom et al. 1985). The structural basis of this phenomenon seems to be a gradual increase in O-glycosylation during red cell differentiation, resulting in increased MN activity (Gahmberg et al. 1984). The reason for the regulation of O-glycosylation remains unclear.

The biosynthesis of glycophorin A is in many respects similar to that of other membrane glycoproteins of similar structure. In cell-free systems a leader sequence was found (Jokinen et al. 1981). Most rewarding has been to use glycophorin A as a model system for O-glycosylation. Few membrane glycoproteins are extensively O-glycosylated, and the presence of several O-glycosidic oligosaccharides in glycophorin A makes it an interesting model for this type of posttranslational modification. In general, much less is known about O-glycosylation than about N-glycosylation Evidently, the innermost N-acetylgalactosamines are attached early to glycophorin A, perhaps in the *cis*-Golgi region (Jokinen et al. 1985b). After a short lag period, the galactosyl and sialic acid residues are rapidly added, well before the protein appears at the cell surface (Jokinen et al. 1979). Whether O-glycosylation is needed for the intracellular transport of glycophorin A is not known.

ABH-ACTIVE RED CELL MEMBRANE GLYCOPROTEINS

For a long time it was believed that red cell ABH antigens were exclusively glycolipids. This was because blood group ABH–active, low-molecular-weight glycolipids were relatively easy to isolate. With the advance in methods of methylation and mass spectrometry, the structures of such glycoconjugates were firmly established. Later, high-molecular-weight, ABH-active glycolipids, megalo- or macroglycolipids, were identified and isolated from red cell membranes (Gardas and Koscielak 1973).

The obstacles to dealing with integral membrane proteins long remained too big for rewarding analysis of such components. But with the technical developments in handling membrane proteins in the 1970s, rapid development took place. Most important was the introduction of various detergents useful for membrane solubilization, cell-surface radioactive labeling techniques, lectin affinity chromatography, and the availability of purified blood group–specific glycosyl transferases.

In 1976 we found that the anion transport protein, band 3, contains an unusual type of oligosacccharide (Gahmberg et al. 1976). When isolated from normal red cells, it had an apparent molecular weight of 7.5 kDa when liberated by hydrazinolysis. Furthermore, the oligosaccharide of band 3 from En(a−) cells had an apparent molecular weight of about 11 kDa. Later, Järnefelt (1978) and Krusius (1978) and their colleagues showed that red cell membranes contain large amounts of oligosaccharides consisting of repeating D-galactose-β1-4-N-acetyl-D-glucosamine-β1-3 disaccharides. Most of them apparently originate from band 3 and the 4.5 proteins, which include the red cell glucose transport protein. These oligosaccharides contained ABH activity. The structures of these lactosaminoglycans (erythroglycans) have been further studied by Fukuda and associates (1979). Interestingly, the same oligosaccharide backbone is found in some leukocyte cell surface glycoproteins (Fukuda et al. 1985) and in lysosomal membrane glycoproteins (Carlsson et al. 1988).

Furthermore, the linear type of lactosaminoglycan, having blood group i activity, is found in K562 erythroleukemia cells and in erythroblasts obtained from fetuses and newborns. Erythroblasts from adults contain the branched galactose-β1-4-N-acetylglucosamine-β1-3D-galactose unit (Fukuda 1985).

Only a fraction of the polylactosamine type of oligosaccharides in AB cells were found to contain terminal α-N-acetyl-D-galactosamine/α-D-galactose at their nonreducing termini (Viitala et al. 1981). These A,B-active oligosaccharides have substantially higher molecular weights than the A,B-negative oligosaccharides, reflecting internal differences. Interestingly, individual ABH-active glycopeptides from AB red cells contain either A or B antigenic determinants, but not both, although the three to four branches found in these oligosaccharides would make hybrid A/B structures possible. This raises the interesting possibility that the intracellular glycosyl transferases responsible for the biosynthesis of the terminal portions of these oligosaccharides are topographically separated.

Early work on the identification of ABH-active glycoproteins in the red cell membrane was complicated by the fact that the glycoprotein fractions were contaminated with various amounts of large glycolipids. Therefore, other means of unequivocally identifying ABH-active glycoproteins became necessary.

One approach was to use blood group A− or B−specific glycosyl transferases to transfer α-N-acetylgalactosamine or galactose, respectively, from the corresponding uridine diphosphate sugars to blood group O cell acceptors. These glycosyltransferases are rather easily purified from plasma. Kobata and co-workers obtained evidence that glycophorin A molecules gained blood group A activity (Takasaki and Kobata 1976).

We purified α-N-acetylgalactosaminyl transferase from A_1 plasma, and used it to transfer radioactive N-acetylgalactosamine to blood group O cells. After this the labeled glycoproteins were visualized by fluorography

(Gahmberg and Karhi 1986). The major acceptors were band 3 and the 4.5 proteins. Indeed, some radioactivity was also incorporated into glycophorin A. This result does not prove that the visualized glycoproteins are blood group A positive. Obviously, this artificial incorporation from the outside of the cell is not physiologic. In fact, affinity chromatography of the labeled glycoproteins using the blood group A–specific lectin from *Vicia cracca* showed that only band 3 and the 4.5 proteins absorbed to the column; glycophorin A did not. That artifacts are introduced easily is also shown by the fact that when B cells were incubated with A-transferase and UDP-N-acetylgalactosamine, blood group A activity was found in B-active oligosaccharides (unpublished data). As pointed out above, normal AB cells do not seem to contain A and B activity in the same oligosaccharides.

Blood group A/B–specific lectins were useful for the identification of the blood group–active glycoproteins. We used galactose oxidase/NaB^3H_4 or lactoperoxidase/^{125}I-labeled red cell membranes and studied the A-positive glycoproteins by affinity chromatography using the *V. cracca* lectin coupled to sepharose (Karhi and Gahmberg 1980). Radioactive material, bound and eluted with N-acetylgalactosamine, was obtained only from blood group A–positive membranes. Polyacrylamide gel electrophoresis again showed that band 3 and the 4.5 proteins were the main A-active components.

Finne (1980) used ^{125}I-labeled blood group–specific lectins in blotting experiments. Band 3 and the 4.5 proteins were positive, but so was glycophorin A. This discrepancy could be due to the fact that acid-labile sialic acids are released during fixation, exposing subterminal α-N-acetylgalactosamines in the O-glycosidic oligosaccharides.

The important questions of what proportion of the total ABH-active molecules is glycoprotein and how much is found in high-molecular-weight glycolipids and in low-molecular-weight glycolipids remain unclear. All approaches have their drawbacks, but an educated guess is that the glycoproteins quantitatively constitute the most important fraction.

THE RH ANTIGENS

Among the Rhesus antigens, the Rh(D) antigen is clinically the most important and biochemically the best characterized molecule. In addition to Rh(D), this system contains the antithetical c and C anigens and e and E antigens. The c/C and e/E antigens are inherited in linkage with Rh(D) but are less immunogenic. Rh(D) incompatibility is the major cause of jaundice of the newborn. Fortunately, in many cases this disease can be prevented by the passive administration of anti-Rh(D) antibodies to the mother.

Whereas the clinical features of Rh(D) isoimmunization and Rh(D) serology are relatively well understood, the molecular nature of the Rh antigen system long remained obscure. Early work indicated that the Rh(D) antigen is an external membrane *protein*, because protease treatment could destroy antigen activity. Treatment with various glycosidases had no effect. On the other hand, extraction with lipid solvents also often destroyed the antigen activity, indicating the involvement of lipids. Several proteins expressed at the human red cell surface have been proposed to carry the Rh(D) antigen, but for a long time no consensus was reached.

This topic was reviewed by Gahmberg in 1988, but since that time some new important results have been obtained. Table 1.1 lists the most significant discoveries in Rh research.

Moore et al. (1982) and Gahmberg (1982) independently showed that surface-exposed proteins of M_r 28 to 33 kDa could specifically be immunoprecipitated with anti-Rh sera from human red cells labeled by ^{125}I-lactoperoxidase catalyzed iodination. The Rh(D) polypeptide was obtained only from Rh(D)-positive cells, and no specific band was seen in immunoprecipitates from Rh(D)-negative cells. Furthermore, polyacrylamide electrophoresis gels of —D—/—D— membranes, containing an increased number of Rh(D) antigenic sites, showed a strongly labeled band in the 30 kDa-molecular-weight region. The c and E antigens had similar molecular weights.

We previously developed radioactive surface-labeling techniques for externally exposed galactose/N-acetylgalactosamine– and sialic acid–containing glycoproteins and glycolipids. These are based on the oxidation of surface-exposed sugar by galactose oxidase or mild periodate, respectively, followed by a reduction with tritiated borohydride (Gahmberg and Hakomori 1973; Gahmberg and Andersson 1977). Naturally we used these techniques, but when the methods were applied to label the Rh(D) antigen, no radioactive band was obtained. This result indicated that the protein does not contain complex-type N-glycosidic oligosaccharides or common-type O-glycosidic sugar.

Further studies showed that the Rh(D) protein did not bind to any of several lectins studied. Mild alkaline treatment under conditions that would liberate O-glycosidic oligosaccharide did not change its apparent molecular weight on gel electrophoresis in the presence of sodium dodecyl sulfate. In addition, treatment with various glycosidases did not affect its electrophoretic mobility (Gahmberg 1983). These results strongly indicated that the Rh(D) protein does not contain carbohydrate. This would make it exceptional among mammalian cell-surface proteins, because to my knowledge no other such example has been described. The recent cloning and sequence analysis of an Rh polypeptide supports this finding, because there is no consensus sequence for N-glycosylation (Chérif-Zahar et al. 1990; Avent et al. 1990). However, it is possible that the Rh antigens are complexed to cell surface *glyco*proteins, and some evidence for this has been obtained. In fact, Moore and Green found ABH-active

Table 1.1. Important events in the history of Rh research

Year	Finding	Reference
1938	Description of hemolytic disease of the newborn	Darrow 1938
1939	Suggestion that fetal red cells are destroyed by maternal antibodies	Levine and Stetson 1939
1940	Antisera made in rhesus monkeys reacted with red cells from part of the human population	Landsteiner and Wiener 1940
1941	Full description of hemolytic disease of the newborn	Levine et al. 1941
1960–1963	Introduction of preventive measures against isoimmunization using anti-Rh(D) antisera	Stern and Berger 1960; Finn et al. 1961; Clarke et al. 1963
1972	Demonstration that lipids are needed for Rh(D) activity	Green 1972
1975	Solubilization and reconstitution of Rh(D) activity	Lorusso and Green 1975
1982	Molecular identification of the Rh(D) antigen	Gahmberg 1982; Moore et al. 1982
1983	Molecular characterization of the Rh(D) molecule	Gahmberg 1983
1984	Demonstration of an association of the Rh(D) molecule with the membrane skeleton	Gahmberg and Karhi 1984; Ridgwell et al. 1984
1987–1988	Demonstration of Rh antigen–specific polypeptides	Moore and Green 1987; Blanchard et al. 1988
1988	Determination of the NH_2-terminal sequence of Rh(D)	Bloy et al. 1988; Saboori et al. 1988
1988	Demonstration of fatty acid acylation in Rh(D)	de Vetten and Agre 1988
1990	Cloning of an Rh molecule	Chérif-Zahar et al. 1990; Avent et al. 1990

Source: Gahmberg, 1988.

glycoproteins bound to Rh antigens. This would then resemble the situation with β_2-microglobulin, which is not a bilayer-spanning protein but is nonglycosylated and specifically binds to the heavy chain of class I transplantation antigens.

Drawing on the behavior of the Rh(D) antigen on gels, I proposed that the protein is unusually hydrophobic, behaving as a proteolipid (Gahmberg 1983). This may be partially explained by the fact that the protein is a major fatty acid–acylated protein in the red cell membrane (de Vetten and Agre 1988). The polypeptide was readily labeled with radioactive fatty acids by the incubation of red cells with the labeled compounds. The acylation was reversible, and did not require protein synthesis. The function of the fatty acid is not known, but it could be involved in anchoring the Rh(D) polypeptide to the lipid bilayer. The deduced amino acid sequence also predicts an extremely hydrophobic protein.

When the Rh(D), c, and E antigens were immunoprecipitated and studied by gel electrophoresis, their apparent molecular weights were similar but not identical (Blanchard et al. 1988). Peptide mapping showed that the polypeptides were structurally related but contained distinct specific peptides. Furthermore, the Rh− polypeptide purified from Rh(D)− red cells was found to be related to the Rh(D)+ polypeptide.

Two groups recently determined the NH_2-terminal amino acid sequence of Rh polypeptides (Bloy et al. 1988; Saboori et al. 1988). The sequence was identical for the protein purified from Rh(D)+ and Rh(D)− cells: Ser-Ser-Lys-Tyr-Pro-Arg-Ser-Val-Arg-Arg-Xaa-Leu-Pro-Leu-Trp-Ala-Leu-Thr-Leu-Glu-. The Xaa was then provisionally assigned as cysteine. A computer search found no homology with previously sequenced proteins. Using the available amino acid sequence, investigators prepared oligonucleotides and screened cDNA libraries. This enabled the cloning of an Rh polypeptide (Chérif-Zaher et al. 1990; Avent et al. 1990), although which polypeptide is not known. Surprisingly, the DNA codes for a polypeptide that is larger than expected, 417 amino acids long. The NH_2-terminal methionine is removed during processing, and the predicted NH_2-terminal amino acids correspond to the published amino acid sequence. The eleventh amino acid was found to be cysteine. This would result in a protein of about 45.5 kDa molecular weight, considerably exceeding the observed value obtained by gel electrophoresis. Two main possibilities for this discrepancy remain: the COOH-terminal is shortened during processing, or the hydrophobic nature of the protein makes it move relatively fast on polyacrylamide gels in the presence of sodium dodecyl sulfate. A combination of both alternatives may also be possible. Importantly, the Rh protein is predicted to contain 13 amphipathic sequences, spanning the membrane. Because there is no obvious leader sequence, this would mean that, if the rest of the molecule after the first methionine remains intact, the COOH-terminal could be on the outside of the cell.

Membrane proteins structurally related to the Rh antigens have been purified from red cells of animals (Saboori et al. 1989). These proteins gave peptide maps partially identical to that obtained from human Rh(D). This conservation during evolution indicates an important role of this group of proteins in cellular physiology. An educated guess would be that the protein functions in transport processes. Figure 1.3 shows a schematic comparison between the probable dispositions of band 3 (anion transporter), the 4.5 protein (glucose transporter), and the cloned Rh protein. They all contain 12 to 14 hydrophobic sequences, suggesting that the Rh proteins may also be transport proteins. The location of the important antigenic site(s) is not presently known, but must, of course, be in the external hydrophilic peptide segments.

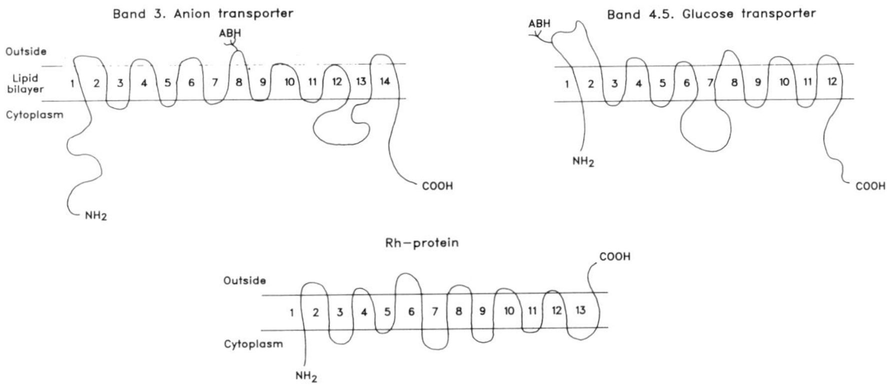

Figure 1.3. A comparison of band 3, the 4.5 protein, and the Rh protein.

The red cell membrane skeleton can be defined as the insoluble residue remaining after the treatment of membranes with nonionic detergents such as Triton X-100. This is a common procedure to solubilize integral membrane proteins for subsequent studies. When this was done and the distribution of the Rh(D) polypeptide studied, investigators observed that most of the Rh(D) polypeptides remained associated with the membrane skeleton (Gahmberg and Karhi 1984; Ridgwell et al. 1984). In contrast, the majority of the glycophorin A and band 3 molecules were solubilized. The membrane skeleton is indeed important for the stability of the Rh(D) antigen. Paradis and associates (1986) found that when Rh(D)-positive red cell membranes were solubilized with Triton X-100 and centrifuged, more than 90 percent of the antigen activity remained insoluble. Treatment with low-ionic-strength buffer solubilized the antigen from the remaining membrane skeleton in antigenically active form. However, the antigen was inactivated if isolated membranes were treated first with the low-ionic-strength buffer and then with Triton X-100.

Rh_{null} cells, apparently lacking all Rh-antigen polypeptides, are more fragile than normal red cell membranes. Furthermore, red cells from patients with hereditary spherocytosis have decreased amounts of Rh(D) antigen in their membranes (Szymanski et al. 1989). Membranes of such red cells often also contain lower-than-normal amounts of membrane skeletal proteins such as spectrin and ankyrin. These findings indicate an important role of Rh(D) and other Rh polypeptides in the stability and shape of the normal red cell membrane.

FUTURE RESEARCH

Nobody knows why we have such a large structural diversification at the red blood cell surface made up by the blood group substances. Is it chance or necessity? Is it typical of most types of cells, and we simply know best what the red cell membrane looks like? With the exception of identical siblings, the chances are low that individuals with identical red cells have ever existed. ABH blood group substances are present on epithelial cells, and in fact phylogenetic and oncogenetic studies have shown that the ABH antigens evolved earlier on epithelial cells than on blood cells (Hakomori and Kobata 1975). Therefore, it may well be that these substances had important functions early in human development, and their presence on red cells reflects remnants of earlier times.

Hakomori and co-workers showed that only four amino acids, at positions 176, 235, 266, and 268, differ between the A and B transferases (Yamamoto et al. 1990). Perhaps even more interesting was the fact that O– individuals possess a DNA sequence with one consistent base deletion, as compared to the *A*– transferase gene. This results in a frame-shift, and no functional protein can evidently be produced. In one case the *O*– gene also contained several additional base substitutions. This indicates that the additional mutations accumulated in *O* alleles, because the gene became nonfunctional through the frame-shift. *A* and *B* alleles probably diverged later.

Some correlations have been made between certain diseases and blood groups, but this issue is rather controversial and poorly understood. Thus, O– individuals may express "incompatible A antigens" in adenocarcinomas. This finding may be linked to the fact that cancer occurs less frequently in O– individuals than in A– individuals.

Interestingly, some microbes use the blood group determinants as receptors, but this does not mean that the receptor sites are physiologically important. On the contrary, no specific cellular function has been ascribed to specific blood groups. Certainly, the blood group–carrying proteins are important for cellular functions, but these seem to be due to the nonvariable molecular portions.

We have to remember that more general functions are not known for cell-surface carbohydrates. Therefore, it is not surprising that it has been difficult to find such activities for blood group–active carbohydrates. One possibility could be that specific interactions between various cells, and between soluble ligands and cells, would involve the blood group–active portions of cell-surface glycoconjugates. This does not, however, explain why different individuals have different structures in these molecules.

Perhaps we should not consider relatively simple mono- or bimolecular interactions, but instead the possibility that the variable regions together form macromolecular assemblies endowed with specific functions. This hypothesis is difficult to test, and probably needs the purification and reconstitution of molecular mixtures in vitro. Another approach would be to make transgenic animals with new blood groups, or to specifically delete blood group antigens. The elucidation of still-unknown functions makes blood group research exciting.

The Rh blood groups must be defined by specific amino acid sequences, because no sugar is found in these proteins. The recent cloning of one Rh protein should soon solve this problem. The Rh polypeptides seem important for the normal red cell because Rh_{null} cells lacking all Rh antigens are less resistant to hypoosmotic lysis. Furthermore, they have abnormal shapes. The strong association of the Rh(D)-polypeptides with the membrane skeleton is probably important in this respect.

We also have to remember that the mature human red cell lacks several important cellular functions and contains no intracellular organelles. Therefore, a major possibility to keep in mind is that essential blood group–associated functions are most important in immature erythroid cells and nonerythroid organs. However, this area of research is still very poorly developed at the molecular level.

ACKNOWLEDGMENTS

The original work was supported by the Academy of Finland and the Sigrid Jusélius Foundation. I thank Yvonne Heinilä for expert secretarial assistance.

REFERENCES

Anderson, R. A., and V. T. Marchesi. 1985. Regulation of the association of membrane skeletal protein 4.1 with glycophorin by a polyphosphoinositide. *Nature* 318:295–98.

Andersson, L. C., K. Nilsson, and C. G. Gahmberg. 1979. K562: A human erythroleukemic cell line. *Int. J. Cancer* 23:143–47.

Anstee, D. 1990. Blood group-active surface molecules of the human red blood cell. *Vox Sang.* 58:1–20.

Avent, N. D., K. Ridgwell, M. J. A. Tanner, and D. J. Anstee. 1990. cDNA cloning of the 30kDa erythrocyte membrane protein associated with Rh (Rhesus)-blood-group-antigen expression. *Biochem. J.* 271:821–25.

Blanchard, D., C. Bloy, P. Hermand, J.-P. Cartron, A. M. Saboori, B. L. Smith, and P. Agre. 1988. Two-dimensional iodopeptide mapping demonstrates that erythrocyte Rh D, c, and E polypeptides are structurally homologous but nonidentical. *Blood* 72:1424–27.

Bloy, C., D. Blanchard, W. Dahr, K. Beyreuther, C. Salmon, and J.-P. Cartron. 1988. Determination of the N-terminal sequence of human red cell Rh(D) polypeptide and demonstration that the Rh(D), (c) and (E) antigens are carried by distinct polypeptide chains. *Blood* 72:661–66.

Bormann, B.-J., W. J. Knowles, and V. T. Marchesi. 1989. Synthetic peptides mimic the assembly of transmembrane glycoproteins. *J. Biol. Chem.* 264:4033–37.

Bretscher, M. S. 1971. Major human erythrocyte glycoprotein spans the cell membrane. *Nature New Biol.* 231:229–32.

Carlsson, S. R., J. Roth, F. Piller, and M. Fukuda. 1988. Isolation and characterization of human lysosomal membrane glycoproteins, h-lamp-1 and h-lamp-2: Major sialoglycoproteins carrying polylactosaminoglycan. *J. Biol. Chem.* 263:18911–19.

Cartron J.-P., Y. Colin, S Kudo, and M. Fukuda. 1990. Molecular genetics of human erythrocyte sialoglycoproteins: Glycophorin A, B, C and D. In *Blood cell biochemistry*. Vol. 1, *Erythroid cells*, ed. J. R. Harris, 299–335. New York: Plenum Publishing.

Chérif-Zahar, B., C. Bloy, C. L. van Kim, D. Blanchard, P. Bailly, P. Hermand, C. Salmon, J.-P. Cartron, and Y. Colin. 1990. Molecular cloning and protein structure of a human blood group Rh polypeptide. *Proc. Natl. Acad. Sci. U.S.A.* 87:6243–47.

Clarke, C. A., W. T. A. Donohoe, R. B. McConnell, J. C. Woodrow, R. Finn, J. R. Krevans, W. Kulke, D. Lehane, and P. M. Sheppard. 1963. Further experimental studies on the prevention of Rh haemolytic disease. *B.M.J.* 1:979–84.

Darrow, R. 1938. Icterus gravis (erythroblastosis) neonatorum. *Arch. Pathol.* 25:378–417.

de Vetten, M. P., and P. Agre. 1988. The Rh polypeptide is a major fatty acid–acylated erythrocyte membrane protein. *J. Biol. Chem.* 263:18193–96.

Ekblom, M., C. G. Gahmberg, and L. C. Andersson. 1985. Late expression of M and N antigens on glycophorin A during erythroid differentiation. *Blood* 66:233–46.

Finn, R., C. A. Clarke, W. T. A. Donohoe, R. B. McConnell, P. M. Sheppard, D. Lehane, and W. Kulke. 1961. Experimental studies on the prevention of Rh haemolytic disease. *B.M.J.* 1:1486–90.

Finne, J. 1980. Identification of the blood-group ABH-active glycoprotein components of human erythrocyte membrane. *Eur. J. Biochem.* 104:181–89.

Fukuda, M. 1985. Cell surface glycoconjugates as oncodifferentiation markers in hematopoietic cells. *Biochim. Biophys. Acta* 780:119–50.

Fukuda, M., B. Bothner, P. Ramsamooj, A. Dell, P. R. Tiller, A. Varki, and J. C. Klock. 1985. Structures of sialylated fucosyl polylactosaminoglycans isolated from chronic myelogenous leukemia cells. *J. Biol. Chem.* 260:12957–67.

Fukuda, M., M. N. Fukuda, and S. Hakomori. 1979. Developmental change and genetic defect in the carbohydrate structure of band 3 glycoprotein of human erythrocyte membrane. *J. Biol. Chem.* 254:3700–3793.

Furthmayr, H. 1978. Structural comparison of glycophorins and immunochemical analysis of genetic variants. *Nature* 271:519–24.

Gahmberg, C. G. 1982. Molecular identification of the human Rh_o(D) antigen. *FEBS Lett.* 140:93–97.

——— 1983. Molecular characterization of the human red cell Rh_o(D) antigen. *EMBO J.* 2:223–27.

——— 1988. Molecular characteristics of the blood group Rh_o(D) molecule. In *Subcellular biochemistry*. Vol. 12, ed. J. Harris, 95–117. New York: Plenum Publishing.

Gahmberg, C. G., and L. C. Andersson. 1977. Selective radioactive labeling of cell surface sialoglycoproteins by periodate-tritiated borohydride. *J. Biol. Chem.* 252:5888–94.

Gahmberg, C. G., M. Ekblom, and L. C. Andersson. 1984. Differentiation of human erythroid cells is associated with an increased O-glycosylation of the major sialoglycoprotein, glycophorin A. *Proc. Natl. Acad. Sci. U.S.A.* 81:67525–26.

Gahmberg, C. G., and S. Hakomori. 1973. External labeling of cell surface galactose and galactosamine in glycolipid and glycoprotein of human erythrocytes. *J. Biol. Chem.* 248:4311–17.

Gahmberg, C. G., M. Jokinen, and L. C. Andersson. 1978. Expression of the major sialoglycoprotein (glycophorin) on erythroid cells in human bone marrow. *Blood* 52:379–87.

——— 1979. Expression of the major red cell sialoglycoprotein, glycophorin A, in the human leukemic cell line K562. *J. Biol. Chem.* 254:7442–48.

Gahmberg, C. G., and K. K. Karhi. 1984. Association of Rh_o(D) polypeptides with the membrane skeleton in Rh_o(D)-positive human red cells. *J. Immunol.* 133:334–37.

——— 1986. Chemistry of ABH/Ii, MN/Ss, and Rh_o(D) blood group–active proteins of the human red-cell membrane. In *Receptors in cellular recognition and developmental processes,* ed. R. M. Gorczynski, 251–66. San Diego: Academic Press.

Gahmberg, C. G., G. Myllylä, J. Leikola, A. Pirkola, and S. Nordling. 1976. Absence of the major sialoglycoprotein in the membrane of human En(a−) erythrocytes and increased glycosylation of band 3. *J. Biol. Chem.* 251:6108–16.

Gardas, A., and J. Koscielak. 1973. New form of A-, B-, and H-blood-group-active substances extracted from erythrocyte membranes. *Eur. J. Biochem.* 32:178–87.

Green, F. A. 1972. Erythrocyte membrane lipids and Rh antigen activity. *J. Biol. Chem.* 247:881–87.

Hakomori, S., and A. Kobata. 1975. Blood group antigens. In *The antigens.* Vol. 2, ed. M. Sela, 79–140. San Diego: Academic Press.

Järnefelt, J., J. Rush, Y.-T. Li, and R. A. Laine. 1978. Erythroglycan, a high molecular weight glycopeptide with the repeating structure (galactosyl(1-4)-2-deoxy-2-acetamidoglucosyl(1-3)) comprising more than one third of the protein-bound carbohydrate of human erythrocyte stroma. *J. Biol. Chem.* 253:8006–9.

Jokinen, M., L. C. Andersson, and C. G. Gahmberg. 1985a. Biosynthesis of the major human red cell sialoglycoprotein, glycophorin A: O-glycosylation. *J. Biol. Chem.* 260:11314–21.

Jokinen, M., C. Ehnholm, V. Väisänen-Rhen, T. K. Korhonen, R. Pipkorn, N. Kalkkinen, and C. G. Gahmberg. 1985b. Identification of the major human sialoglycoprotein from red cells, glycophorin A^M as the receptor for *Escherichia coli* IH11165 and characterization of the receptor site. *Eur. J. Biochem.* 147:47–52.

Jokinen, M., C. G. Gahmberg, and L. C. Andersson. 1979. Biosynthesis of the major human red cell sialoglycoprotein, glycophorin A, in a continuous cell line. *Nature* 279:604–7.

Jokinen, M., I. Ulmanen, L. C. Andersson, L. Kääriäinen, and C. G. Gahmberg. 1981. Cell-free synthesis and glycosylation of the major human red cell sialoglycoprotein, glycophorin A. *Eur. J. Biochem.* 114:393–97.

Karhi, K. K., and C. G. Gahmberg. 1980. Identification of blood group A–active glycoproteins in the human erythrocyte membrane. *Biochim. Biophys. Acta* 622:344–54.

Krusius, T., J. Finne, and H. Rauvala. 1978. The poly (glycosyl) chains of glycoproteins: Characterization of a novel type of glycoprotein saccharides from human erythrocyte membranes. *Eur. J. Biochem.* 92:289–300.

Landsteiner, K., and A. S. Wiener. 1940. An agglutinable factor in human blood recognised by immune sera for Rhesus blood. *Proc. Soc. Exp. Biol. Med.* 43:223.

Levine, P., L. Burnham, W. M. Katzin, and P. Vogel. 1941. The role of iso-immunization in the pathogenesis of erythroblastosis fetalis. *Am. J. Obstet. Gynecol.* 42:925–37.

Levine, P., and R. E. Stetson. 1939. An unusual case of intra-group agglutination. *J.A.M.A.* 113:126–27.

Lorusso, D. J., and F. A. Green. 1975. Reconstitution of Rh(D) antigen activity from human erythrocyte membranes solubilized by deoxycholate. *Science* 188:66–67.

Mäkelä, O., and K. Cantell. 1958. Destruction of M and N blood group receptor of human red cells by some influenza viruses. *Ann. Med. Exp. Biol. Fenn.* 36:366–74.

Marchesi, V. T., H. Furthmayr, and M. Tomita. 1976. The red cell membrane. *Annu. Rev. Biochem.* 45:667–98.

Martin, P., and T. Papayannopoulou. 1982. HEL cells: A new human erythroleukemia cell line with spontaneous and induced globin expression. *Science* 216:1233–34.

Moore, S., and C. Green. 1987. The identification of specific Rhesus polypeptide blood group ABH active glycoprotein complexes in the human red cell membrane. *Biochem. J.* 244:735–42.

Moore, S., C. F. Woodrow, and D. B. L. McClelland. 1982. Isolation of membrane components associated with human red cell antigens Rh(D), (c), (E) and Fya. *Nature* 295:529–31.

Paradis, G., R. Bazin, and R. Lemieux. 1986. Protective effect of the membrane skeleton on the immunologic reactivity of the human red cell Rh_o(D) antigen. *J. Immunol.* 137:240–44.

Ridgwell, K., M. J. A. Tanner, and D. J. Anstee. 1984. The Rhesus (D) polypeptide is linked to the human erythrocyte cytoskeleton. *FEBS Lett.* 174:7–10.

Saboori, A. M., B. M. Denker, and P. Agre. 1989. Isolation of proteins related to the Rh polypeptides from nonhuman erythrocytes. *J. Clin. Invest.* 83:187–91.

Saboori, A. M., B. L. Smith, and P. Agre. 1988. Polymorphism in the Mr 32,000 Rh protein purified from Rh(D)-positive and -negative erythrocytes. *Proc. Natl. Acad. Sci. U.S.A.* 85:4042–45.

Siebert, P. D., and M. Fukuda. 1986. Isolation and characterization of human glycophorin A cDNA clones by a synthetic oligonucleotide approach: Nucleotide sequence and mRNA structure. *Proc. Natl. Acad. Sci. U.S.A.* 83:1665–69.

Springer, G. F., and N. J. Ansell. 1958. Inactivation of human erythrocyte agglutinogens M and N by influenza viruses and receptor-destroying enzyme. *Proc. Natl. Acad. Sci. U.S.A.* 44:182–89.

Steck, T. L. 1974. The organization of proteins in the human red blood cell membrane: A review. *J. Cell Biol.* 62:1–19.

Stern, K., and M. Berger. 1960. Experimental isosensitization to hemoantigens in man. Presented at the Thirteenth Annual Meeting of the American Association of Blood Banks, San Francisco.

Szymanski, I. O., P. Araskiewicz, P. Odgren, and L. M. Snyder. 1989. Decreased amount of the Rh D antigen in hereditary spherocytosis. *Br. J. Haematol.* 73:537–40.

Takasaki, S., and A. Kobata. 1976. Chemical characterization and distribution of ABO blood group active glycoprotein in human erythrocyte membrane. *J. Biol. Chem.* 251:3610–15.

Tanner, M. J. A., and D. J. Anstee. 1976. Membrane change in En(a−) human erythrocytes: Absence of major sialoglycoprotein. *Biochem. J.* 153:271–77.

Tomita, M., and V. T. Marchesi. 1975. Amino acid sequence and oligosaccharide attachment sites of human erythrocyte glycophorin. *Proc. Natl. Acad. Sci. U.S.A.* 72:2964–68.

Viitala, J., K. K. Karhi, C. G. Gahmberg, J. Finne, J. Järnefelt, G. Myllylä, and

T. Krusius. 1981. Blood group A and B determinants are located in different polyglycosyl peptides isolated from human blood group AB erythrocytes. *Eur. J. Biochem.* 113:259–65.

Wasniowska, K., Z. Drzeniek, and E. Lisowska. 1977. The amino acids of M and N blood group glycopeptides are different. *Biochem. Biophys. Res. Commun.* 76:385–90.

Yamamoto, F., H. Clausen, T. White, J. Marken, and S. Hakomori. 1990. Molecular genetic basis of the histo-blood group ABO system. *Nature* 345:229–33.

2

THE MOLECULAR BIOLOGY OF THE RH ANTIGENS

Peter C. Agre, M.D.
and Jean-Pierre Cartron, Ph.D.

The Rh blood group antigens are of much clinical importance because of their involvement in hemolytic disease of newborns, in transfusion medicine, and in autoimmune hemolytic anemia (reviewed by Race and Sanger 1975; Mollison et al. 1987; Petz and Garratty 1980). The historic discovery of the Rh D antigen was made just over 50 years ago by Levine and Stetson (1939), who examined the serum of a mother of a stillborn infant. Soon after childbirth, the woman had received a transfusion of blood donated by her husband, and had experienced an immediate and severe transfusion reaction. The investigators detected an antibody that agglutinated red cells from the husband and 80 percent of randomly selected type O donors. This specificity was identical to that of agglutinating antibodies raised in rabbits injected with red cells from Rhesus monkeys, and hence called *anti-Rhesus* or *anti-Rh* (Landsteiner and Wiener 1940). Ironically, *Rh* is in fact a misnomer, since the surface antigens detected by the human and rabbit antibodies were not identical but resulted from the coexpression of an antigen recognized by the rabbit antibody, which was subsequently named *LW* in honor of Landsteiner and Wiener (Levine et al. 1961).

The large number of blood transfusions performed during World War II made it apparent that Rh is very complicated with multiple antigenic variants. Because of limited communication across the Atlantic at that time, a controversy arose over whether Rh is a single complex protein that contains multiple antigens (referred to as Rh_o, rh′, hr′, etc.), as proposed by Wiener in the United States (1944), or whether there exist multiple closely linked alleles each coding for independent proteins specific for the different Rh antigens (C/c, D/d, and E/e), as proposed by Fisher and Race in Britain (Race 1944). Table 2.1 compares these systems.

The Fisher-Race system does not explain all of the complexities of Rh, but is easier to communicate and is more compatible with current molecular studies. D is the major Rh antigen detected on the surface of red

Table 2.1. Abbreviated Rh nomenclature

Rosenfield	Fisher-Race (CDE)	Wiener (Rh-Hr)
Rh1	D	Rh_o
Rh2	C	rh′
Rh3	E	rh″
Rh4	c	hr′
Rh5	e	hr″

Source: Data from Mollison et al. 1987.

Table 2.2. Rh gene frequencies in selected ethnic groups

Gene	Whites	Blacks	Asians
CDe	0.41	0.10	0.55
cde	0.39	0.15	0.10
cDE	0.14	0.10	0.35
cDe	0.03	0.60	<0.01
CDE	<0.01	<0.01	<0.01

Source: Data from Mollison et al. 1987.

cells obtained from individuals with the presumed genotypes *D*/*d* or *D*/*d*, and is commonly referred to as *Rh positive.* The antithetical antigen d is not detectable immunologically and is probably not even expressed, hence *Rh negative.* Whether from Rh-positive or Rh-negative individuals, virtually all normal red cells bear the antithetical antigens C and/or c in addition to E and/or e. The C/c and E/e antigens are all immunologically detectable and are presumed to be products of the *C*/*c* and *E*/*e* alleles. Interestingly, the expression of Rh antigens is very different between ethnic groups (Table 2.2).

Exceedingly rare individuals contain none of the Rh antigens (lacking D, C, c, E, and e) and are referred to as Rh_{null} (reviewed by Nash and Shojania 1987). Rh_{null} red cells contain multiple abnormalities (Schmidt and Vos, 1967) presumably stemming from mutations within the Rh locus (amorph type) or mutations that affect the expression of Rh (regulator type). Rh_{null} red cells have a curious stomatocyte-spherocyte morphology (Fig. 2.1) as well as other membrane pathology, indicating that the Rh antigens are of physiologic importance (Sturgeon, 1970). Identifying the molecular basis of the Rh antigens has proven to be a very difficult problem in membrane biology, and unfortunately many early research efforts proved to be false leads. Rh antigenic reactivity is lost after membranes are solubilized or transferred onto immunoblots. Most biochemical methods therefore actually kill the antigenic reactivity that iden-

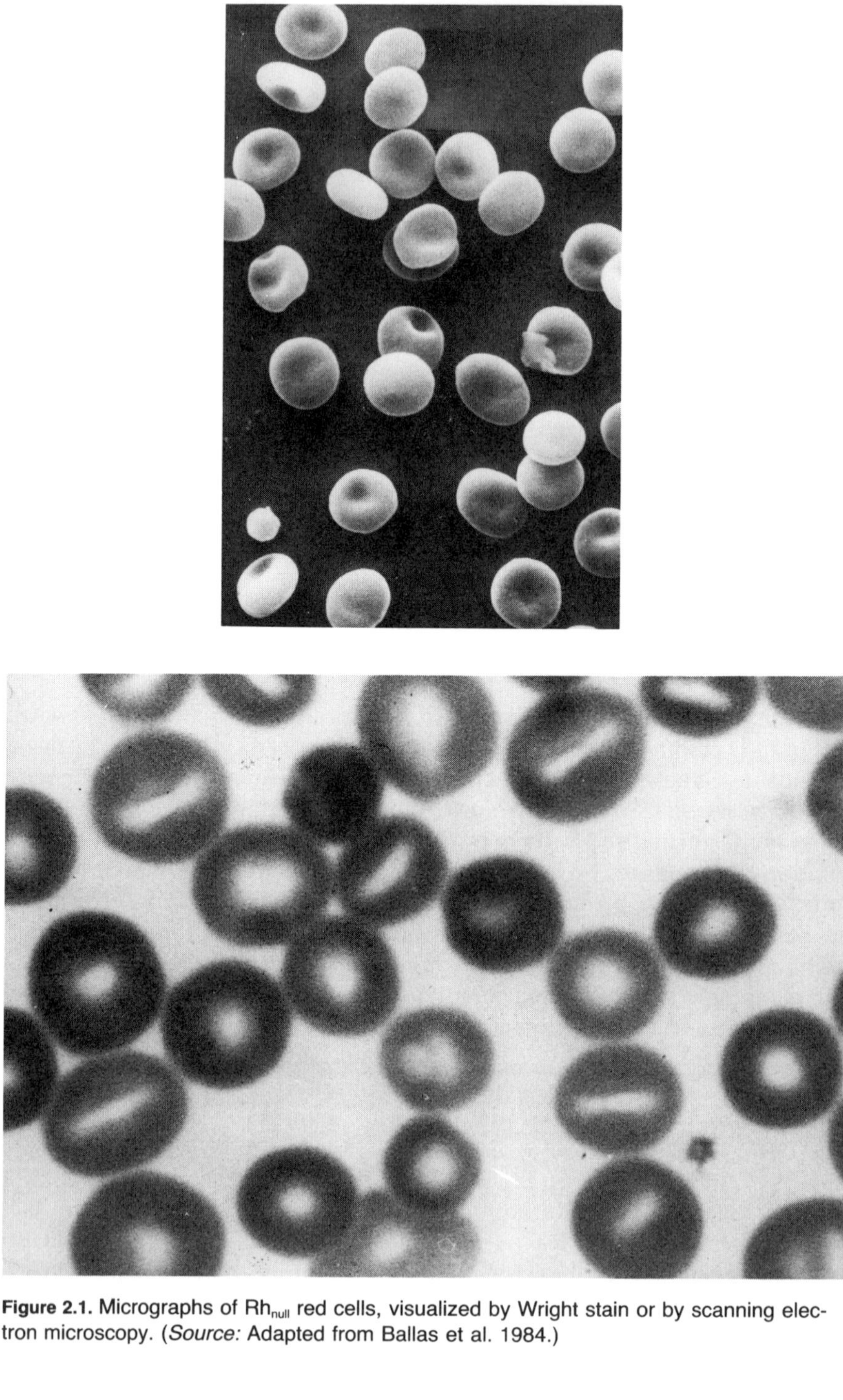

Figure 2.1. Micrographs of Rh_{null} red cells, visualized by Wright stain or by scanning electron microscopy. (*Source:* Adapted from Ballas et al. 1984.)

tifies and defines the Rh antigens. Until recently, there was little agreement about the physical size, composition, or molecular identity of the Rh antigens. Because of the lack of agreement, most of these early studies have not been cited here. Nevertheless, pioneering efforts of certain early investigators proved to be entirely consistent with current molecular studies, and several provided the motivation for recent advances.

THE RH POLYPEPTIDES

A major advance in the molecular understanding of the Rh antigens was provided by two reports published in the winter of 1982. Stephen Moore and colleagues in Edinburgh (1982) and Carl Gahmberg in Helsinki (1982) independently observed a previously unrecognized protein on the extracellular surface of intact red cells by using lactoperoxidase-catalyzed ^{125}I labeling. Although the glycophorins and the band 3 anion transporter were also labeled, membranes from Rh-positive red cells (obtained from individuals with presumed genotype *D/D* or *D/d*) were noted by autoradiography to have a strongly labeled but diffuse band of approximately 28 to 33 kDa. A similar but much fainter band was seen in membranes from typical Rh-negative red cells (Fig. 2.2).

The ^{125}I-labeled band was immunoprecipitated only if anti-D antibodies were added to the membranes before detergent solubilization. This confirmed a relationship of the protein to the Rh antigens. In addition, anti-c immunoprecipitated a similar but less heavily radiolabeled band from red cell membranes of individuals with presumed genotype *cDE/cDE* but not from *CDe/CDe* red cells, whereas anti-E permitted the converse immunoprecipitation (Moore et al. 1982). These new bands are now referred to as the *Rh polypeptides.*

The Rh polypeptides were found to be atypical red cell membrane proteins (Gahmberg 1983). They contained no detectable carbohydrate when examined with methods for labeling terminal sialic acid, galactose, or N-acetylgalactosamine residues with $NaB[^3H]_4$ (Gahmberg 1983). The isolated Rh polypeptide also failed to adsorb to *Ricinus communis*, wheat germ, or lentil lectin columns. The Rh polypeptides were not degraded by endoglycosidase H, endo-β-galactosidase, or alkaline hydrolysis, which normally removes O-linked oligosaccarides. While the existence of a cryptic O-linked glycosylation was not disproved, there is no evidence suggesting that such oligosaccharides exist on the Rh polypeptides. The apparent lack of carbohydrate was indeed an extraordinary finding, since all blood group antigens and virtually all mammalian transmembrane proteins are glycoproteins.

The Rh polypeptides were also found to have other unusual properties. Their electrophoretic mobility was decreased in SDS-PAGE (sodium dodecyl sulfate–polyacrylamide gel electrophoresis) gels of higher acry-

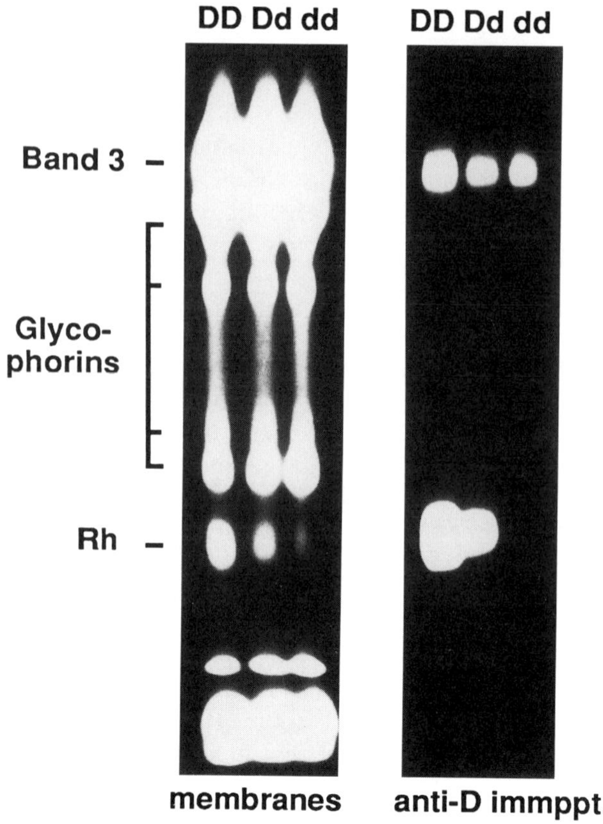

Figure 2.2. Autoradiograph of radiolabeled Rh polypeptides on membranes of intact red cells (left panel) or immunoprecipitated with anti-D (right panel). Intact red cells from individuals with the presumed Rh genotypes *cDE/cDE* (DD), *CDe/cde* (Dd), and *cde/cde* (dd lanes) were ^{125}I-labeled using Iodogen. Note the strong surface labeling of Rh polypeptides on DD red cells, intermediate labeling on Dd red cells, and weak labeling on dd red cells. The anti-D immunoprecipitates are from five volumes of the same red cells. Note the absolute lack of Rh in the immunoprecipitates from dd red cells. A small amount of band 3 was nonspecifically immunoprecipitated from all preparations. (*Source:* From Agre et al. 1987.)

lamide concentrations, behaving as a M_r 33-kDa protein in 12 percent gels and M_r 28 kDa in 8 percent gels. This was thought to represent an extreme example of increased binding of SDS, which is known to occur to very hydrophobic proteins (Helenius and Simons 1975). Also of note, despite the presence of an extracellular domain containing the surface ^{125}I-labeled tyrosine, the Rh polypeptides were resistant to degradation when intact red cells were digested with pronase or trypsin, a feature also shared by the Rh antigens. Attempts to detect endogenous phosphorylation by the addition of ^{32}P to whole cells failed to demonstrate any incorporation.

MEMBRANE SKELETON LINKAGE?

The red cell membrane skeleton is known to be the source of the shape and deformability of the cell. It is also the intracellular structure to which certain transmembrane proteins are attached (reviewed by Bennett 1989). The membrane skeleton is a complex of spectrin, actin, and several associated proteins that are insoluble in low concentrations on nonionic detergents such as 1 percent Triton X-100 (Yu et al. 1973). This operational definition of the membrane skeleton will not distinguish proteins that are insoluble owing to tight association with skeleton components from proteins that are inherently insoluble in these detergents. Moreover, the band 3 anion transporter exists in two forms: a minor subpopulation (approximately 15 percent) that is linked to the membrane skeleton by ankyrin, and a major portion that is unlinked and therefore soluble in the detergent (Bennett 1982).

Masouredis and colleagues at the University of California at San Diego provided several early observations about the distribution of Rh antigens on the surface of red cells by immunoelectron microscopy employing ferritin-labeled antibodies. These observations are especially interesting in view of our present understanding of the membrane skeleton. Although one early report concluded that the Rh immune complexes were randomly distributed on the red cell surface (Nicolson et al. 1971), subsequent statistical analysis of the same data led investigators to the conclusion that the D antigens were spaced a mean distance of 64 nm from the nearest neighbors on the red cell membranes of presumed Rh D homozygotes, whereas the mean distance was 92 nm in heterozygotes (James and James 1978). These are interesting dimensions, given that the approximate length of a spectrin molecule is approximately 100 nm (Shotton et al. 1979). Studies performed with saturating amounts of Rh antibodies demonstrated a lattice-like distribution on the membrane surface with fenestrations of approximately 100 nm (Masouredis et al. 1976). When complexed with Rh antibodies, the Rh antigens had previously been noted to resist complement-mediated lysis, presumably owing to the inability of the antigen to diffuse laterally through the membrane, so IgG molecules would not be spaced appropriately for binding and activation of the complement cascade.

Linkage of the Rh polypeptide to the membrane skeleton would be a plausible explanation for these observations, but such linkage has not been directly established. Under certain conditions the Rh polypeptides were found to precipitate with the membrane skeleton (Gahmberg and Karhi 1984; Ridgwell et al. 1984; Paradis et al. 1986). Moreover, certain other glycoproteins, including LW (Mallinson et al. 1986) and the BRIC

69 and 125 glycoproteins, also behave as if linked to the membrane skeleton (Avent et al. 1988a); these are known to be deficient in Rh_{null} red cells.

The Rh polypeptides are in fact partially soluble in 1 percent (v/v) Triton X-100. The initial reports described immunoprecipitation of Rh polypeptide from Triton-solubilized membranes (Moore et al. 1982); Gahmberg 1982, 1983), conditions in which the spectrin-actin membrane skeleton is insoluble (Yu et al. 1973). The increased solubility of Rh polypeptide when complexed with anti-D may result from the water-soluble immunoglobulin rather than a secondary effect upon the membrane skeleton. When assessed quantitatively, 70 to 80 percent of the Rh polypeptides were still associated with the insoluble membrane skeleton after incubation in up to 5 percent (v/v) Triton X-100 at 0°C for 15 minutes, whereas glycophorin A, a non–skeleton–linked protein, was largely soluble (Gahmberg and Karhi 1984). Similar findings were reported by others (Ridgwell et al. 1984). The membrane skeleton was also shown to preserve Rh antigenic activity when membranes were solubilized in nonionic detergents (Paradis et al. 1986).

The apparent membrane skeleton linkage actually reflects the relative insolubility of the Rh polypeptides in nonionic detergents, such as Triton X-100. Subsequent investigators demonstrated that physical shaking of intact red cell membranes in 5 percent (w/v) Triton X-100 produces an altogether different result, with less than 30 percent of the Rh polypeptide remaining with the insoluble membrane skeletons (Bloy et al. 1987). When Triton X-100 extractability of the Rh polypeptide from whole red cell membranes was compared with extractability from spectrin-depleted membrane vesicles, the solubilities were similar, suggesting that the membrane skeleton is not a major constraint (Smith and Agre, unpublished data). In addition, a subtype of hereditary elliptocytosis inherited in linkage with Rh phenotype was shown to result not from a defective physical association of Rh polypeptides with the membrane skeleton but from defects within the membrane skeleton protein 4.1, which coincidentally resides near the Rh locus on the short arm of chromosome 1 (McGuire et al. 1988). Nevertheless, a relatively weak interaction between the Rh polypeptides and the membrane skeleton may exist.

THE RH POLYPEPTIDES ARE ACYLPROTEINS

Early research by Floyd Green at the State University of New York in Buffalo and N.C. Hughes-Jones at St. Mary's Hospital in London demonstrated an unusual relationship between membrane lipids and Rh antigenic reactivity. Rh D reactivity was eluted from red cell membranes with butanol (Green 1968), but was restored with exogenous phosphatidylcholine (Green 1972). Digestion of intact red cells with phospholipase A_2 removes the fatty acid from the second carbon of outer leaflet phospholipids, and this produced increased fluorescence intensity of a membrane sulfonate probe in normal red cells but not those of the Rh_{null} phenotype (Smith et al. 1973). Phospholipase A_2 digestion also produced partial loss of Rh D antigenic reactivity (Hughes-Jones et al. 1975), and this could be prevented by the prior addition of anti-D (Green et al. 1984), whereas the antibody provided no protection against phospholipase C. Alterations in the membrane cholesterol–phospholipid ratio by cholesterol enrichment or depletion produced an enhancement or reduction, respectively, of Rh antigenic reactivity (Shinitzky and Souroujon 1979; Basu et al. 1980). These findings all indirectly suggest a strong association of the Rh antigens and membrane lipids.

The Rh polypeptide was shown to be a major fatty acylated membrane protein in human red cells (de Vetten and Agre 1988). Mammalian red cell membranes were known to contain two major acylproteins of approximately M_r 55 kDa and 30 kDa, which both become ^{3}H-palmitylated when intact red cells are incubated with ^{3}H-palmitate (Staufenbiel and Lazarides 1986; Staufenbiel 1988). When human red cells of different Rh phenotypes were incubated with ^{3}H-palmitate, approximately six membrane proteins became labeled, and two proteins of M_r 55 kDa and M_r 32 kDa were intensely and comparably ^{3}H-palmitylated in Rh D-negative and -positive red cells (de Vetten and Agre 1988). The M_r 32-kDa protein was immunoprecipitated by anti-D antibody only from the latter cells. The M_r 32-kDa band was labeled negligibly in the membranes of Rh_{mod} cells, a variant of Rh_{null} in which Rh antigens are severely depressed but not entirely absent (Fig. 2.3).

Palmitic acid is covalently attached to the Rh polypeptide by thioester linkages onto free sulfhydryls on certain cysteine residues within the Rh polypeptide. It was found that the ^{3}H-palmitate can be eluted from the Rh polypeptide and other red cell acylproteins with 1 M hydroxylamine at neutral pH, and the attached ^{3}H-palmitate was not metabolically degraded to another molecular species (Hartel-Schenk and Agre 1992). Moreover, the fatty acylation was not reduced by inhibitors of protein synthesis. The fatty acylation was also found to be reversible and was entirely removed during chase with unlabeled palmitate (de Vetten and Agre 1988).

The ^{3}H-palmitylation of Rh polypeptides within mature red cells is most likely the result of continuous exchange of free palmitate for esterified palmitate attached to the Rh polypeptide and a few other red cell membrane proteins. The acylation of the Rh polypeptide was shown to occur at sites near the inner leaflet of the phospholipid bilayer. In the presence of Mg^{2+}, ATP, and coenzyme A, inside-out red cell membrane vesicles incorporated ^{3}H-palmitate nearly exclusively onto the Rh polypeptides (Hartel-Schenk and Agre 1992). Despite the apparently large evolutionary diversity, nonhuman Rh homologs have been identified (Saboori et al. 1989) and retain the capacity to become fatty acylated (Hartel-

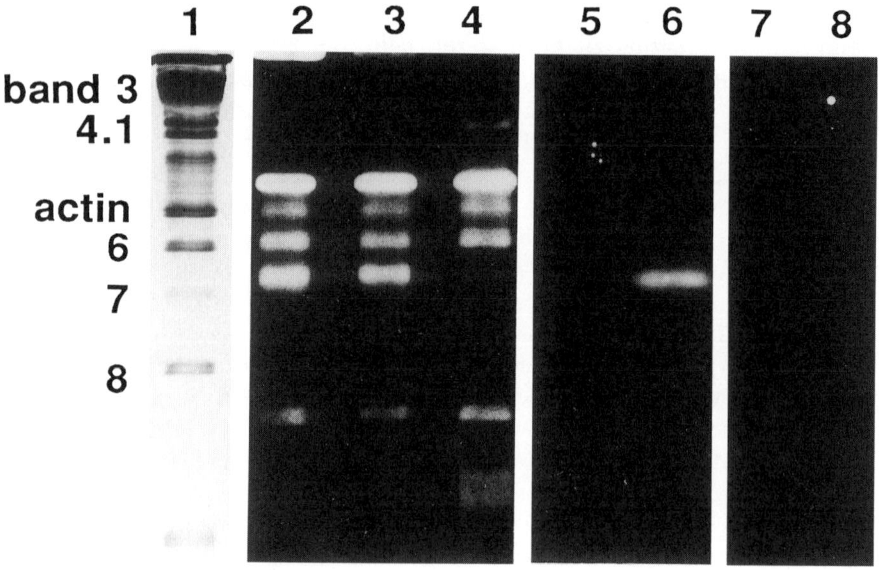

Figure 2.3. Autoradiograph of membranes and anti-D immunoprecipitates from red cells incubated with ^{3}H-palmitic acid. Intact red cells were incubated overnight in tissue culture medium containing up to 1 mCi ^{3}H-palmitic acid. The cells were washed, and membranes were prepared by hypotonic lysis. A portion of the membranes was incubated with anti-D antibody or nonimmune globulin, and immunoprecipitates collected. Coomassie stained SDS-PAGE of red cell membranes (lane 1), autoradiograph of membranes (lanes 2–4), Rh D immunoprecipitated with anti-D (lanes 5 and 6), or nonimmune globulin (lanes 7 and 8) from red cells of presumed genotype *cde/cde* (lanes 1, 2, 5, and 7), *CDe/cDE* (lanes 3, 6, and 8), and the Rh_{mod} phenotype (lane 4). (*Source:* From de Vetten and Agre 1988.)

Schenk and Agre 1992). The existence of selective palmitylation of human Rh polypeptides and nonhuman homologs suggests that this posttranslational modification is of some functional significance, since numerous other sulfhydryls in other red cell membrane proteins are not palmitylated.

EXOFACIAL FREE SULFHYDRYL

Other early research by Green established the important observation that Rh D and c antigenic reactivities were dependent upon an exofacial free sulfhydryl. Employing a variety of sulfhydryl-reactive probes, Green found that the oxidation of a single sulfhydryl led to a loss of antigen sites, which could be reversed by the electrochemical reduction of disulfides and could be prevented by prior incubation with anti-D antibodies (Green 1965, 1967, 1983b).

Rh polypeptides were found to contain exofacial free sulfhydryl(s). Using a radiolabeled impermeant maleimide, two membrane proteins of M_r 32 and 34 kDa were labeled on normal red cells, but not on membranes of Rh_{null} red cells of the regulator type (Ridgwell et al. 1983); the sulfhydryl oxidation apparently destroyed the Rh antigenic activity of the labeled proteins. Nevertheless, the electrophoretic mobilities were identical to ^{125}I-labeled Rh polypeptides, the 32-kDa band corresponding to the Rh D polypeptide, and the 34-kDa band corresponding to the Rh polypeptides immunoprecipitated with the R6A monoclonal antibody (possibly the C/c or E/e polypeptides).

ISOLATION OF THE RH POLYPEPTIDES

RH MONOCLONAL ANTIBODIES

Human monoclonal antibodies were subsequently developed by investigators in the Institut National de Transfusion Sanguine (INTS) in Paris using human B cells obtained from individuals with circulating anti-Rh antibodies. The B cells were immortalized with Epstein-Barr virus transformation, providing human monoclonal cell lines specific for Rh D, c, and E antigens (Goossens et al. 1987). Investigators at the University of Bristol and the South Western Regional Blood Transfusion Centre in Britain also developed panels of murine monoclonal antibodies reacting with nonpolymorphic determinants in the Rh polypeptides (Avent et al. 1988a).

Monoclonal antibodies permitted improved quantitation of the number of Rh antigen sites per red cell. It was determined that individuals with presumed genotype *cDE/cDE* have red cells each containing 0.32×10^5 c, 0.43×10^5 D, and 0.38×10^5 E antigens (Bloy et al. 1988b). Also, using the ^{125}I-labeled anti-D monoclonal antibody, it was estimated that there are 1.09×10^5 D antigens on each red cell from individuals with presumed genotype *—D—/—D—*, and 0.32×10^5 from *CDe/CDe* (Bloy et al. 1987). The Bristol monoclonal antibody provided a similar estimate (Merry et al. 1984). These data together indicate that red cells bear a total of approximately 10^5 Rh antigens (C/c + D + E/e), although these numbers are somewhat higher than estimates previously made with polyclonal antisera (Rochna and Hughes-Jones 1965; Hughes-Jones et al. 1971; Masouredis 1960; Masouredis et al. 1976).

PURIFICATION OF THE RH POLYPEPTIDES

Biochemical studies of the Rh polypeptides were made possible by the development of immunologic and nonimmunologic methods for their purification. Immunoprecipitations with polyclonal anti-D antibodies permitted successful small-scale isolations of surface ^{125}I-labeled Rh D polypeptide (Moore et al. 1982; Gahmberg 1982, 1983). By adding large quantities of the monoclonal anti-D to membranes from red cells that had been surface-^{125}I-labeled, the Paris investigators immunoprecipitated the Rh D polypeptide from red cells of individuals with the presumed Rh genotypes *—D—/—D—*, *cDE/cDE*, and *CDe/CDe*, but not from *cde/cde* or Rh_{null} red cells (Bloy et al. 1987). The Rh D polypeptide was further purified to homogeneity by SDS-PAGE. Investigators at the New York Blood Center used a similar strategy to isolate Rh polypeptides employing polyclonal anti-D antibodies, and this denatured Rh polypeptide was then used to raise a rabbit polyclonal antibody reacting with Rh polypeptides on immunoblots (Suyama and Goldstein 1988).

Investigators at Johns Hopkins were simultaneously isolating Rh polypeptides from Rh D-positive human red blood cells by a nonimmune method. Membrane skeletons were prepared from red cells and solubilized in sodium dodecylsulfate (SDS). A tiny amount of immunoprecipitated ^{125}I-surface labeled Rh D polypeptide was added as a radiolabeled tracer, and the solubilized membranes were fractionated by hydroxylapatite chromatography, gel filtration, and preparative SDS polyacrylamide gel electrophoresis (Agre et al. 1987). This nonimmune method led to a nearly 200-fold purification but only a 2.6 percent recovery. Nevertheless, this permitted calculation of the number of Rh polypeptides in the native red cell membrane to be 60,000, about two thirds of the numbers of combined Rh C/c + D + E/e antigens titrated with monoclonal antibodies. The nonimmune method was subsequently improved by starting with red cell membrane vesicles stripped of cytoskeletal components. The vesicles contained transmembrane proteins that were quantitatively solubilized in SDS, and the Rh polypeptide was isolated in one step owing to its unusually strong adsorbance to hydoxylapatite columns (Saboori et al. 1988).

The amino acid composition obtained from the nonoclonal immunoprecipitated Rh D polypeptide (Bloy et al. 1987) and the nonimmune (hydroxylapatite) purified Rh polypeptides (Agre et al. 1987) were very similar. The amino acid composition was similar to that of other transmembrane proteins, but clearly did not entirely explain the hydrophobic nature of the protein.

THE RH POLYPEPTIDES ARE POLYMORPHIC

The M_r 32-kDa protein is known to comprise multiple species (hence "Rh polypeptides"). These proteins contain the polymorphisms underlying the Rh antigen system. Careful analysis of one-dimensional SDS-PAGE gels of immunoprecipitated Rh polypeptides revealed a small but reproducible difference in the mobilities of the different polypeptides: D migrated with an M_r of 31.9 kDa whereas c and E migrated with an M_r of 33.1 kDa (Moore and Green 1987). These values probably correspond to the two membrane proteins labeled with the impermeant sulfhydryl reagent (Ridgwell et al. 1983). In other studies, red cells of different Rh phenotypes were surface ^{125}I-labeled and the M_r 32-kDa Rh polypeptides were cut from preparative SDS-PAGE gels (Krahmer and Prohaska 1987) or immunoprecipitated with Rh-specific monoclonal antibodies (Bloy et al.

1988b), digested with proteases, and analyzed by one-dimensional SDS-PAGE autoradiography. Variations in the degradation patterns indicated that Rh D is distinct from the C/c and E/e polypeptides. Moreover, it was concluded that the surface ^{125}I-labeled tyrosine resided near the C-terminus of the Rh polypeptide (Krahmer and Prohaska 1987; Bloy et al. 1990a).

Rh polypeptides isolated by the nonimmune approach also showed distinct polymorphisms when Rh-negative (presumed genotype *cde/cde*) and Rh-positive (*CDe/cDE*) preparations were compared by two-dimensional iodopeptide maps (Saboori et al. 1988). This technique provided a "fingerprint" whereby the Rh polypeptides were compared (Elder et al. 1977). All tyrosines within the denatured purified protein were ^{125}I-labeled. After thorough digestion with proteases, the radiolabeled fragments (the "iodopeptides") were compared by two-dimensional analysis, electrophoresis, and thin-layer chromatography.

Distinct variations were noted when iodopeptide maps of the different immunopurified Rh polypeptides were compared. Rh polypeptides were immunoprecipitated from a single unit of blood from an individual with presumed Rh genotype *cDE/cDE* with monoclonal antibodies specific for c, D, and E. The immunoprecipitates were compared by two-dimensional iodopeptide maps (Fig. 2.4), and the Rh c, D, and E polypeptides were found to be highly related, although distinct polymorphisms were found (Blanchard et al. 1988). The c and E polypeptides were nearly identical, with only one additional spot seen in E, while 12 iodopeptides were common to both preparations. The D polypeptide was definitely related although less similar, approximately eight iodopeptides being identical to those in the c and E preparations. Of note, the composite of the two-dimensional iodopeptide maps prepared from the individually precipitated Rh c, D, and E polypeptides corresponded to the two-dimensional iodopeptide map prepared from the Rh polypeptide isolated by hydroxylapatite chromatography (Fig. 2.4, lower right). Using this approach, investigators also found that a single iodopeptide could be ^{125}I-labeled on the surface of intact red cells, and this iodopeptide was conserved among the c, D, and E polypeptides, although it labeled the strongest in the D polypeptide (Fig. 2.4, arrow).

Although the Rh polypeptides for the c, D, and E antigens are different proteins, the overall similarity is considerable, and the antiserum to denatured purified Rh D polypeptide produced strong cross-reactivity with the Rh c and e polypeptides on immunoblots (Suyama and Goldstein 1988). Moreover, digestion of intact red cells with phospholipase A_2 followed by digestion with papain resulted in partial degradation of the Rh D polypeptide but not of the Rh C/c or E/e polypeptides, confirming an inherent difference between these Rh polypeptides (Suyama and Goldstein 1990).

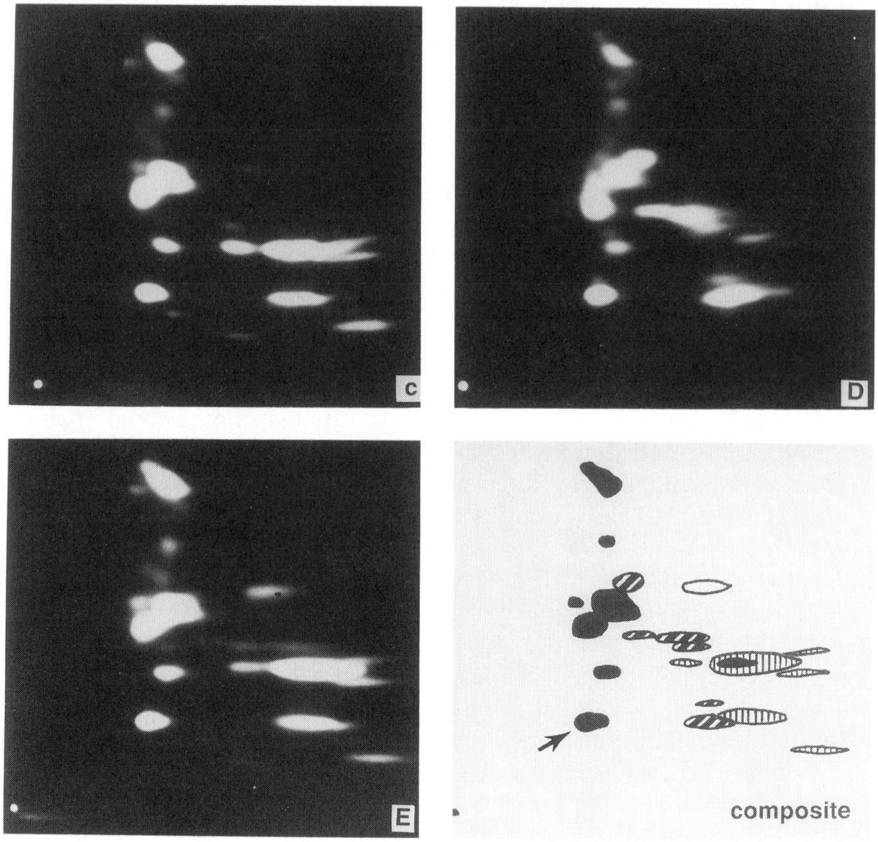

Figure 2.4. Two-dimensional iodopeptide map of Rh c, D, and E polypeptides showing that they are highly related but not identical. Autoradiograph of two-dimensional iodopeptide maps prepared from Rh c, D, or E polypeptides separately immunoprecipitated from the red cells of a single individual (presumed Rh genotype *cDE/cDE*) with human monoclonal antibodies specific for c, D, or E, respectively. The SDS-denatured purified proteins were first radiolabeled with ^{125}I by chloramine T oxidation, then were completely digested with alpha-chymotrypsin, and finally spotted on thin-layer plates and analyzed in two dimensions: (1) electrophoresis, and (2) thin-layer chromatography. A composite drawing (lower right panel) shows the iodopeptide corresponding to an extracellular domain of the protein (arrow). Specific iodopeptides are indicated: those shared by the Rh c, D, and E polypeptides (solid spots), iodopeptides unique for Rh D (diagonal stripes), iodopeptide unique for E (open figure), and iodopeptides unique to c and E (vertical pattern). (*Source:* From Blanchard et al. 1988.)

NONHUMAN HOMOLOGS OF THE RH POLYPEPTIDES

Despite the name, the Rh D antigen is strictly a human antigen, and not even in all humans (Table 2.2). An antigen that is related to the Rh c antigen exists on the red cells of certain higher-order primates but not other species (Wiener et al. 1966). Using the nonimmune method, investigators isolated proteins with elution behaviors similar to the Rh polypeptides from membranes of monkey, cow, cat, and rat red cells (Saboori et al. 1989). When these proteins were compared by one-dimensional SDS-PAGE, they displayed electrophoretic mobilities identical to those of the human Rh polypeptide. Nevertheless, when two-dimensional iodopeptide maps were compared, the nonhuman proteins were found to share only two of approximately one dozen iodopeptides found in the human preparation. Interestingly, the iodopeptide corresponding to the surface ^{125}I-labeled extracellular domain was not found in the nonhuman preparations (Saboori et al. 1989).

MOLECULAR CLONING OF THE RH POLYPEPTIDES

As described previously, human antibodies to Rh D and other Rh antigens are commercially available, but react with the Rh antigens only within the native membrane. None of these antibodies reacts with denatured Rh polypeptides, thereby precluding immunologic identification of Rh polypeptides expressed from cDNAs in recombinant libraries. Determination of the N-terminal amino acid sequence by classic Edman degradation of the isolated Rh polypeptides ultimately permitted the isolation of an Rh cDNA.

Three research groups each employing different methods to isolate the Rh polypeptides determined overlapping amino acid sequences (Saboori et al. 1988; Bloy et al. 1988a; Avent et al. 1988b). The amino acid sequence for the first 20 residues was determined from Rh polypeptides isolated by the nonimmune method. Moreover, identical sequences were obtained from Rh polypeptides isolated from red cells from individuals with multiple different Rh D-negative and -positive phenotypes, indicating that different Rh polypeptides shared the same N-terminal sequence (Saboori et al. 1988). This sequence contained the amino acid sequence determined for the first 16 residues from the Rh D polypeptide isolated by immunoprecipitation from Rh D-positive red cells with human monoclonal anti-D antibodies (Bloy et al. 1988a). In addition, several short segments of internal amino acid sequences were determined from proteolytic fragments of Rh polypeptide (Cherif-Zahar et al. 1990).

The Bristol investigators employed the murine R6A Rh monoclonal antibody and the human anti-D monoclonal antibody to immunopurify Rh polypeptides and were able to determine the N-terminal amino acid sequences (Avent et al. 1988b, 1990). The amino acid sequence of two

Rh polypeptides, the M_r 32-kDa R6A polypeptide (possibly derived from the C/c or E/e antigens) and the M_r 30-kDa Rh D polypeptide, were sequenced to the forty-first and fifty-fourth residues, respectively (Fig. 2.5). The sequences of the two Rh polypeptides were identical to each other as far as sequenced.

A family of glycosylated proteins (referred to here as *Rh glycoproteins*) were discovered to co-precipitate with the Rh polypeptides. The N-terminal amino acid sequence was determined from the glycoproteins that co-precipitated with the R6A and anti-D monoclonal antibodies and was found to contain a unique sequence (see Fig. 2.5). However, when the amino acid sequences of the Rh polypeptides and the Rh glycoproteins were compared, 11 of 39 residues were found to be identical, suggesting that the two proteins were descendants of a common ancestor.

The research groups in Paris (Cherif-Zahar et al. 1990) and Bristol (Avent et al. 1990) each isolated a cDNA corresponding to one species of Rh polypeptide. Both groups had failed in previous attempts that used the traditional method of screening recombinant libraries with oligonucleotides. This probably resulted from the low abundance of the Rh cDNA and because of codon degeneracy for the amino acids identified in the N-terminal sequence. Both groups ultimately succeeded using the polymerase chain reaction (PCR) with oligonucleotide primers derived from proximal and distal segments of the N-terminal amino acid sequence to amplify the intervening segment from cDNA templates prepared from RNA

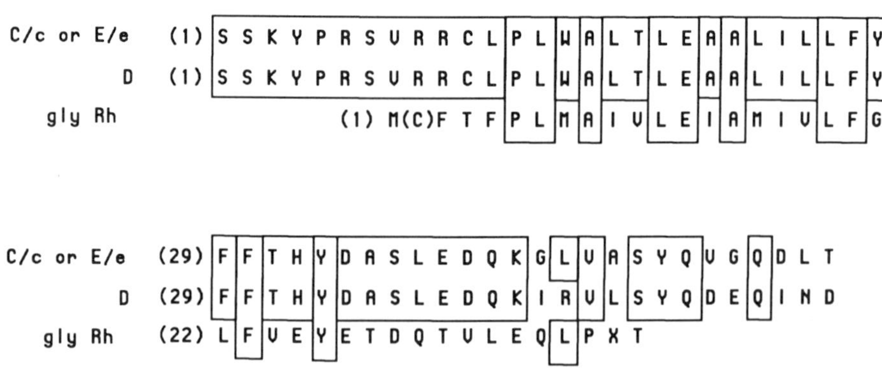

Figure 2.5. N-terminal amino acid sequence determined from purified polypeptides of Rh specificities. The presumed C/c or E/e polypeptides isolated by R6A immunoprecipitation were sequenced to the forty-first residue; subsequent sequence was derived from cloned cDNA (Cherif-Zahar et al. 1990; Avent et al. 1990). Amino acid sequences for the presumed D polypeptide (Avent et al. 1990) and the glycosylated Rh D_{50} protein (Avent et al. 1988b) were entirely determined by sequencing the purified protein. Identical residues are contained within boxes. Note that the amino acid sequence of the presumed C/c or E/e polypeptide diverges from the D polypeptide at the forty-second residue and that the D_{50} polypeptide bears a partial homology. (*Source:* From Agre and Cartron 1991.)

isolated from red cell progenitors and reticulocytes. The PCR products were radiolabeled and used to select plaques from lambda libraries constructed from human bone marrow, and both groups isolated clones of approximately 1.4 kb.

The Rh mRNA may be restricted to cells of erythroid lineage. The isolated Rh clone was used to search for poly(A)+ RNA from several cell lines by Northern analysis, and major 1.7-kb and minor 3.5-kb signals were found in preparations from adult erythroblasts (Charif-Zahar et al. 1990). The 1.7-kb Rh transcript was also found in RNA preparations from HEL and K562 erythroid cell lines and the MEG01 megakaryocytic line, as well as human fetal liver. Expression of Rh transcripts was not identified in adult human liver or kidney, or in the Jurkat lymphoblastic or HL60 promyelocytic cell lines.

THE PRIMARY STRUCTURE OF THE RH POLYPEPTIDES

ANALYSIS OF THE DEDUCED AMINO ACID SEQUENCE

The coding sequences of the cDNAs isolated by the Paris and Bristol groups were identical (Cherif-Zahar et al. 1990; Avent et al. 1990). Ironically, both groups had obtained commercially available cDNA libraries that had been prepared from the marrow of the same individual, explaining the lack of heterogeneity. Nevertheless, a search of existing data banks failed to identify any related sequences, confirming the novelty of the cloned Rh cDNA.

The open reading frame of the Rh cDNA encodes 416 amino acids plus an initiating methionine that is removed from the mature protein. The primary amino acid sequence is notable for the lack of potential surface N-glycosylation sites, consistent with the studies of Gahmberg (1983). The calculated molecular weight of the deduced protein is 45.5 kDa, but the Rh polypeptide has a mobility of approximately 32 kDa upon SDS-PAGE. The most likely explanation is that the rapid electrophoretic mobility results from increased SDS binding, which is characteristic of extremely hydrophobic proteins (Helenius and Simons 1975).

Analysis of the deduced amino acid sequence for the Rh polypeptide demonstrated an astonishing degree of hydrophobicity (Cherif-Zahar et al. 1990; Avent et al. 1990). Most of the polypeptide is predicted to reside between the leaflets of the phospholipid bilayer (Fig. 2.6). There are probably 13 bilayer spanning domains with only very short connecting regions extending outside the cell or protruding into the cytoplasm. Certain spanning domains may turn while still between the leaflets of the bilayer, thereby crossing the bilayer twice with no extra- or intracellular connecting loops (see Fig. 2.6). While most of the bilayer spanning domains are exclusively hydrophobic, four of the first five domains contain acidic residues that may be functionally important.

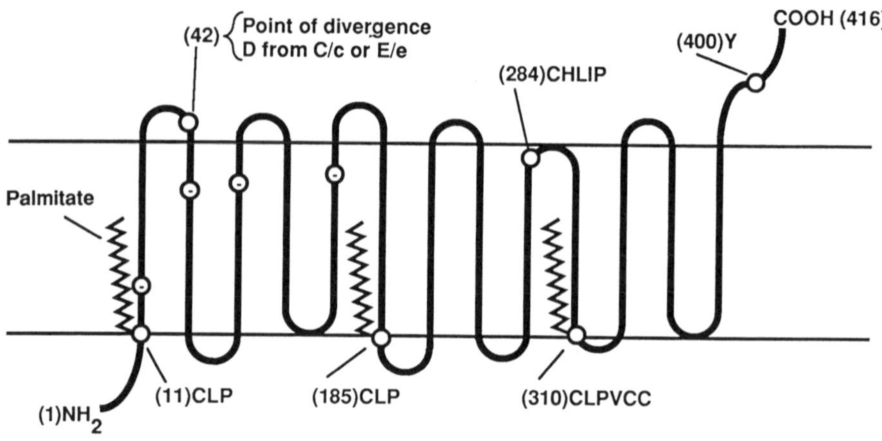

Membrane topology of Rh polypeptide

Figure 2.6. Model of Rh polypeptide topology within the membrane lipid bilayer based upon hydropathy analysis of cDNA sequence (Cherif-Zahar et al. 1990; Avent et al. 1990). The N-terminus (NH_2) of the mature protein is localized within the cell, and the C-terminus (COOH) faces outward. Locations of selected deduced amino acid sequences are indicated, including cysteines (residues 11, 185, 284, 310), an extracellular tyrosine (400), a point where the sequences of D diverge from C/c or E/e (42), and negatively charged residues located within the first, second, third, and fifth bilayer spanning domains (–) (see text). (*Source:* From Agre and Cartron 1991.)

The N-terminus appears to be located intracellularly, since there is no cleavable leader peptide, and the flanking charge differences are consistent with those described by Hartmann et al. (1989). The Bristol investigators found that the tyrosine at position number 4 did not contain radioactivity after red cells were surface-labeled with ^{125}I (Avent et al. 1988a).

The location of the C-terminus was deduced by biochemical studies. Digestion of the Rh polypeptide from surface ^{125}-labeled red cells with carboxypeptidase Y established that an extracellular tyrosine exists at an extracellular location very near the C-terminus, consistent with the model in Figure 2.6 (Krahmer and Prohaska 1987; Bloy et al. 1990b). Two sets of interesting sequence repeats were noted in the cDNA sequence (Avent et al. 1990). Although the importance is not clear, an identical 13 nucleotide sequence (TGGTGCTGGTGGA) was found in the 5′ noncoding sequence (−38 to 26) and in the coding sequence (425 to 437). Also, related seven amino acid sequences were found beginning at residues 392 and 407 (Avent et al. 1990b). The latter sequences are predicted to reside at an extracellular site near the C-terminus.

THE IDENTIFICATION OF AN RH ISOFORM

The isolated Rh cDNA sequence does not correspond to the Rh D polypeptide. The Paris group used oligonucleotide primers flanking amino acids 8 through 26 and isolated a single 90-bp product containing the intervening sequence that corresponded exactly to the amino acid sequence determined from sequencing purified Rh polypeptide (Cherif-Zahar et al. 1990). The Bristol group, however, used oligonucleotide primers flanking amino acids 29 to 46 from the amino acid sequence they determined for the first 54 residues of Rh polypeptide immunoprecipitated with an anti-D monoclonal antibody (see Fig. 2.5). The PCR amplification gave an 88-bp product that was found to contain two internal sequences. One sequence corresponded exactly to the Rh D sequence, and the other was a related sequence in which only eight of 11 amino acids were identical (see Fig. 2.5). When the PCR products were used together to screen the library, the isolated clone corresponded to the latter sequence (Avent et al. 1990).

The cloned Rh cDNA sequence reported by both the Paris and Bristol groups probably corresponds to the Rh C/c or E/e sequences. The different Rh polypeptides diverge at the forty-second residue. Of the 54 residues determined from sequencing the Rh D polypeptide, only five of the last 13 residues correspond to those deduced from the Rh cDNA (see Fig. 2.5). Moreover, the eight variant residues represent nonconservative substitutions. The existence of tyrosines in the flanking sequence suggests that this region of the Rh polypeptides may correspond to the variant iodopeptides specific for the Rh c, D, and E iodopeptides (described above and in Fig. 2.4). The extent of the divergence in more distal sequence is being investigated.

THE TOPOLOGY OF CYSTEINE RESIDUES

Six cysteine residues are predicted by the deduced amino acid sequence (Cherif-Zahar et al. 1990; Avent et al. 1990), and their locations and the identity of surrounding amino acids have proven to be interesting. Residue 284 is a cysteine that is predicted to lie very near the outer leaflet of the lipid bilayer. The existence of exofacial sulfhydryls is known to be involved in the immunoreactivity of Rh D and c antigens (discussed above) and is entirely consistent with the location of this residue in the model in Figure 2.6.

The other five cysteines are predicted to lie near the inner leaflet of the bilayer and exist in the interesting sequence motif CLP (cysteine-leucine-proline), except the last, which is CLPVCC (see Fig. 2.5). These CLP motifs are also flanked by multiple basic amino acids (not shown). In all cases these CLP motifs precede or follow a region of presumed alpha helix entering or emerging from the inner leaflet of the phospholipid bilayer. Each cysteine is adjacent to a leucine that may provide a hydrophobic side chain within a structural kink in the tertiary structure resulting from the following proline.

The CLP motifs are likely to be the palmitylation sites on the Rh polypeptide (Hartel-Schenk and Agre 1992). The motif would be predicted to be a suitable site for the addition of fatty acids from preformed fatty acyl–coenzyme A complex. While the palmitylation of certain other mammalian and viral glycoproteins has been established, no consensus sequence has been identified. Nevertheless, the topology of the cysteines in these established palmitylation sites of these other acylproteins resembles that of the cysteines within the Rh polypeptide, being located within a few residues of the inner leaflet of the bilayer with adjacent basic amino acids and glycine or proline helix breakers (reviewed by Schmidt 1989).

THE ORGANIZATION OF THE RH GENE(S)

Recent studies have demonstrated that the Rh D antigen is likely to have evolved from a duplicated Rh polypeptide (Colin et al. 1991). Using the isolated Rh cDNA as a probe for Southern blot analyses, the Paris investigators demonstrated evidence for two Rh genes in DNA from several individuals with Rh D-positive phenotypes (including —D—, which contains D but not C, c, E, or e), whereas DNA from several Rh D-negative individuals apparently contains only one Rh gene. These findings are in agreement with theoretical analysis of Rh genetics which predicted two separate but closely linked loci corresponding to *D* and *CcEe* (Tippett 1986). While the Rh c and E polypeptides are indeed closely related, they were shown to be distinct proteins. The Rh C, c, E, and e polypeptides may all be products of a single Rh gene with divergence arising from alternate splicing of mRNA, different transcriptional initiation sites, or differential mRNA stability (reviewed by Leff et al. 1986). The chromosomal location of the Rh cDNA has been confirmed on the short arm of chromosome 1, the site of the Rh locus as established by linkage studies (Cherif-Zahar et al. 1991).

RH-ASSOCIATED GLYCOPROTEINS

Although the M_r 32-kDa Rh polypeptides were found to lack carbohydrate (Gahmberg 1983), subsequent investigation by Moore and Green (1987) revealed that a glycosylated protein (or proteins) co-precipitated with Rh polypeptides. Terminal galactose residues on glycoproteins may be labeled upon the surface of red cells labeled with NaB^3H_4 and galactose oxidase (Gahmberg 1976). Rh polypeptides immunoprecipitated from such ^3H-labeled red cells were analyzed by fluorography, and a large, heterogeneous band of M_r 45 to 100 kDa, "D_{50}," was shown to be immunoprecipitated along with the Rh D polypeptide by anti-D, while similar bands of M_r 35 to 60 kDa were precipitated along with the Rh c polypeptide by anti-c and along with the Rh E polypeptide by anti-E. These higher-molecular-weight bands are a subpopulation of "band 4.5," an electrophoretically described group of membrane glycoproteins that includes the glucose transporter and several as yet uncharacterized membrane glycoproteins. These Rh-associated glycoproteins were susceptible to endo-β-galactosidase digestions, characteristic of the polylactosaminoglycans, a family of complex asparagine-linked carbohydrates containing numerous Gal-GlcNAc repeating units (Fukuda et al. 1979).

The studies did not include quantitative immunoprecipitations, and the existence of an Rh complex remains to be established (see below). Nevertheless, the investigators showed that the glycoproteins were precipitated specifically (Moore and Green 1987). Polylactosaminoglycans are known to carry ABH blood group determinants, and the Rh polypeptides were immunoprecipitated from A-positive red cells with anti-A antibodies. Moreover, when immunoblots were decorated with anti-A, Rh immunoprecipitates from A-positive but not O-positive red cells gave a strong reaction corresponding to these higher-molecular-weight glycoproteins. Interestingly, the Rh-associated glycoproteins were still immunoprecipitated with Rh antibodies after the glycosidase digestion, indicating that the Rh antigenic reactivity is not simply the result of the attached glycan.

The initial confusion of Rh and LW antigens resulted from the partially linked expression of the two antigens. Higher levels of LW antigen expression exist in Rh D-positive red cells than in Rh D-negative red cells. LW antigens are altogether missing from Rh_{null} red cells. Employing a monoclonal antibody with LW specificity, an M_r 37 to 47 kDa glycoprotein was identified on normal red cells but not on Rh_{null} or LW-negative membranes, and the LW antigenic reactivity was reported to be destroyed by endoglycosidase F (digests all asparagine-linked oligosaccharides) but not by endo-β-galactosidase (Mallinson et al. 1986). The biology of the LW antigen is complex and the antigenic reactivity does not require glycosylation. The chelation of Mg^{2+} by EDTA has recently been shown to block LW antigenic reactivity, and a functional role has been suggested (Bloy et al. 1990b). While it had been speculated that LW is a glycosylated form of the Rh polypeptide, two-dimensional iodopeptide maps of purified Rh polypeptide and purified LW glycoprotein maps conclusively demonstrated that the Rh and LW are distinctly different proteins (Bloy et al. 1990b).

Rh_{null} red cells were shown to partially or totally lack several distinct glycoproteins and are pathologically affected. Glycophorin B was shown to be reduced to approximately 30 percent of the normal level (Dahr et al. 1987). In addition, one of the Duffy antigens (Fy^5) as well as U-related antigens are also deficient in Rh_{null} red cells (reviewed by Issitt 1985).

Two murine monoclonal antibodies developed by the Bristol investigators revealed that at least two other membrane glycoproteins may be associated with the Rh polypeptides and are distinct from the LW and Duffy antigens (Avent et al. 1988a). The BRIC 125 monoclonal antibody reacts with an M_r 47 to 52 kDa glycoprotein on normal red cells but is greatly reduced in Rh_{null} red cells. The BRIC 125 antibody reacts with a glycoprotein that contains asparagine-linked carbohydrate and migrated as an M_r 28.5-kDa band after digestion with endoglycosidase F and peptide-N-glycosidase. The BRIC 125 glycoprotein is not restricted to red cells and was found in several tissues including kidney and liver as well as myeloid, lymphoid, and megakaryocytic cell lines. Interestingly, although red cells from Rh_{null} individuals have reduced expression of the BRIC 125 glycoprotein, immunohistochemical staining of their lymphocytes was normal.

The BRIC 69 monoclonal antibody was found to resemble the Rh-related R6A monoclonal antibody (Anstee and Edwards 1982). Both antibodies precipitate a broad complex of M_r 35 to 52 kDa glycoprotein as well as an M_r 31-kDa Rh polypeptide that was shown by immunoblot to be missing from Rh_{null} red cells. Digestion of the higher-molecular-weight BRIC 69 glycoprotein reduces it entirely to the M_r 31-kDa polypeptide that is similar to the Rh polypeptides (Avent et al. 1988a, 1988b). Immunohistochemical studies with the BRIC 69/R6A antibodies indicated that the corresponding proteins are restricted to erythroid tissues.

A MACROMOLECULAR RH MEMBRANE COMPLEX

The current feeling among most investigators is that the native Rh antigen may exist as a large membrane complex or cluster that contains the Rh polypeptides as well as certain glycoproteins and possibly lipids. Most evidence for this is indirect, since several membrane proteins are now known to be reduced or absent from Rh_{null} red cell membranes (see above). The existence of a putative Rh complex does not appear to involve interchain disulfides, since reduction does not affect the electrophoretic mobility of the Rh polypeptides (Gahmberg 1983). It is conceivable that palmitylation of the Rh polypeptides contributes to a multisubunit assembly. Nevertheless, the components of the putative Rh complex do not appear to be tightly associated, since Rh D antigenic reactivity is lost after red cell membranes are solubilized in detergents, quite possibly because the Rh complex is easily dissociated.

Because of instability in the isolated state, the size of the putative Rh complex has never been accurately measured. Early investigation showed that Rh D antigenic reactivity transiently survived solubilization in deoxycholate roughly estimated by ultrafiltration to have an M_r of less than 300 kDa (Lorusso and Green 1975). Using radiation inactivation as a measure of molecular size, two different investigators estimated the Rh complex to be M_r 60 kDa and 174 kDa (Green et al. 1983a; Folkerd 1977).

Other investigations also indicated that the Rh polypeptides may be complexed with a membrane glycoprotein (Gahmberg 1983). Whole membranes from ^{125}I-labeled red cells were solubilized in nondenaturing detergent and added to various lectin-sepharose affinity columns, and the Rh polypeptide was found to adsorb to the column containing *Ricinus communis* lectin (Gal and GalNAc specific), but not when the isolated Rh polypeptide by itself was added to the columns (Gahmberg 1983). Moreover the coprecipitation of higher-molecular-weight proteins with antibodies specific for Rh c, D, and E (Moore and Green 1987), and the detection of several glycoproteins missing from Rh-deficient red cells (see above), both suggest that the Rh polypeptides and other proteins exist within a larger membrane complex.

The fact that the M_r 30 to 32 kDa Rh polypeptides are not glycosylated suggests that they may be translated and processed in association with a specific glycoprotein. This appears to be necessary for the expression of the β_2 microglobulin, a nonglycosylated protein associated with the membrane histocompatibility complex (Ploegh 1979; Lee 1980). The D_{50} and $R6A_{45}$ glycoproteins that co-precipitate with Rh-specific antibodies have N-terminal amino acid sequences distantly related to the N-terminus of the Rh polypeptides and might therefore be considered likely components of a multisubunit Rh complex.

While glycoproteins including the LW antigen, BRIC 125 glycoprotein, glycophorin B, and Duffy (Fy^5) may exist within the putative Rh complex, this has not been proven. These proteins are all deficient or totally missing from Rh_{null} cells, but the converse is not true. Cells lacking glycophorin B (S-s-U), LW, and Duffy blood groups are phenotypically normal and are not deficient in Rh. Moreover, certain of these other glycoproteins are clearly not immunoprecipated by anti-D along with the Rh polypeptides. However, although quantitative immuno-precipitations are lacking, anti-LW can precipitate at least some M_r 32 kDa Rh polypeptides (Bloy et al. 1989). Monoclonal antibodies apparently reacting with the Rh complex including a glycoprotein were recently identified (Von dem Borne et al. 1990).

Using ^{3}H-palmitylation to label the Rh polypeptides, investigators recently demonstrated that the Triton solubilized membrane vesicles contain Rh polypeptides that behaved as a macromolecular complex with a sedimentation coefficient of 8.6 S, Stokes' radius of 52Å, and calculated M_r of 170 kDa (Hartel-Schenk and Agre 1992). These values are regarded as approximate and include correction for binding of a large amount of detergent (approximately 0.7 mg detergent per mg protein) as well as inaccuracies inherent to Stokes' radius determinations in the presence of detergent.

WHY IS RH D SO ANTIGENIC?

After ABH, the Rh D antigen is the most immunogenic of all the red cell antigens, although the basis of this extreme antigenic reactivity remains very poorly understood. Isolation of the Rh polypeptide cDNA has provided only small insight into the basis of the Rh antigenic reactivity. Most of the Rh polypeptide is predicted to reside between the leaflets of the lipid bilayer, with minimal projection into the extracellular space (see Fig. 2.6). Rh antigenic reactivities are also easily destroyed by biochemical methods, including the oxidation of free sulfhydryls and solubilization in detergents. Interestingly, a sulfhydryl exists near the surface of the red cell that is critical to the antigenic reactivity of Rh D and c antigens (Green 1965). A candidate cysteine has been identified at residue number 284 in the deduced amino acid sequence in the recently isolated Rh cDNA (see Fig. 2.6). This cysteine is therefore probably distinct from the palmitylation sites located near the inner leaflet of the phospholipid bilayer (Hartel-Schenk and Agre 1992).

All existing information suggests that the Rh D antigenic epitope is not a simple peptide sequence but is likely to be a precise surface conformation resulting from the cooperative interactions of at least one of the Rh polypeptides with surrounding glycoprotein and/or lipid structures. Anti-D antibodies react with Rh polypeptides on the surface of red cells but not on immunoblots (Agre et al. 1987). The Rh antigenic reactivities on intact red cells are not degraded with proteases. Indeed, serologists have long employed this characteristic to actually enhance Rh antigenic reactivity by degrading other membrane glycoproteins that apparently partially obscure the Rh antigenic site. Recent work has demonstrated that the digestion of intact red cells first with phospholipase A_2, and then with high concentrations of trypsin or chymotrypsin, will degrade the Rh D polypeptide to fragments of 17 and 13 kDa, the larger which still forms an immune complex with anti-D (Suyama and Goldstein 1990).

As noted above, membrane lipid has a role in Rh antigenic reactivity, presumably by supporting other components of the Rh antigenic complex. Extraction of membrane phospholipids reduces Rh antigenic reactivity, which may be partially restored by the addition of exogenous phospholipid (Green 1972). Alteration of the cholesterol composition of the membrane significantly alters the Rh antigenic reactivity, which is enhanced by the addition of membrane cholesterol but is reduced by depletion (Shinitzky and Souroujon 1979; Basu et al. 1980).

Inherent differences between Rh D, c, and E antigenic reactivities indicate that the epitopes of these different Rh antigens are structurally dissimilar. Rh c and E polypeptides are highly related (see Fig. 2.4), whereas D is much less similar (Blanchard et al. 1988). While Rh D antigenic reactivity is lost, Rh c and E antigenic reactivities survive solubilization in nonionic detergent. Moreover, by competitive radioimmunoassay, the c and E structures show a small degree of overlap (Cartron 1987).

Because of their lability, attempts to reconstitute the Rh antigens biochemically are likely to be exceedingly difficult. The actual demonstration of the components needed for Rh antigenicity may ultimately require the expression of specific genetic material by transfection. The genetic polymorphism underlying the Rh antigens appears to lie within the gene(s) that encodes the Rh polypeptides, and the nucleotide and deduced amino acid sequences should soon be identified. Nevertheless, the determination of exactly which structures together constitute the Rh antigen ensemble may not be easily determined. Since multiple associated structural components may be required, the simultaneous transfection and expression of Rh polypeptide cDNAs, Rh glycoprotein cDNAs, and possibly cDNAs for other structural components may be needed.

Except for instances of spontaneous or drug-induced autoimmunity, Rh D is immunogenic only for individuals who are Rh D-negative. Since the latter are phenotypically normal, there is no obvious evolutionary advantage for being Rh D-positive or -negative. However, hemolytic disease of the newborn affects Rh D-positive infants of Rh-negative mothers, an occurrence that would theoretically affect one in seven pregnancies among multiparous women in the United States. Such a negative factor would be expected to result in greater uniformity within a genetically isolated population (see Table 2.2). Indeed, 99 percent of Japanese are Rh D-positive (Race and Sanger 1965), and their family sizes are small. Hemolytic disease of the newborn and Rh transfusion incompatibilities are therefore much less frequently encountered in Japan than in the United States or Europe.

Recent work by the group in Paris has demonstrated that Rh D-positive individuals have two Rh polypeptide genes, presumably *D* and *CcEe*, whereas Rh D-negative individuals only have one gene, *ce* (Colin et al. 1991). It is therefore possible that the *D* gene represents an ancient genetic accident during which an ancestral Rh gene was possibly duplicated. The explanation for evolutionary selection of the *D* gene may have resulted from a reproductive advantage by Rh D-positive mothers, since they are immune from Rh D sensitization and their offspring will not suffer hemolytic disease. Some Rh D-negative mothers will become sensitized by their Rh D-positive fetuses. In subsequent pregnancies, many of the Rh D-positive fetuses would have developed hydrops fetalis and would have died in utero. However, in ancient times, stillborn hydropic infants and their mothers would probably both have perished owing to the lack of obstetric care, thereby canceling the selection against Rh D-positive infants. Once introduced into a population, the Rh D-positive phenotype might have predominated over the Rh D-negative phenotype because of the extreme antigenic reactivity associated with Rh D.

THE PHYSIOLOGIC FUNCTION(S) OF RH

Several lines of evidence indicate that the Rh polypeptides have a fundamental role in the physiology of red cell membranes that is unrelated to their antigenic reactivities. Such a notion is consistent with observations of other blood group antigens that are often functionally important structures. The multiple bilayer spanning domains of the membrane model of the Rh polypeptide (see Fig. 2.6) are reminiscent of known membrane transporters. Nevertheless, the function of this polypeptide is not obvious. Examination of Rh polypeptide distribution by Northern analyses suggests that it is an erythroid-specific gene product (Cherif-Zahar et al. 1990).

The red cells from humans of all of the frequent Rh phenotypes are obviously normal. The Rh polypeptides within the red cell membranes from individuals with presumed *CDe/cDE* genotype must therefore function identically to those of *cde/cde* individuals. Although the Rh antigens are unique to humans and higher primates, homologous proteins have been identified and isolated from the red cells of several nonhuman species (Saboori et al. 1990). Although they are of similar size and chromatographic characteristics, the nonhuman Rh homologs were quite dissimilar when analyzed by two-dimensional iodopeptide maps. Nevertheless, fatty acylation appears to be conserved among widely divergent mammalian species, suggesting a functional significance (Hartel-Schenk and Agre 1992). All human Rh polypeptides and the nonhuman homologs may therefore function equivalently.

THE PATHOLOGY OF THE RH_{NULL} PHENOTYPE

Red cells from individuals with the rare Rh_{null} phenotype bear several membrane defects and provide certain clues to the functional importance of Rh. Rh_{null} patients suffer from a chronic hemolytic anemia that is usually of mild to moderate clinical severity (reviewed by Nash and Shojania 1987). The lack of severe clinical manifestations suggests that Rh may be a fine-tuning mechanism in red cell membrane physiology, and a lack of Rh polypeptides is therefore not lethal. Rh_{null} red cells are pleomorphic but always have some degree of stomatocytosis and spherocytosis (see Fig. 2.1) and have increased sensitivity to osmotic lysis. Rh_{null} membranes have characteristically hyperactive Na,K-ATPase and Mg-ATPase activities (Lauf and Joiner 1976), reduced red cell cation and water contents, and a relative deficiency of membrane cholesterol (Ballas et al. 1984). Rh_{null} red cells therefore suffer from both reduced membrane surface area and dehydration. Physiologic roles in membrane stability and volume regulation have been suggested for Rh, but specific details about such roles are still lacking.

PHOSPHATIDYLSERINE FLIPPASE?

Phospholipids are known to be asymmetrically distributed between the leaflets of the red cell lipid bilayer, with phosphatidylcholine (PC) being enriched in the outer leaflet, while phosphatidylethanolamine (PE) is enriched in the inner leaflet and phosphatidylserine (PS) is located entirely in the inner leaflet (Bretscher 1972; Verkleij 1973; Gordesky and Marinetti 1973; Zwaal et al. 1975). Phosphatidylserine is a co-factor in blood coagulation, and cells with PS in the outer leaflet are rapidly cleared from the bloodstream (Schroit et al. 1985). An ATP-dependent phosphatidylserine translocase ("PS flippase") that is inactivated by sulfhydryl oxidation has been identified as the enzyme responsible for this (Seigneuret and Devaux 1984); Daleke and Huestis 1985; Zachowski et al. 1986).

A variety of phosphatidylserine analogs were found to inhibit PS translocation. When photoactivatable, radiolabeled PS analogs were incubated with red cells, they were nearly exclusively cross-linked onto an M_r 27 to 32 kDa membrane skeleton–associated transmembrane protein, which was therefore regarded as a likely candidate to be the PS flippase (Schroit and Madsen 1987; Zachowski et al. 1989; Connor and Schroit 1988). These reports, together with the previous observation that PE distribution may be abnormal in Rh_{null} membranes (Kuypers et al. 1984) and the recognition of abundant palmitylation of the Rh polypeptide, led to the speculation that Rh and the PS flippase may be the same (de Vetten and Agre 1988; Schroit et al. 1990).

The role of Rh in PS flippase and overall membrane phospholipid organization is currently being debated. Phosphatidylserine flippase activity was studied in intact red cells by Daleke and colleagues at Stanford and Indiana Universities. The generation of echinocytes or stomatocytes was monitored after the addition of PC or PS, which located in the outer or inner leaflet of the bilayer, respectively. Rh_{null} and control cells were not different and Rh antibodies did not interfere with flippase activity in normal red cells, observations that led these investigators to conclude that flippase is not related to the Rh polypeptide (Smith and Daleke 1990).

Schroit and colleagues at the University of Texas, M.D. Anderson Cancer Center, sought to identify the M_r 32-kDa protein labeled with the photoactivatable PS analogs. The PS-labeled protein was specifically immunoprecipitated by Rh monoclonal antibodies (Schroit et al. 1990). Surprisingly, the same investigators studied red cells from several Rh_{null} patients and found that the PS analogs were cross-linked to a similar M_r 32-kDa band. Moreover, PS flippase activity was found to be normal in these Rh_{null} red cells, which was interpreted as showing that Rh_{null} red cells may contain mutant Rh polypeptides that are devoid of Rh antigenic reactivity but may still contribute to PS transbilayer movements. In addition to several glycoproteins (described above), Rh_{null} red cells were previously shown to have severely reduced if not absent Rh polypeptides, as detected by labeling the exofacial sulfhydryl (Ridgwell et al. 1983), surface ^{125}I-labeling (Gahmberg 1983), immunoblot with polyclonal antisera to denatured Rh polypeptides (Suyama and Goldstein 1988), and ^{3}H-palmitylation (de Vetten and Agre 1988). Nevertheless, the use of isotopic amounts of photoactivatable PS analog may not distinguish reduced from normal levels of Rh polypeptides. The creation of truly null Rh mutants by genetic knockouts of murine Rh genes may therefore be needed to demonstrate the importance of Rh in vivo.

It is also possible that the Rh polypeptides may be noncatalytic subunits of the PS flippase. The deduced amino sequence of the cloned Rh polypeptide does not contain the consensus sequence characteristic of ATPases (Walker et al. 1982), and the likely existence of large Rh complexes in the membrane suggests the possibility that the Rh polypeptides may be associated with catalytic subunits in a complex. A candidate protein with Mg–ATPase activity and of greater than M_r 100 kDa has been identified (Morrot et al. 1990). Alternatively, Rh polypeptides may be structures that passively restrain PS in the favored inner leaflet locations and are entirely independent of PS flippase activity. Rapid PS flippase activities would therefore be measured to be normal, while long-term maldistributions of phospholipids may occur. Multiple covalently linked palmitic acids on sites of the Rh polypeptide near the inner leaflet of the lipid bilayer may function to directly influence the surrounding phospholipid organization.

OTHER POSSIBLE ROLES

Several different glycoproteins are deficient or absent from Rh_{null} membranes that do not appear to be associated with Rh polypeptides in a membrane complex (described above). This suggests that the Rh polypeptides may regulate the glycosylation or possibly the translation or membrane insertion of these other glycoproteins. The Rh polypeptide may therefore confer stability to certain other membrane components that are missing from Rh_{null} red cell membranes but may not be directly associated with the Rh polypeptides in the mature red cell plasma membrane. Analysis of Rh expression made with fluorescence-activated cell sorting demonstrated that some Rh antigens are already located in the plasma membrane in CFU-E, committed red cell progenitors, although the more primitive BFU-E cells were devoid of Rh (Falkenburg et al. 1985). This suggests a physiologic need for Rh rather early in the differentiating red cell. Despite these lines of evidence, the actual physiologic role of Rh remains to be defined and is likely to be an active area of research in the 1990s.

ACKNOWLEDGMENTS

Supported in part by NATO Collaborative Research Grant 0556/88, the National Institutes of Health, and Institut National de la Sante et de la Recherche Medicale. Dr. Agre is an Established Investigator of the American Heart Association.

The authors thank Drs. Floyd Green, David Anstee, Michael Tanner, Peter Issitt, Alan Schroit, and David Daleke for information and valuable discussions.

This chapter was written in honor of Professor C. Lockard Conley, Emeritus Director of the Johns Hopkins Hematology Division, and Professor Charles Salmon, Emeritus Director of the Institut National de Transfusion Sanguine.

An abridged version of this chapter appeared as an invited review in *Blood* 1991; 78:551–63.

REFERENCES

Agre, P., A. M. Saboori, A. Asimos, and B. L. Smith. 1987. Purification and partial characterization of the M_r 30,000 integral membrane protein associated with the erythrocyte Rh(D) antigen. *J. Biol. Chem.* 262:17497–503.

Anstee, D. J., and P. A. W. Edwards. 1982. Monoclonal antibodies to human erythrocytes. *Eur. J. Immunol.* 12:228–32.

Avent, N. D., P. A. Judson, S. F. Parsons, G. Mallinson, D. J. Anstee, M. J. A. Tanner, P. R. Evans, E. E. Hodges, A. G. Maciver, and C. Holmes. 1988a. Monoclonal antibodies that recognize different membrane proteins that are deficient in Rh_{null} human erythrocytes. *Biochem. J.* 251:499–505.

Avent, N. D., K. Ridgwell, W. J. Mawby, M. J. A. Tanner, D. J. Anstee, and B. Kumpel. 1988b. Protein-sequence studies of Rh-related polypeptides suggest the presence of at least two groups of proteins which associate in the human red-cell membrane. *Biochem. J.* 256:1043–48.

Avent, N. D., K. Ridgwell, M. J. A. Tanner, and D. J. Anstee. 1990. cDNA cloning of a 30 kDa erythrocyte membrane protein associated with Rh (Rhesus)-blood-group-antigen expression. *Biochem. J.* 271:821–25.

Ballas, S., M. R. Clark, N. Mohandas, H. F. Colfer, M. S. Caswell, M. O. Bergen, H. A. Perkins, and S. B. Shohet. 1984. Red cell membranes and cation deficiency in Rh null syndrome. *Blood* 63:1046–55.

Basu, M. K., M. Flamm, D. Schacter, J. F. Bertles, and A. Maniatis. 1980. Effects of modulating erythrocyte membrane cholesterol. *Biochem. Biophys. Res. Commun.* 95:887–93.

Bennett, V. 1982. Isolation of an ankyrin-band 3 oligomer from human erythrocyte membranes. *Biochim. Biophys. Acta* 689:475–84.

——— 1989. The spectrin-actin junction of the erythrocyte membrane-skeleton. *Biochim. Biophys. Acta* 988:107–21.

Blanchard, D., C. Bloy, P. Hermand, J.-P. Cartron, A. M. Saboori, B. L. Smith, and P. Agre. 1988. Two-dimensional iodopeptide mapping demonstrates erythrocyte Rh D, c, and E polypeptides are structurally homologous but nonidentical. *Blood* 72:1424–27.

Bloy, C., D. Blanchard, W. Dahr, K. Beyreuther, C. Salmon, and J.-P. Cartron. 1988a. Determination of the N-terminal sequence of human red cell Rh(D) polypeptide and demonstration that the Rh(D), (c) and (E) antigens are carried by distinct polypeptide chains. *Blood* 72:661–66.

Bloy, C., D. Blanchard, P. Lambin, D. Goossens, P. Rouger, C. Salmon, and J.-P. Cartron. 1987. Human monoclonal antibody against Rh(D) antigen: Partial characterization of rh Rh(D) polypeptide from human erythrocytes. *Blood* 69:1491–97.

Bloy, C., D. Blanchard, P. Lambin, D. Goossens, P. Rouger, C. Salmon, S. P. Masouredis, and J.-P. Cartron. 1988b. Characterization of the C, c, E, and G antigens of the Rh blood group system with human monoclonal antibodies. *Mol. Immunol.* 25:925–30.

Bloy, C., D. Blanchard, P. Hermand, M. Kordowicz, H. H. Sonneborn, and J.-P. Cartron. 1989. Properties of the blood group LW glycoprotein. *Mol. Immunol.* 26:1013–19

Bloy, C., P. Hermand, D. Blanchard, B. Cherif-Zahar, D. Goossens, and J.-P Cartron. 1990b. Surface orientation and antigen properties of Rh and LW polypeptides of the human erythrocyte membrane. *J. Biol. Chem.* 265:21482–87.

Bloy, C., P. Hermand, B. Cherif-Zahar, H. Sonneborn, and J.-P. Cartron. 1990a. Comparative analysis by two-dimensional iodopeptide mapping of the RhD protein and LW glycoprotein. *Blood* 75:2245–51.

Bretscher, M. 1972. Asymmetric lipid bilayer structure for biological membranes. *Nature* 236:11–13.

Cartron, J.-P. 1987. Recent advances in the biochemistry of blood group Rh antigens. In *Monoclonal antibodies against human red blood cell and related antigens*, eds. P. Rouger and C. Salmon. 69–97. Paris: Arnette.

Cherif-Zahar, B., C. Bloy, C. Le Van Kim, D. Blanchard, P. Bailly, P. Hermand, C. Salmon, J.-P. Cartron, and Y. Colin. 1990. Molecular cloning and protein structure of a human blood group Rh polypeptide. *Proc. Natl. Acad. Sci. U.S.A.* 87:6243–47.

Cherif-Zahar, B., M. F. Mattei, C. Le Van Kim, P. Bailly, J.-P. Cartron, and Y. Colin. 1991. Localization of the human Rh blood group gene structure to chromosome lp34.3-1p36.1 region by in situ hybridization. *Hum. Genet.* 86:398–400.

Colin, Y., Cherif-Zahar, B., Le Van Kim, C., Raynal, V., Van Huffel, V., and Cartron, J.-P. 1991. Genetic basis of the Rh-D positive and Rh-D negative polymorphism. *Blood* 78:2747–52.

Connor, J., and A. J. Schroit. 1988. Transbilayer movement of phosphatidylserine in erythrocytes: Inhibition of transport and preferential labeling of a 31,000-dalton protein by sulfhydryl reactive reagents. *Biochemistry* 27:848–51.

Dahr, W., M. Kordowicz, J. Moulds, W. Gielen, L. Lebeck, and J. Krueger. 1987. Characterization of the Ss sialoglycoprotein and its antigens in Rh_{null} erythrocytes. *Blut* 54:13–24.

Daleke, D. L., and W. H. Huestis. 1985. Incorporation and translocation of aminophospholipids in human erythrocytes. *Biochemistry* 24:5406–16.

de Vetten, M. P., and P. Agre. 1988. The Rh polypeptide is a major fatty acid acylated erythrocyte membrane protein. *J. Biol. Chem.* 263:18193–96.

Elder, J. H., R. A. Pickett, H. Hampton, and R. A. Lerner. 1977. Radioiodination of proteins in single polyacrylamide gel slices. *J. Biol. Chem.* 252:6510-15.

Falkenburg, J. H. F., W. E. Fibbe, N. van der Vaart-Duinkerken, M. E. Nichols, P. Rubinstein, and J. Jansen. 1985. Human erythroid progenitor cells express rhesus antigens. *Blood* 66:660–63.

Folkerd, E. J., J. C. Ellory, and N. C. Hughes-Jones. 1977. A molecular size determination of Rh(D) antigen by radiation inactivation. *Immunochemistry* 14:529–31.

Fukuda, M., M. N. Fukuda, and S. Hakomori. 1979. Developmental change and genetic defect in the carbohydrate structure of band 3 glycoprotein of human erythrocyte membrane. *J. Biol. Chem.* 254:5458–65.

Gahmberg, C. G. 1976. External labeling of erythrocyte glycoproteins. *J. Biol. Chem.* 251:510–15.

——— 1982. Molecular identification of the human Rh_o(D) antigen. *FEBS Lett.* 140:93–97.

——— 1983. Molecular characterization of the human red cell Rh_o(D) antigen. *EMBO J.* 2:223–27.

Gahmberg, C. G., and K. K. Karhi. 1984. Association of Rh_o(D) polypeptides with the membrane skeleton in Rh_o(D)-positive human red cells. *J. Imunol.* 133:334–37.

Goossens, D., G. Champomier, P. Rouger, and C. Salmon. 1987. Human monoclonal antibodies against blood group antigens. *J. Immunol. Methods* 101:193–200.

Gordesky, S. E., and G. V. Marinetti. 1973. The asymmetric arrangement of phospholipids in the human erythrocyte membrane. *Biochem. Biophys. Res. Commun.* 50:1027–33.

Green, F. A. 1965. Studies on the Rh(D) antigen. *Vox Sang.* 10:32–53.

——— 1967. Erythrocyte membrane sulfhydryl groups and Rh antigen activity. *Immunochemistry* 4:247–57.

——— 1968. Phospholipid requirement for Rh antigen activity. *J. Biol. Chem.* 243:5519–25.

——— 1972. Erythrocyte membrane lipids and Rh antigen activity. *J. Biol. Chem.* 247:881–87.

Green, F. A., H. L. Hui, L. A. D. Green, P. Heubusch, and W. Pudlak. 1984. The phospholipid requirement for Rh_o(D) antigen activity. *Mol. Immunol.* 21:433–38.

Green, F. A., N. A. Owens, H. L. Hui, C. Y. Hung, and J. Cuppoletti. 1983a. Molecular size of the Rh_o(D) antigen of the human erythrocyte in situ by radiation inactivation. *Mol. Immunol.* 20:361–65.

——— 1983b. The mode of attenuation of erythrocyte membrane Rh_o(D) antigen activity by 5,5′-dithiobis-(2-nitrobenzoic acid) and protection against loss of activity by bound anti-Rh_o(D) antibody. *Mol. Immunol.* 20:769–75.

Hartel-Schenk, S., and P. Agre. 1992. Mammalian red cell membrane Rh polypeptides are selectively palmitoylated subunits of a macromolecular complex. *J. Biol. Chem.* 267:5569–74.

Hartmann, E., T. A. Rapoport, and H. F. Lodish. 1989. Predicting the orientation of eukaryotic membrane-spanning proteins. *Proc. Natl. Acad. Sci. U.S.A.* 86:5786–90.

Helenius, A., and K. Simons. 1975. Solubilization of membranes by detergents. *Biochim. Biophys. Acta* 415:29–79.

Hughes-Jones, N. C., B. Gardner, and P. J. Lincoln. 1971. Observations of the number of available c, D, and E antigen sites on red cells. Vox Sang. 21:210–16.

Hughes-Jones, N. C., E. J. Green, and V. A. Hunt. 1975. Loss of Rh antigen activity following the action of phospholipase A_2 on red cell stroma. *Vox Sang.* 29:184–91.

Issitt, P. D. 1985. *Applied blood group serology*, 3rd ed. Miami: Montgomery Scientific Publications.

James, N. T., and V. James. 1978. Nearest neighbour analyses on the distribution of Rh antigens on erythrocyte membranes. *Br. J. Haematol.* 40:657–59.

Krahmer. M., and R. Prohaska. 1987. Characterization of human red cell Rhesus-specific polypeptides by limited proteolysis. *FEBS Lett.* 226:105–10.

Kuypers, F., M. van Linde-Sibenius-Trip, B. Roelofsen, M. J. A. Tanner, D. J.

Anstee, and J. A. F. Op den Kamp. 1984. Rh_{null} human erythrocytes have an abnormal membrane phospholipid organization. *Biochem. J.* 221:931–33.
Landsteiner, K., and A. S. Wiener. 1940. An agglutinable factor in human blood recognized by immune sera for rhesus blood. *Proc. Soc. Exp. Biol. Med.* 43:223.
Lauf, P. K., and C. H. Joiner. 1976. Increased potassium transport and ouabain binding in human Rh null red blood cells. *Blood* 48:457–68.
Lee, J. S., J. Trowsdale, and W. F. Bodener. 1980. Synthesis of HLA antigens from membrane-associated mRNA. *J. Exp. Med.* 152:3s–10s.
Leff, S. E., M. G. Rosenfeld, and R. M. Evans. 1986. Complex transcriptional units: Diversity in gene expression by alternative RNA processing. *Ann. Rev. Biochem.* 55:1091–1107.
Levine, P., M. Celano, R. Fenichel, W. Pollack, and H. A. Singher. 1961. A "D-like" antigen in rhesus monkey, human Rh positive and human Rh negative red blood cells. *J. Immunol.* 87:6–10.
Levine, P., and R. E. Stetson. 1939. An unusual case of intragroup agglutination. *J.A.M.A.* 113:126–27.
Lorusso, D. J., and F. A. Green. 1975. Reconstitution of Rh(D) antigen activity from human erythrocyte membranes solubilized by deoxycholate. *Science* 188:66–67.
Mallinson, G., P. G. Martin, D. J. Anstee, M. J. A. Tanner, A. H. Merry, D. Tillis, and H. H. Sonneborn. 1986. Identification and partial characterization of the human erythrocyte membrane component(s) which express the antigens of the LW blood group system. *Biochem. J.* 234:649–52.
Masouredis, S. P. 1960. Relationship between Rh_o(D) genotype and quantity of ^{131}I anti-Rh_0(D) bound to red cells. *J. Clin. Invest.* 39:1450–60.
Masouredis, S. P., E. J. Sudora, L. Mahan, and E. J. Victoria. 1976. Antigen site densities and ultrastructural distribution patterns of red cell Rh antigens. *Transfusion* 16:94–102.
McGuire, M., B. L. Smith, and P. Agre. 1988. Distinct variants of erythrocyte protein 4.1 inherited in linkage with elliptocytosis and Rh type in three Caucasian families. *Blood* 72:287–93.
Merry, A. H., E. E. Thomson, D. J. Anstee, and F. Stratton. 1984. The quantification of erythrocyte antigen sites with monoclonal antibodies. *Immunol.* 51:793–800.
Mollison, P. L., C. P. Engelfriet, and M. Contreras. 1987. *Blood transfusion in clinical medicine*, 8th ed. Oxford: Blackwell.
Moore, S., C. F. Woodrow, and D. B. L. McClelland. 1982. Isolation of membrane components associated with human red cell antigens Rh_o(D), (c), (E), and Fy^a. *Nature* 295:529–31.
Moore, S., and C. Green. 1987. The identification of specific Rhesus polypeptide blood group ABH active glycoprotein complexes in the human red cell membrane. *Biochem. J.* 244:735–42.
Morrot, G., A. Zachowski, and P. F. Devaux. 1990. Partial purification and characterization of the human erythrocyte Mg-ATPase: A candidate aminophospholipid translocase. *FEBS Lett.* 266:29–32.
Nash, R., and A. M. Shojania. 1987. Hematological aspect of Rh deficiency syndrome: A case report and review of the literature. *Am. J. Hematol.* 24:267–75.
Nicolson, G. L., S. P. Masouredis, and S. J. Singer. 1971. Quantitative two-dimensional ultrastructural distribution of Rh_o(D) antigenic sites on human erythrocyte membranes. *Proc. Natl. Acad. Sci. U.S.A.* 68:1416–20.
Paradis, G., R. Bazin, and R. Lemieux. 1986. Protective effect of the membrane

skeleton on the immunologic reactivity of the human red cell Rh_o(D) antigen. *J. Immunol.* 137:240–44.
Petz, L. D., and G. Garratty. 1980. *Acquired immune hemolytic anemia.* New York: Churchill Livingstone.
Ploegh, H. L., L. E. Cannon, and J. L. Strominger. 1979. Cell-free translation of the mRNAs for the heavy and light chains of HLA-A and HLA-B antigens. *Proc. Natl. Acad. Sci. U.S.A.* 76:2273–77.
Race, R. R. 1944. An incomplete antibody in human serum. *Nature* 153:771–72.
——— 1965. Modern concepts of the blood group systems. *Ann. N.Y. Acad. Sci.* 127:884–91.
Race, R. R., and R. Sanger. 1975. *Blood groups in man*, 6th ed. Oxford: Blackwell.
Ridgwell, K., S. J. Roberts, M. J. A. Tanner, and D. J. Anstee. 1983. Absence of two membrane proteins containing extracellular thiol groups in Rh_{null} human erythrocytes. *Biochem. J.* 213:267–169.
Ridgwell, K. M. J. A. Tanner, and D. J. Anstee. 1984. The Rhesus(D) polypeptide is linked to the human erythrocyte cytoskeleton. *FEBS Lett.* 174:7–10.
Rochna, E., and N. C. Hughes-Jones. 1965. The use of purified ^{125}I-labelled antiglobulin in the determination of the number of D antigen sites on red cells of different phenotypes. *Vox Sang.* 10:675–80.
Saboori, A., B. M. Denker, and P. Agre. 1990. Isolation of proteins related to the Rh polypeptides from non-human erythrocytes. *J. Clin. Invest.* 83:187–91.
Saboori, A. M., B. L. Smith, and P. Agre. 1988. Polymorphism in the M_r 32,000 Rh protein purified from Rh(D) positive and negative erythrocytes. *Proc. Natl. Acad. Sci. U.S.A.* 85:4042–45.
Schmidt, M. F. G. 1989. Fatty acylation of proteins. *Biochim. Biophys. Acta* 988:411–26.
Schmidt, P. J., and G. H. Vos. 1967. Multiple phenotypic abnormalities associated with Rh_{null} (—/—. *Vox Sang.* 13:18–20.
Schroit, A. J., C. Bloy, J. Connor, and J.-P. Cartron. 1990. Involvement of Rh blood group polypeptides in the maintenance of aminophospholipid asymmetry. *Biochemistry* 29:10303–6.
Schroit, A. J., and J. Madsen. 1987. Radioiodinated, photoactivatable phosphatidylcholine and phosphatidylserine: Transfer properties and differential photoreactive interaction with human erythrocyte membrane proteins. *Biochemistry* 26:1812–19.
Schroit, A. J., J. W. Madsen, and Y. Tanaka. 1985. *In vivo* recognition and clearance of red blood cells containing phosphatidylserine in their plasma membranes. *J. Biol. Chem.* 260:5131–38.
Seigneuret, M., and P. F. Devaux. 1984. ATP-dependent asymmetric distribution of spin-labeled phospholipids in the erythrocyte membrane. *Proc. Natl. Acad. Sci. U.S.A.* 81:3751–55.
Shinitzky, M., and M. Souroujon. 1979. Passive modulation of blood group antigens. *Proc. Natl. Acad. Sci. U.S.A.* 76:4438–40.
Shotton, D. M., B. E. Burke, and D. M. Branton, 1979. The molecular structure of human erythrocyte spectrin: Biophysical and electron microscopic studies. *J. Mol. Biol.* 131:303–29.
Smith, J. A., F. V. Lucas, A. P. Martin, D. A. Senhauser, and M. L. Vorveck. 1973. Lipid-protein interactions of erythrocyte membranes. *Biochem. Biophys. Res. Commun.* 54:1015–20.
Smith, R. E., and D. L. Daleke. 1990. Phosphatidylserine transport in Rh_{null} erythrocytes. *Blood* 76:1021–27.

Staufenbiel, M. 1988. Fatty acids covalently bound to erythrocyte proteins undergo a differential turnover in vivo. *J. Biol. Chem.* 263:13615–22.

Staufenbiel, M., and E. Lazarides. 1986. Ankyrin is fatty acid acylated in erythrocytes. *Proc. Natl. Acad. Sci. U.S.A.* 83:318–22.

Sturgeon, P. 1970. Hematological observations on the anemia associated with blood type Rh_{null}. *Blood* 36:310–20.

Suyama, K., and J. Goldstein. 1988. Antibody produced against isolated Rh(D) polypeptide reacts with other Rh-related antigens. *Blood* 72:1622–26.

——— 1990. Enzymatic evidence for differences in the placement of Rh antigens within the red cell membrane. *Blood* 75:255–60.

Tippett, P. 1986. A speculative model for the Rh blood groups. *Ann. Hum. Genet.* 50:241–47.

Verkleij, A. J., R. F. A. Zwaal, B. Roelofsen, P. Comfurius, D. Kastelijn, and L. L. M. van Deenen. 1973. The asymmetric distribution of phospholipids in the human red blood cell membrane. *Biochim. Biophys. Acta* 323:187–93.

Von dem Borne, A. E. G., M. J. E. Bos, C. Lomas, P. Tippett, C. Bloy, P. Hermand, J.-P. Cartron, L. G. Admiraal, J. van de Graaf, and M. A. M. Overbeeke. 1990. Murine monoclonal antibodies against a unique determinant of erythrocytes related to Rh and U antigens. *Br. J. Haematol.* 75:254–61.

Walker, J. E., M. Saraste, J. Runswick, and N. J. Gay. 1982. Distantly related sequences in the alpha and beta subunits of ATP synthase, myosin, kinases and other ATP-requiring enzymes and a common nucleotide binding fold. *EMBO J.* 8:945–51.

Wiener, A. S. 1944. The Rh series of allelic genes. *Science* 100:595–97.

Wiener, A. S., J. Moor-Jankowski, E. B. Gordon, and C. H. Kratochvil. 1966. Individual differences in chimpanzee blood, demonstrable with absorbed human anti-Rh_0 sera. *Proc. Natl. Acad. Sci. U.S.A.* 56:458–62.

Yu, J., D. A. Fischman, and T. L. Steck. 1973. Selective solubilization of proteins and phospholipids from red blood cell membranes by nonionic detergents. *J. Supramol. Struct.* 1:233–48.

Zachowski, A., E. Favre, S. Cribier, P. Herve, and P. Devaux. 1986. Outside-inside translocation of aminophospholipids in the human erythrocyte membrane is mediated by a specific enzyme. *Biochemistry* 25:2585–90.

Zachowski, A., Henry, J. P., and Devaux, P. F. 1989. Control of transmembrane lipid asymmetry in chromaffin granules by an ATP-dependent protein. *Nature* 340:75–76.

Zwaal, R. F. A., B. Roelofsen, P. Comfurious, and L. L. M. van Deenen. 1975. Organization of phospholipids in red blood cell membranes as detected by various purified phospholipases. *Biochim. Biophys. Acta* 406:83–96.

3

THE KELL ANTIGENS AND McLEOD RED CELLS

Colvin M. Redman, Ph.D.
and W. Laurence Marsh, Ph.D.

After ABO and Rh, Kell antigens are the most immunogenic of the major blood group systems. Indeed, within a few weeks of the application of their new antiglobulin test Coombs and colleagues detected a novel antibody which caused hemolytic disease in a new born infant (Coombs 1946). Named Kell after the proposita, the antigens are a complex of several sets of autosomal co-dominant alleles at the Kell locus. The expression of Kell is modified by an independent x-linked gene named *Xk* that encodes the Kx antigen protein.

Most antigens of the Kell system have good immunogenicity, with K1 (Kell), the first antigen to be discovered, having the highest potency. About one in 20 K: −1 recipients given a transfusion of one unit of K1 blood will make anti-K1. Fortunately, the K1 antigen has a frequency of only 9 percent in Caucasians and even lower in other populations, and compatible blood is easy to find. Kell system antibodies are usually IgG proteins and may cause severe hemolytic disease in antigen-positive newborns or severe reactions if incompatible blood is transfused. Since it was first described (Coombs et al. 1946), the system has been shown to include 24 associated antigens (Table 3.1). Kell is largely a system of high-frequency antigens with, in several instances, low-frequency alternates. The common phenotype is K: −1, 2, −3, 4, 5, −6, 7, −8, 9, −10, 11, 12, 13, 14, 15, 16, −17, 18, 19, 20, −21, 22, −23, −24. A number of antigens in the system have allelic relationships (*K1–K2*; *K3–K4*; *K6–K7*; *K11–K17*) with autosomal co-dominant inheritance, but the Kell gene has not yet been mapped.

Kell has interesting anthropologic variations, for different populations show considerable differences in phenotype frequency. For example, K6 is restricted to aboriginal African people, while K1 is essentially an antigen of Caucasians. All known antigens of the Kell complex except for Kx(K15) appear to be products of a single Kell gene and are markers on a 93-kDa transmembrane red cell membrane glycoprotein that is linked to the

Table 3.1. The Kell Blood Group System: Nomenclature and Antigen Frequency

Kell Number	Colloquial Name and Letter(s)	Antigen Frequency (%)
K1	Kell, K	9.0
K2	Cellano, K	99.8
K3	Penny, Kp^a	2.0
K4	Ratenberg, Kp^b	> 99.9
K5	Peltz, Ku	> 99.9
K6	Sutter, Js^a	< 1.0 in whites, 19.5 in blacks
K7	Matthews, Js^b	> 99.9
K8	—, kw	5.0
K9	Claas, KL	> 99.9
K10	Karhula, Ul^a	2.6 in Finns, > 0.1 in others
K11	Coté	> 99.9
K12	Bockman	> 99.9
K13	Szro	> 99.9
K13	—	> 99.9
K14	Santini	> 99.9
K15*	—, Kx	> 99.9
K16	—, K-like	99.8
K17	Weeks, Wk^a	0.3
K18	Marshall	> 99.9
K19	Sublett	> 99.9
K20	—, Km	> 99.9
K21	Levay, Kp^c	< 0.1
K22	Ikar	> 99.9
K23	—	< 0.1
K24	—, cls	< 2.0

*K15 or Kx is usually listed in the Kell blood group system, but it is different from all other Kell blood group antigens in that it resides on a separate protein.
Source: Adapted from Marsh and Redman 1990.

underlying red cell cytoskeleton (Marsh and Redman 1987). Kx is an associated antigen carried on a 37-kDa protein, coded by an independent gene, named *Xk*, present on the short arm of the X chromosome at Xp21 (Bertelson et al. 1988).

Two variant Kell phenotypes, Ko (null) and McLeod, demonstrate the serologic relationship between Kell and Kx blood group antigens. The Ko red cell has normal morphology and lacks all known Kell antigens, but has enhanced expression of Kx. Kx appears to be present on red blood cells from most individuals and is absent only on rare occasions. About 60 persons are known who lack Kx antigen and have an associated marked depression of Kell antigen activity. This phenotype is called McLeod. McLeod red cells, in addition to an absence of Kx, are characterized by abnormal morphology, usually manifested as acanthocytosis, and reduced in vivo survival (Fig. 3.1). Individuals of the McLeod type have a permanent hemolytic state, which is usually compensated by erythropoietic hyperplasia. Since the McLeod gene is X-linked, all known

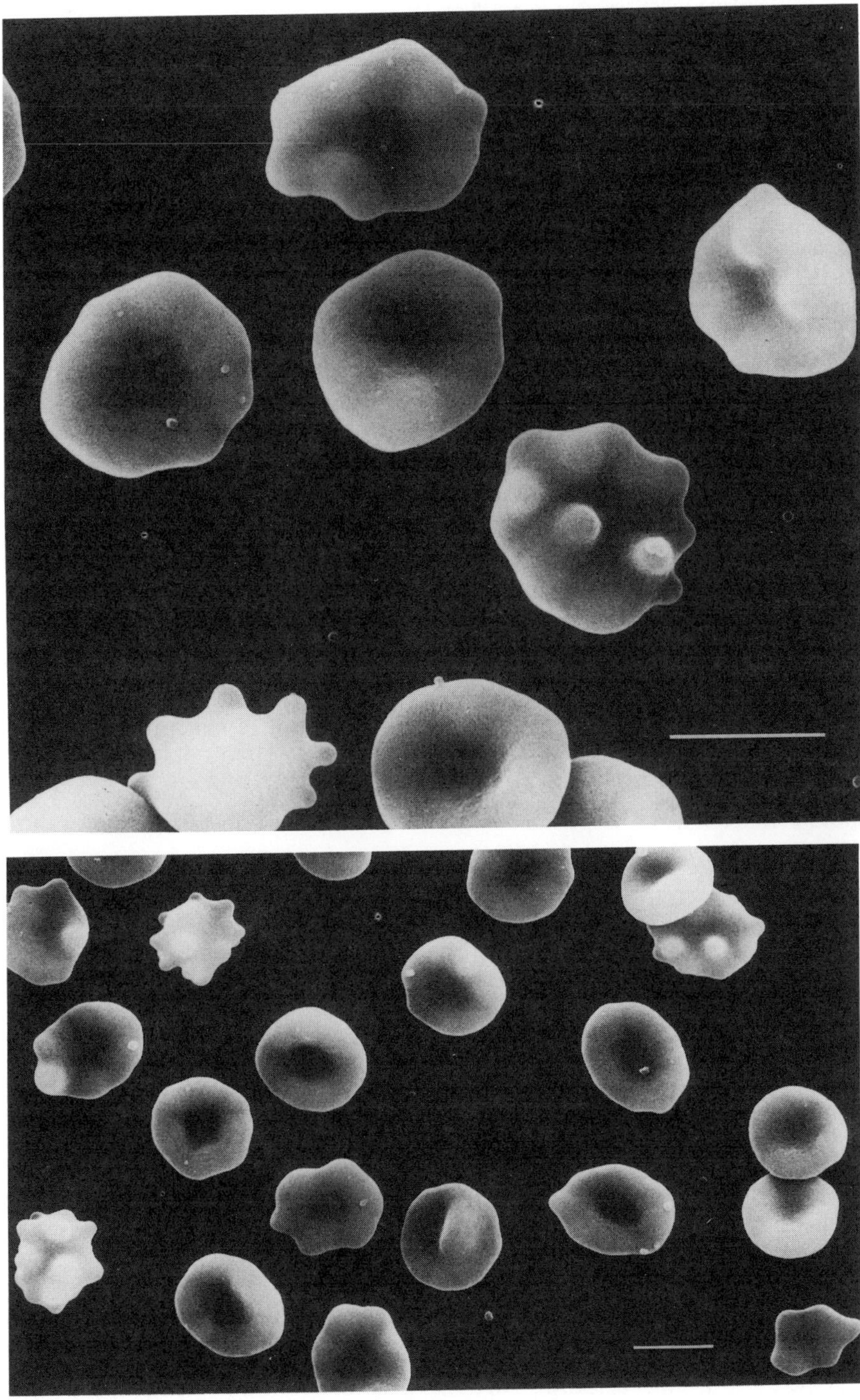

Figure 3.1. A scanning electron micrograph of McLeod red cells. The bar equals 10 μm. (*Source:* Tellervo Huima, New York Blood Center.)

McLeod individuals are male. The expression of the gene is suppressed by X-chromosome inactivation; as a result, female carriers exhibit red cell mosaicism with a double population of McLeod acanthocytes and normocytes of common Kell type in their peripheral blood. The mosaicism is best recognized by flow cytometric analysis using a selected Kell antibody and may be greatly unbalanced, favoring either the McLeod or the common Kell cell population.

The serologic relationship between Kell and Kx therefore is as follows: Ko red cells lack Kell antigens and have enhanced Kx antigen, while McLeod red cells lack Kx and have diminished Kell antigens. Because of the serologic association noted above, Kell and Kx are usually grouped and discussed together. However, it should be noted at the outset that Kell and Kx antigens are coded by different genes and carried on different proteins: Kell antigen on a 93-kDa glycoprotein and Kx on a 37-kDa protein.

Some boys with X-linked chronic granulomatous disease (CGD) have red cells of the McLeod type. The CGD and McLeod genes are in close proximity on the X-chromosome and in some boys a cytogenetic deletion spanning both regions is responsible (Bertelson et al. 1988).

Transfusion of blood of common Kell type to Ko or McLeod individuals produces different patterns of alloimmunization. Ko individuals make an antibody called anti-Ku (anti-K5) that reacts with all except Ko red cell samples. Immunoprecipitation with this antibody yields the Kell 93-kDa glycoprotein. McLeod individuals with CGD mount an alloimmune response to Kell protein (nonreactive with Ko cells) and also make anti-Kx.

THE McLEOD SYNDROME

A notable characteristic of the McLeod phenotype is the clinical syndrome that accompanies it. In addition to the erythropoietic changes, McLeod subjects have elevated levels of serum creatine kinase of MM isoenzyme type, derived from skeletal or cardiac muscle. Areflexia can usually be demonstrated early in life. By the fifth decade there is usually a slow progression to cardiomegaly, followed sometimes by cardiomyopathy and skeletal muscle wasting, and choreiform and dystonic movements (Marsh et al. 1981; Marsh and Redman 1987).

In family studies involving McLeod subjects, inheritance of the muscular and neurologic defects is always concomitant with the McLeod phenotype, while other kindred are normal. It appears that the multiple tissue abnormalities are a pleiotropic effect of the same X-linked gene.

In some subjects, McLeod syndrome is associated with X-linked CGD. McLeod syndrome in some boys is also concomitant with Duchenne muscular dystrophy (DMD) (Swash et al. 1983). This coincidental occurrence proved useful in the localization of the McLeod locus (XK), by deletion analysis, to the Xp21 region of the X-chromosome. The McLeod gene is located between the CGD and DMD genes, within a 500-kb interval, distal to the CGD locus (Bertelson et al. 1988).

A salient feature of the McLeod syndrome is marked acanthocytosis of red cells, reduced red cell survival, and a compensated hemolytic state. The proportion of red cells that are acanthocytes varies, but usually about 30 percent are distinctly acanthocytic, while the remainder, when examined carefully by scanning electron microscopy, also exhibit aberrant morphology, often appearing with wavy or ruffled surfaces (see Fig. 3.1). Since Ko (null) red cells have normal morphology and normal in vivo survival, it is unlikely that the reduced number of Kell antigens is responsible for the abnormality of cell shape, but rather that the absence of Kx protein may be associated with the morphologic defect present in McLeod red cells.

McLeod red cells, although grossly distorted in shape, have a near normal composition of membrane lipid and protein (Symmans et al. 1979; Tang et al. 1981; Glaubensklee et al. 1982), and normal levels of glycolytic and nonglycolytic enzymes (Tang et al. 1981). Few biochemical and physiologic defects have been described. Hexokinase activity is slightly elevated, which would be expected, as McLeod subjects have a mild hemolytic condition accompanied by an elevated reticulocyte count (for review, see Marsh and Redman 1987). McLeod red cells have increased phosphorylation of some proteins and phospholipids, predominantly band 3, spectrin, phosphatidic acid, and the polyphosphoinositides (Tang et al. 1981); enhanced exchangeability of membrane phosphatidylcholine with an exogenous source (Kuypers et al. 1985); and a 30 percent decrease in cell membrane water permeability (Wimer et al. 1977; Galey et al. 1978). McLeod red cells have normal osmotic fragility (Wimer et al. 1977), but the cell membrane appears to be more rigid than that of normal red cells (Ballas et al. 1990).

Red cell acanthocytosis can be corrected by inserting lipids, or other compounds, into the inner layer of the lipid membrane (Khodadad et al. 1989). Phosphatidylserine, a normal component of the inner leaflet of the membrane, is transported from the outside to the inner layer of the membrane by an enzymatic process, causing changes in cell shape that can be used as a measure of uptake and transport (Daleke and Huestis 1985). A 31- to 32-kDa protein, which is similar in size to Kx protein, has been proposed as a transport carrier for phosphatidylserine (Conner and Schroit 1989). However, McLeod red cells transport phosphatidylserine across the membrane normally, and the entry of phosphatidylserine corrects the shape of McLeod acanthocytes (Redman et al. 1989a), indicating that Kx protein is not the transporter of phosphatidylserine.

The factors that regulate the shape of the red cell have not been clearly defined. An attractive hypothesis is that disturbances to any components of the cytoskeletal system or to either of the two membrane lipid bilayers cause changes in the cell shape (Sheetz and Singer 1974; Elgsaeter et al. 1983; Lange and Steck 1984). Thus, a number of factors, such as aberrancies in the protein components of the cytoskeletal system, or variation in ATP metabolism or in lipid content, can affect cell morphology. How Kx affects these or other parameters that influence the cell shape is an open question, but the fact that a lack of Kx in red cells is always accompanied by distorted cell morphology suggests that Kx has a role in maintaining cell shape. Also, the observation that people with McLeod syndrome have associated muscular and neurologic disorders indicates that Kx is also present in nonerythroid tissue and has a similar role in these cells.

The absence of Kx antigen is the salient feature of McLeod red cells. Unfortunately, little is known about the protein that carries Kx antigens, mostly because it is present in small amounts in red cells and there is limited availability of specific antibodies to Kx that could be used in its isolation. Nevertheless, immunoprecipitation, from surface-iodinated Ko (null) and from normal red cells, with a human alloimmune antibody to Kx yielded a 37-kDa radioactive protein. This protein has not been isolated from McLeod red cells (Redman et al. 1988). The yield of 37-kDa protein was 10 percent of that obtained when compared with the isolation of Kell protein by a similar procedure. Since there are only 5000 Kell antigen sites per red cell, this suggests that Kx is a minor component of the red cell membrane.

KELL BLOOD GROUP PROTEIN

The first studies on the biochemistry of Kell noted conditions that led to inactivation of the antigen. Kell antigens are inactivated by reagents that react with disulfide groups such as a-aminoethylisothiouronium bromide (AET) (Advani et al. 1982), and high concentrations of dithiothreitol (DTT) (Branch et al. 1983), but are difficult to inactivate by treatment with proteolytic enzymes. Trypsin or chymotrypsin by itself has little effect on Kell activity, but the two enzymes together inactivate Kell (Judson and Anstee 1977). Mixtures of reducing reagents (DTT) and proteolytic enzymes (papain) immediately destroy Kell antigens (Branch and Petz 1982). These early studies suggested that Kell antigens reside on a protein that is present on the outer surface of the membrane and is tightly folded by disulfide bonds, and that opening the protein structure by reducing sulfhydryl bonds unravels the protein and allows proteolysis to occur.

Immunoprecipitation of surface-labeled red cells with monospecific human alloimmune antibodies (Redman et al. 1984) or with mouse (Redman et al. 1986) or human (Jaber et al. 1989) monoclonal antibodies yielded a 93-kDa glycoprotein. These antibodies appear to react with conformation-dependent structures, as they do not immunoprecipitate Kell protein from a detergent-solubilized membrane preparation or react on Western blots with red cell membrane proteins. All Kell antigens are part of the same, or very similar, 93-kDa protein, since all 93-kDa proteins immunoprecipitated by different Kell antibodies react, by Western blot, with a rabbit polyclonal antibody prepared by the administration of K7 protein to rabbits. In addition, chymotryptic peptide fingerprint maps of Kell protein isolated by anti-K14 and anti-K7 are practically indistinguishable (Redman et al. 1986). However, small differences in amino acid sequence or in carbohydrate content may go unnoticed by these procedures. Kell protein, isolated by immunoprecipitation with mouse monoclonal antibody to K:14, is not homogeneous and has several isoforms. These isoforms, all of which are basic, also exist in the deglycosylated form. At present we do not know the biochemical basis for the various antigenic determinants in the Kell system. The differences may be due to variation in amino acid sequences or in carbohydrate content. Elucidation must await the characterization of the Kell gene and of the expressed protein from persons of different phenotypes.

Ko (null) red cells do not express any antigens coded by the Kell gene, while McLeod red cells have weak expression of Kell antigens. Western blot studies on total red cell membrane proteins with a rabbit polyclonal antibody to Kell protein, which reacts with multiple epitopes throughout the 93-kDa glycoprotein, have shown that Kell protein is not present in the membrane of Ko red cells and is greatly diminished in McLeod red cell membranes (Redman et al. 1988). This indicates that a deficiency of Kell antigens is due not to a modification of surface structure or to an occlusion of the protein in the membrane but to an absence or reduction of protein. The causes for this are not yet understood.

Kell is a glycoprotein composed of about 12 percent carbohydrates by weight. Deglycosylation with N-glycanase yields a protein that, based on its mobility on SDS polyacrylamide gel electrophoresis, has a molecular size of 79 to 80 kDa (Redman et al. 1989b). There are no O-linked sugars, since treatment with O-glycanase does not affect the protein's mobility on SDS-PAGE and carbohydrate analysis did not detect significant amounts of neuraminic acid or N-acetylglucosamine, which are usual components of O-linked glycans (Jaber et al. 1989). Based on these analyses, it was calculated that the 93-kDa Kell protein has four to six N-linked oligosaccharides of the biantennary type. Recent determination of the primary structure of Kell protein, deduced from its cDNA, demonstrated that the extracellular domain of Kell has six putative N-glycosylation sites. Two of the carbohydrate chains are close together just outside of the membrane-spanning domain (asparagines in positions 94 and 115), two are in the middle of the extracellular segment (residues 191 and 345), and the other two are near the C-terminus (residues 627 and 724) (Lee et al. 1991). At present we do not know whether the carbohydrates participate in Kell immunodeterminants or whether different Kell phenotypes vary in carbohydrate content and sequence.

Early attempts, using a rabbit polyclonal antibody to Kell protein and a λgtll human bone marrow cDNA library, to clone Kell cDNA were unsuccessful and suggest that Kell, like some other membrane proteins, is not easily expressed in these systems. Therefore, to successfully clone Kell, investigators isolated and purified the protein, and obtained amino acid sequences to synthesize Kell-specific oligonucleotides with which to screen an appropriate cDNA library. Kell protein was isolated by immunoprecipitation with mouse monoclonal antibody to K14, separated by SDS-PAGE, and eluted from the gels. Further purification was by high-performance liquid chromatography (HPLC) (Redman et al. 1988). Kell protein, as isolated, has a blocked N-terminus, which did not allow amino acid sequence analysis from the amino terminal end of the protein. Therefore, amino acid sequences were obtained from tryptic peptides derived from purified Kell protein (Redman et al. 1988). The cloning strategy was as follows: an exact oligonucleotide sequence, corresponding to the amino acid sequences of one of the Kell peptides, was obtained using polymerase chain reaction (PCR) technology. This Kell-specific oligonucleotide was then used to screen a λgt10 human bone marrow cDNA library. Four positive clones, from about 1.6×10^6 plaques, were obtained. Only one of these clones had a full-length open-reading frame coding for Kell protein. The cDNA insert in this clone had two internal EcoRI sites and was isolated as three fragments. At the 5′ end a 0.5-kb segment contained a 121-bp untranslated region followed by an initiation codon and an open-reading frame. The 0.5-kb fragment was contiguous with a 1.9-kb fragment. The 1.9-kb fragment had a large open-reading frame that coded the bulk of Kell protein, and had a termination codon and a polyadenylation signal near the 3′ end. The 1.9-kb was contiguous with a third fragment (3kb) that represents a large untranslated 3′ region. Northern blot analysis of human bone marrow mRNA demonstrated that the major Kell transcripts are about 2.6 kb (Lee et al. 1991). As will be discussed later, Kell has structural similarities with common acute lymphoblastic leukemia antigen (CALLA), and CALLA also has a large 3′ untranslated segment (Shipp et al. 1988). The CALLA gene has been characterized: it spans more than 80 kb and is composed of 24 exons (D'Adamio et al. 1989).

As deduced from its cDNA, Kell protein consists of 732 amino acids with a calculated molecular weight of 82,802. It is a basic protein with an estimated isoelectric point of 8.68 (Table 3.2). The amino acid sequence deduced from its cDNA contains all the known Kell sequences obtained from isolated tryptic peptides (Lee et al. 1991) (Fig. 3.2). Kell does not have an identifiable signal sequence. There is an initiation methionine followed by glutamic acid. Posttranslational cleavage of N-

Table 3.2. Amino Acid Composition*

	Number	Percentage
Nonpolar		
Ala	57	7.79
Val	36	4.92
Leu	91	12.43
Ile	23	3.14
Pro	51	6.97
Met	18	2.46
Phe	40	5.46
Trp	12	1.64
Polar		
Gly	39	5.33
Ser	61	8.33
Thr	33	4.51
Cys	16	2.19
Tyr	18	2.46
Asn	23	3.14
Gln	50	6.83
Acidic		
Asp	25	3.42
Glu	44	6.01
Basic		
Lys	22	3.01
Arg	50	6.83
His	23	3.14

*The amino acid composition is deduced by the translation of Kell cDNA.

```
              10        20        30        40        50        60        70
N-  MEGGDQSEEEPRERSQAGGMRTLWSQESTPEERLPVEESRPWAVARRVLTAILILGPLLCFSVLLFYNFQ
              80        90       100       110       120       130       140
    NCGPRPCETSVCLDLRDHYLASGNTSVAPCXDFFSFACGRAKETNNSFQELATKNKNRLRRILEVQNSWH
             150       160       170       180       190       200       210
    PGSGEEKAFQFYNSCMDTLAIEAAGTGPLRQVIEELGGWRISGKWTSLNFNRTLRLLMSQYGHFPFFRAY
             220       230       240       250       260       270       280
    LGPHPASPHTPVIQIDQPEFDVPLKQDQEQKIYAQIFREYLTYLNQLGTLLGGDPSKVQEHSSLSISITS
             290       300       310       320       330       340       350
    RLFQFLRPLEQRRAQGKLFQMVTIDQLKEMAPAIDWLSCLQATFTPMSLSPSQSLVVHDVEYLKNMSQLV
             360       370       380       390       400       410       420
    EEMLLKQRDFLQSHMILGLVVTLSPALDSQFQEARRKLSQKLRELTEQPPMPARPRWMKCVEETGTFFEP
             430       440       450       460       470       480       490
    TLAALFVREAFGPSTRSAAMKLFTAIRDALITRLRNLPWMNEETQNMAQDKVAQLQVEMGASEWALKPEL
             500       510       520       530       540       550       560
    ARQEYNDIQLGSSFLQSVLSCVRSLRARIVQSFLQPHPQHRWKVSPWDVNAYYSVSDHVVVFPAGLLQPP
             570       580       590       600       610       620       630
    FFHPGYPRAVNFGAAGSIMAHELLHIFYQLLLPGGCLACDNHALQEAHLCLKRHYAAFPLPSRTSFNDSL
             640       650       660       670       680       690       700
    TFLENAADVGGLAIALQAYSKRLLRHHGETVLPSLDLSPQQIFFRSYAQVMCRKPSPQDSHDTHSPPHLR
             710       720       730
    VHGPLSSTPAFARYFRCARGALLNPSSRCQLW* -C
```

Figure 3.2. The amino acid sequence deduced from the open reading frame of Kell cDNA. The initiation methionine is removed from the protein. The N-terminus is glutamic acid (boxed), which probably exists as pyroglutamate. A hydrophobic segment of 20 amino acids (boxed and lightly shaded) is likely to be the membrane-spanning region. Possible N-glycosylation sites are double underlined. Amino acid sequences, obtained by analyzing tryptic peptides of isolated Kell protein, are also underlined. A likely neutral endoprotease active sequence (HELLH) is shown in a vertical shaded box. The single-letter abbreviation for amino acids is used.

terminal methionine has been described in other membrane-associated proteins, and thus it is likely that the N-terminus of Kell is glutamic acid that has been converted to pyroglutamic acid. Glutamic acid is easily deamidated, even at neutral pH, to form pyroglutamic acid, which is a likely explanation for the observed blocked N-terminus of Kell protein.

Hydropathy analysis (Kyte and Doolittle 1982), with a window of 20 amino acids, suggests one possible membrane-spanning domain at amino acids 48 to 67 (Fig. 3.3). The N-terminal segment that precedes the membrane-spanning region is very hydrophilic and is likely to be a cy-

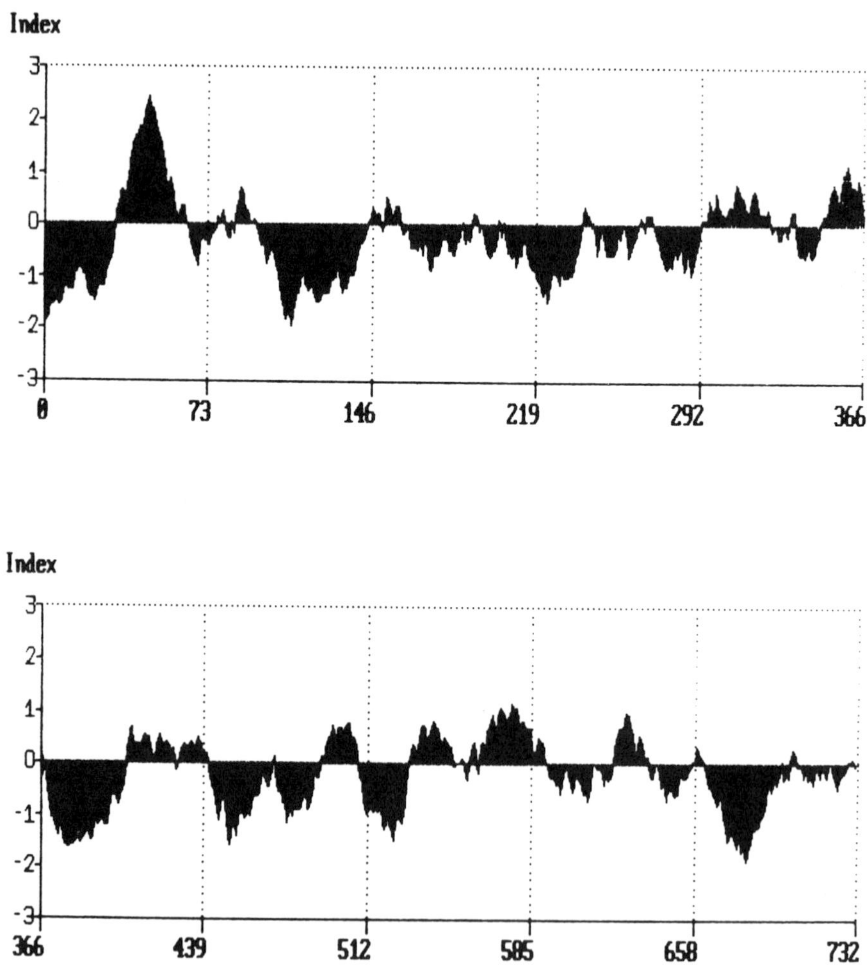

Figure 3.3. Hydropathy analysis of Kell protein. The amino acid sequence of Kell protein, deduced from its cDNA, was analyzed, using a window of 20 amino acid residues, by the method of Kyte and Doolittle (1982). A membrane-spanning segment was noted at residues 48 to 67.

toplasmic domain. The N-terminal cytoplasmic domain is marked by a pair of arginine residues immediately below the membrane-spanning region (see Fig. 3.2). Kell protein conforms with the charge-difference rule suggested by Hartman and associates (1989) to predict the N-terminal cytoplasmic orientation of membrane-spanning proteins.

Kell contains 16 cysteine residues. None of the cysteines is in the cytoplasmic domain, one is in the membrane-spanning region, and the other 15 are in the extracellular segment. The cysteines in the extracellular segment are clustered in two areas, close to the membrane-spanning region and at the C-terminal end (Fig. 3.4). As described earlier, Kell antigens are sensitive to sulfhydryl compounds, and the presence of 16 cysteine residues suggests that Kell is tightly folded extracellularly by disulfide bonds.

In addition to the clusters of cysteines, which are possible zinc-binding sites, Kell protein has three other areas that can bind zinc. These putative sites are at an LPGH, sequence at positions 211 to 214 and at a neighboring histidine at position 219. Another possible zinc-binding site is a pentameric sequence HELLH (position 581 to 585). This pentamer is a consensus sequence HE(ILM)XH that is common to the catalytic sites for zinc endopeptidases present in bacteria and mammals (McKerrow 1987) (Fig. 3.5).

Kell protein has two overlapping leucine-zipper motifs, starting at positions 583 and 590. The heptad array of leucine residues usually presents an α-helix configuration that may participate as oligomerization interfaces in protein–protein interactions. Figure 3.4 indicates the linear arrangement of these residues and motifs on Kell protein.

THE SIMILARITIES OF KELL WITH ZINC ENDOPEPTIDASES

Kell protein shares a pentameric consensus amino acid sequence with a family of zinc metalloendopeptidases. The members of this enzyme family are drawn from a wide number of species. These include bacterial thermolysin, a metallopeptidase of *Serratia*, and the human enkephalinases,

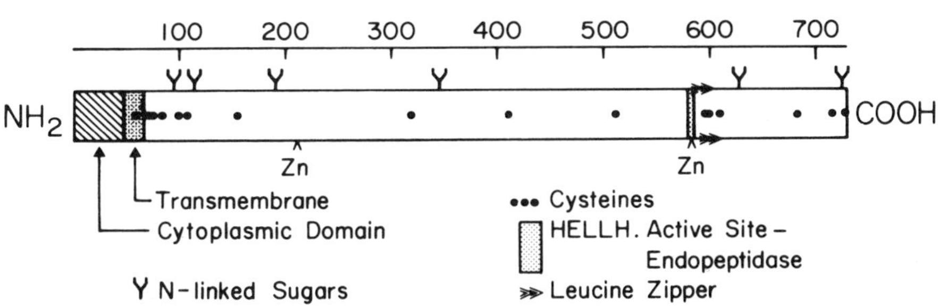

Figure 3.4. The arrangement of Kell protein, showing various pertinent amino acid residues and sequence motifs.

```
GQDLGGQTWYNVNQSNVKHPATEDYGRQTFT HEIGH ALGLSHPTDIGA S protease
:...::.. .. ... ...  .  .  :  .  .  ::.:: .:::::..:..:
GPGIGGDAHFDEDERWTNNFREYNLHRVA-A HELGH SLGLSHSGDYNA Collagenase

NAFWNGSQMVYGDGDGVTFTSLSGGI-DVIG HELTH AVTENSSNLIYQ Thermolysin
  :.  :   .       .  .  .:::  ::: ::.::  .  .:.  :.
IVFPAGILQPPFFSAQQSNSLNYGGIGMVIG HEITH GFDDNGRNFNKD CALLA
 ::::.::::::  .   ....:.:. :  ..  ::.  :  ::  .  .
VVFPAGLLQPPFFHPGYPRAVNFGAAGSIMA HELLH IFYQLLLPGGCL Kell
  550                                           597
```

Figure 3.5. Amino acid sequence similarities between Kell and some zinc metalloendopeptidases. Glutamic acid (E) is the active residue, and the histidine residues are thought to be coordinating sites for zinc binding. The similarities among thermolysin, CALLA, and Kell, and among *Serratia* protease, fibroblast collagenase, and thermolysin, are noted. Identical amino acids are shown by double dots (:), and a match with conservatively replaced amino acids is shown by a single dot (.).

which belong to a large group of physiologically important neutral endopeptidases such as angiotensin-converting enzyme, the enkephalinases, and collagenase. One of these enzymes, thermolysin, has been crystallized and models for the active sites have been derived. There is considerable structural and sequence similarity around the active sites of bacterial thermolysin and mammalian enkephalinases (Benchetrit et al. 1988), and within mammals there is near identity between human CALLA and rat and rabbit neutral endopeptidases (Shipp et al. 1989; Letarte et al. 1988).

Figure 3.5 demonstrates the consensus pentameric sequence at the active sites of *Serratia* protease, bacterial thermolysin, fibroblast collagenase, CALLA, and Kell protein. The glutamic acid residue in the pentameric sequence is thought to be the active residue in the catalytic activity of thermolysin, and the adjacent histidines are coordinating sites for zinc binding. Kell protein has striking sequence and structural similarities with CALLA. In the segment around the putative catalytic active sites there is a 59 percent base identity in a 152-bp region and a 25 percent amino acid identity in a 445–amino acid overlap. Figure 3.5 shows the similarities between CALLA and Kell protein in a smaller 47–amino acid segment near the active site. There is also similarity in this area between *Serratia* protease and fibroblast collagenase (McKerrow 1987) and between thermolysin and CALLA (Benchetrit et al. 1988), but not all of these homologies are shown in Figure 3.5.

In addition to sequence homology close to the active site of these enzymes, there are other similarities between Kell and CALLA. Placing the membrane-spanning domain of these two proteins in juxtaposition aligns four cysteine residues (residues 77, 82, 100 and 108) of Kell protein with four cysteines of CALLA, suggesting that these cysteines have an important role in the structure of both Kell and CALLA. Also to be noted is that both Kell and CALLA have short, hydrophilic N-terminal cytoplasmic domains (Fig. 3.6).

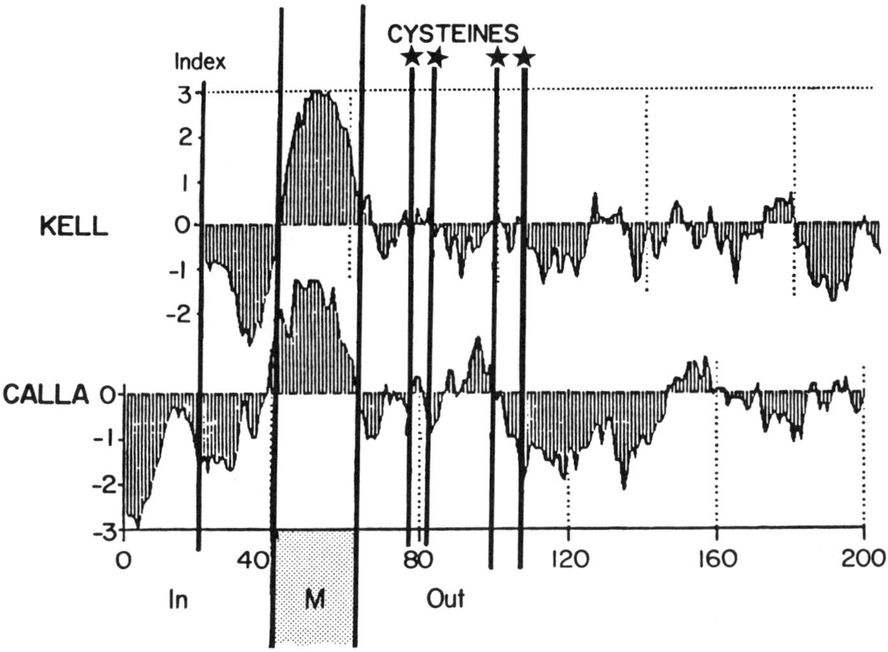

Figure 3.6. A comparison of hydropathy plots of Kell and CALLA, showing the cysteine arrangement near the membrane-spanning region. The membrane-spanning regions of CALLA (lower plot) and Kell (upper plot) are shown in the shaded region marked *M*. The cytoplasmic (In) and extracellular (Out) segments are shown. The alignment of four cysteine residues is marked by stars.

Further similarities between Kell and CALLA occur at the C-terminal segments of these proteins. Alignment of the putative catalytic active endopeptidase sites (H.E.L.L.H., positions 581 to 585 in Kell and H.E.I.T.H., positions 583 to 587 in CALLA) also places four cysteine residues, in both of the proteins, in near alignment. The pertinent cysteine residues are cysteines 610, 682, 717, and 729 in Kell and 620, 694, 734, and 746 of CALLA (Lee et al. 1991). Taken together, these similarities between Kell and CALLA indicate that Kell is a member of the neutral endopeptidase family and that the cysteines mentioned above may have important roles in the structure and function of both Kell and CALLA.

POSSIBLE FUNCTIONS AND FUTURE RESEARCH

The neutral endopeptidases inactivate a number of biologically active peptides, such as glucagon, the enkephalins, neurotensin, oxytocin, bradykinin, substance P, and the chemotactic peptide fMet-Leu-Phe (Gafford et al. 1983; Malfroy et al. 1988; Connelly et al. 1985; Letarte et al. 1988; Shipp et al. 1989). Although not yet demonstrated, it is likely that Kell will share similar endopeptidase enzymatic activity. However, we do not yet know whether this probable enzymatic activity, present on the surface of red cells, has a significant physiologic role. There are only 5000 Kell antigen sites per red cell, but there are about 5×10^9 red cells per milliliter of blood. It is therefore possible that, if Kell enzymatic activity is confirmed, it may play a significant part in inactivating (or activating) biologically active peptides that circulate in blood.

Kell also has structural similarities with a number of membrane receptors. For example, platelet adhesion receptors (Andrews and Fox 1990) and some hormone receptors such as the epidermal growth factor receptor (Ullrich et al. 1984) span the plasma membrane once, and have cysteine-rich domains in the extracellular segment. It is possible that Kell may also be a receptor for an as-yet-unknown ligand and that its proteolytic activity may serve a complementary role in inactivating the bound ligand.

There is a serologic association of Kell with certain other blood group antigens whose absence in red cells is accompanied by abnormal shape. For example, weakened Kell antigens are found in red cells of some individuals of Gerbich-negative type, and weakened Kell antigens always accompany the absence of Kx antigen. Gerbich antigens are markers on glycophorin C, a membrane sialoglycoprotein. Red cells of the rare Leach phenotype lack glycophorin C and have elliptocytic shape (Anstee 1990). These phenotypic associations suggest a close neighbor relationship among Kell, Kx, and glycophorin C, and indicate that the interrelationship in normal individuals plays a part in maintaining normal discoid cell shape. Both Kell protein and glycophorin C are known to be transmembrane proteins in which the cytoplasmic component is complexed with the cell cytoskeleton.

Kell has two leucine zipper motifs in its extracellular segment. Areas such as these act as oligomerization interfaces and may enhance protein–protein interactions. It is possible that some blood group antigens, such as Kell, the glycophorins, and Kx, may exist as clusters on the red cell surface and have cooperative functions in promoting the shape and stability of the membrane. It should be noted, however, that a lack of Kell protein does not itself alter cell morphology, for Ko cells, which lack Kell protein, have normal shape.

Among the human blood groups, a number of phenotypes with reduced antigen expression are known. Most are inherited, but the biochemical basis for the depression is not known. The Kell group includes several such phenotypes. Thus, in the *cis*-modifying Kp^a type, the expression of all other Kell antigens is markedly depressed. Elucidation of the basis for such changes may provide a model for similar changes in other blood group systems and allow an understanding of variation and reduced penetrance at the biochemical and genomic levels.

REFERENCES

Advani H., J. Zamor, W. J. Judd, C. L. Johnson, and W. L. Marsh. 1982. Inactivation of Kell blood group antigens by 2-aminoethylisothiouronium bromide. *Br. J. Haematol.* 51:107–15.

Andrews, R. K., and J. E. B. Fox. 1990. Platelet receptors in hemostasis. *Current Opinion in Cell Biology*. 2:894–901.

Anstee, D. J. 1990. Blood group-active surface molecules of the human red blood cells. *Vox Sang*. 58:1–20.

Ballas, S. K., S. M. Bator, J. P. Aubuchon, W. L. Marsh, D. E. Sharp, and E. M. Toy. 1990. Abnormal membrane physical properties of red cells in McLeod syndrome. *Transfusion* 30:722–27.

Benchetrit, T., V. Bissery, J. P. Mormon, A. Devault, P. Crine, and B. P. Rogues. 1988. Primary structure homologies between two zinc metalloproteases, the neutral endopeptidase 24.11 ("enkephalinase") and thermolysin through clustering analysis. *Biochemistry* 27:592–96.

Bertelson, C. J., A. O. Pogo, A. Chadhuri, C. M. Redman, D. Banerjee, W. A. Symmans, T. Simon, and L. M. Kunkel. 1988. Localization of the McLeod locus (XK) within Xp21 by deletion analysis. *Am. J. Hum. Genet.* 423:703–11.

Branch, D. R., H. A. Muensch, H. L. S. Siok Hian, and L. D. Petz. 1983. Disulfide bonds are a requirement for Kell and Cartwright (Yta) blood group antigen integrity. *Br. J. Haematol.* 54:573–78.

Branch, D. R., and L. D. Petz. 1982. A new reagent (ZZAP) having multiple applications in immunohematology. *Am. J. Clin. Pathol.* 78:161–67.

Connelly, J. C., A. Skidgel, W. W. Schultz, A. R. Johnson, and E. G. Erdos. 1985. Neutral endopeptidase 24.11 in human neutrophils: Cleavage of chemotactic peptide. *Proc. Natl. Acad. Sci. U.S.A.* 82:8737–41.

Conner, J., and A. J. Schroit. 1989. Transbilayer movement of phosphatidylserine in nonhuman erythrocytes: Evidence that the aminophospholipid transporter is a ubiquitous membrane protein. *Biochemistry* 28:9680–85.

Coombs, R. R. A., A. E. Mourant, and R. R. Race. 1946. *In vivo* isosensitization of red cells in babies with haemolytic disease. *Lancet* i:264–266.

D'Adamio, L., M. A. Shipp, E. L. Masteller, and E. L. Reinherz. 1989. Organization of the gene encoding common acute lymphoblastic leukemia antigen (neutral endopeptidase 24.11): Multiple miniexons and separate 5′ untranslated regions. *Proc. Natl. Acad. Sci. U.S.A.* 86:7103–7.

Daleke, D. L., and W. H. Huestis. 1985. Incorporation and translocation of aminophospholipids in human erythrocytes. *Biochemistry* 24:5406–16.

Elgsaeter, A., B. T. Stokke, A. Mikkelsen, and D. Branton. 1983. The molecular basis of erythrocyte shape. *Science* 234:1217–23.

Gafford, J. T., R. A. Skidgel, E. G. Erdos, and L. B. Hersh. 1983. Human kidney "enkephalinase": A neutral metalloendopeptidase that cleaves active peptides. *Biochemistry* 22:3265–71.

Galey, W. R., A. P. Evan, P. S. Van Nice, W. G. Dail, B. M. Wimer, and R. A. Cooper. 1978. Morphology and physiology of the McLeod erythrocyte. I. Scanning electron microscopy and electrolyte and water transport properties. *Vox Sang*. 34:152–61.

Glaubensklee, C. S., A. P. Evan, and W. R. Galey. 1982. Structural and biochemical analysis of the McLeod erythrocyte membrane. I. Freeze fracture and discontinuous polyacrylamide gel electrophoresis analysis. *Vox Sang*. 42:262–71.

Hartmann, E., T. A. Rapoport, and H. F. Lodish. 1989. Predicting the orientation of eukaryotic-membrane spanning proteins. *Proc. Natl. Acad. Sci. U.S.A.* 86:5786–90.

Jaber, A., D. Blanchard, D. Goossens, C. Bloy, P. Lambin, P. Rouger, C. Salmon, and J. P. Cartron. 1989. Characterization of blood group Kell (K1) antigen with a human monoclonal antibody. *Blood* 73:1597–1602.

Judson, P. A., and D. J. Anstee. 1977. Comparative effect of trypsin and chymotrypsin on blood group antigens. *Med. Lab. Sci.* 34:1–6.

Khodadad, J. K., R. S. Weinstein, W. L. Marsh, and T. L. Steck. 1989. Shape determinants of McLeod acanthocytes. *J. Membr. Biol.* 107:213–18.

Kuypers, F. A., M. Van Linde Sibenius, B. Trip, B. Roelofsen, J. A. F. Opdenkamp, M. J. A. Tanner, and D. J. Anstee. 1985. The phospholipid organizations in the membranes of McLeod and Leach phenotype erythrocytes. *FEBS Lett.* 184:20–4.

Kyte, J., and R. F. Doolittle. 1982. A simple method for displaying the hydropathic character of a protein. *J. Mol. Biol.* 157:105–32.

Lange, Y., and T. L. Steck. 1984. The mechanisms of red blood cell acanthocytosis and echinocytosis in vivo. *J. Membr. Biol.* 77:153–59.

Lee, S., E. Zambas, W. L. Marsh, and C. M. Redman. 1991. Molecular cloning and primary structure of Kell blood group protein. *Proc. Natl. Acad. Sci. U.S.A.* 88:6353–57.

Letarte, M., S. Vera, R. Tran, J. B. L. Addis, R. J. Onizuka, E. J. Quackenbush, C. V. Jongeneel, and R. R. McInnes. 1988. Common acute lymphocytic leukemia antigen is identical to neutral endopeptidase. *J. Exp. Med.* 168:1247–53.

Malfroy, B., W.-J. Kuang, P. H. Seeburg, A. J. Mason, and P. R. Schofield. 1988. Molecular cloning and amino acid sequence of human enkephalinase (neutral endopeptidase). *FEBS Lett.* 229:206–10.

Marsh, W. L., N. J. Marsh, A. Moore, W. A. Symmans, C. L. Johnson, and C. M. Redman. 1981. Elevated serum creatine phosphokinase in subjects with McLeod syndrome. *Vox Sang.* 40:403–11.

Marsh W. L., R. Oyen, M. E. Nichols, and F. H. Allen. 1975. Chronic granulomatous disease and the Kell blood groups. *Br. J. Haematol.* 29:247–62.

Marsh, W. L., and C. M. Redman. 1987. Recent developments in the Kell blood group system. *Trans. Med. Rev.* 1:4–20.

McKerrow, J. H. 1987. Human fibroblast collagenase contains an amino acid sequence homologous to the zinc-binding site of *Serratia* protease. *J. Biol. Chem.* 262:5943.

Redman, C. M., G. Avellino, S. R. Pfeffer, T. K. Mukherjee, M. Nichols, P. Rubinstein, and W. L. Marsh. 1986. Kell blood group antigens are part of a 93,000 Dalton red cell membrane protein. *J. Biol. Chem.* 261:9521–25.

Redman, C. M., T. Huima, E. Robbins, S. Lee, and W. L. Marsh. 1989a. Effect of phosphatidylserine on the shape of McLeod red cell acanthocytes. *Blood* 74:1826–35.

Redman, C. M., S. Lee, D. Ten Bokkel Huinink, B. I. Rabin, C. L. Johnson, R. Oyen, and W. L. Marsh. 1989b. Comparison of human and chimpanzee Kell blood group systems. *Transfusion* 29:486–90.

Redman, C. M., W. L. Marsh, K. A. Mueller, G. P. Avellino, and C. L. Johnson. 1984. Isolation of Kell-active protein from the red cell membrane. *Transfusion* 24:176–78.

Redman, C. M., W. L. Marsh, A. Scarborough, and C. L. Johnson, B. I. Rabin, and M. Overbeeke M. 1988. Biochemical studies on McLeod phenotype red cells and isolation of Kx antigen. *Br. J. Haematol.* 68:131–36.

Sheetz, M. P., and S. J. Singer. 1974. Biological membranes as bilayer couples: A molecular mechanism of drug-erythrocyte interactions. *Proc. Natl. Acad. Sci. U.S.A.* 71:4457–61.

Shipp, M. A., N. E. Richardson, P. H. Sayre, N. R. Brown, E. L. Masteller, L. K. Clayton, J. Ritz, and E. L. Reinherz. 1988. Molecular cloning of the common acute lymphoblastic leukemia antigen (CALLA) identifies a type II integral membrane protein. *Proc. Natl. Acad. Sci. U.S.A.* 85:4819–23.

Shipp, M. A., J. Vijayaraghavan, E. V. Schmidt, E. L. Masteller, L. D. D'Adamio, L. B. Hersh, and E. L. Reinherz. 1989. Common acute lymphoblastic antigen (CALLA) is active neutral endopeptidase 24.11 ("enkephalinase"): Direct eivdence by cDNA transfected analysis. *Proc. Natl. Acad. Sci. U.S.A.* 86:297–301.

Swash, M., M. S. Schwartz, N. D. Carter, R. Heath, M. Leak, and K. L. Rogers. 1983. Benign X-linked myopathy with acanthocytes (McLeod syndrome): Its relationship to X-linked muscular dystrophy. *Brain* 106:717–33.

Symmans, W. A., C. S. Shepherd, W. L. Marsh, R. Oyen, S. B. Shohet, and B. J. Linehan. 1979. Hereditary acanthocytosis associated with the McLeod phenotype of the Kell blood group system. *Br. J. Haematol.* 42:575–83.

Tang, L. L., C. M. Redman, D. Williams, and W. L. Marsh. 1981. Biochemical studies on McLeod phenotype erythrocytes. *Vox Sang.* 40:17–26.

Ullrich, A., L. Coussens, J. S. Hayflick, T. J. Dull, A. Gray, A. W. Tam, J. Lee, Y. Yarden, T. A. Leibermann, J. Schlessinger, J. Downward, E. L. Y. Mayes, N. Whittle, M. D. Waterfield, and P. H. Seeburg. 1984. Human insulin receptor and its relationship to the tyropsine kinase family of oncogenes. *Nature* 309:418–25.

Wimmer, B. M., W. L. Marsh, H. F. Taswell, and H. R. Galey. 1977. Haematological changes associated with the McLeod phenotype of the Kell blood group system. *Br. J. Haematol.* 36:219–24.

4

THE LUTHERAN ANTIGENS AND PROTEINS AFFECTED BY LUTHERAN REGULATORY GENES

Marilyn J. Telen, M.D.

The Lutheran (Lu) blood group antigens are a family of human red cell antigens that appear to arise from polymorphisms of two probably related red cell integral membrane proteins. Although of relatively infrequent importance to the clinician concerned with transfusion or hemolytic disease of the newborn, these antigens have played an important part in the history of human genetics, so both clinicians and research scientists should be aware of them. In addition, Lutheran-related regulatory genes, of which two have been identified, also represent important and unique human genes, the study of which is on-going and promises many interesting insights into human genetics.

Lutheran antigens first made genetic history in 1951, when *Lu* was used, along with the *secretor* (*Se*) gene, to propose the first example of autosomal linkage in humans (Mohr 1954). Mohr also suspected the later-proved linkage between *Lu* and *Dm*, the myotonic dystrophy gene (Renwick et al. 1971). These relationships were subsequently confirmed by several groups. Further genetic history was then made when the published observations on the *Lu-Se* linkage, along with some additional data, became the basis for the first documentation of a sex-related difference in the frequency of crossing-over in humans (Cook 1965). Since these observations, *Lu* has been mapped to chromosome 19 by genetic linkage to C3 (the third component of human complement) (Eiberg et al. 1983), and the linkage group has been expanded to include the *LDLR* (the low-density-lipoprotein receptor), *LW* (blood group), and *APOC2* (apolipoprotein C-II) loci (Lewis et al. 1988).

The importance of the Lutheran blood group to geneticists grew even further in 1961, when Crawford and colleagues described a Lutheran-negative phenotype, apparently inherited as a dominant characteristic independent of Lutheran genes (Crawford et al. 1961). The gene responsible for this phenotype was designated *In(Lu)* and became the first such human regulatory gene described (Taliano et al. 1973). More recently, an X-linked Lutheran regulatory gene was discovered, expanding the regulatory repertoire of the Lutheran antigens (Norman et al. 1986). The study of these two regulatory genes has linked the expression of Lutheran antigens to that of several other antigens and proteins also affected by the same regulatory genes; at least one of these proteins (CD44) has well-recognized blood group antigen and functional activity (reviewed in Haynes et al. 1989).

LUTHERAN BLOOD GROUP ANTIGENS

SEROLOGY

The first Lutheran antigen to be described—Lu^a—was identified in 1945 by Callender and associates, who found an antibody that reacted with about 8 percent of all donor samples. The antibody that identified the antithetical antigen, present in more than 99 percent of all persons, was not found until 1956 (Cutbush and Chanarin, 1956). Since that time, 16 Lutheran or so-called para-Lutheran antigens have been described by researchers working with antisera from transfusion recipients or women exposed to antigens on fetal blood cells (Table 4.1). Most of these antigens were identified as being part of the Lutheran blood group system by family studies demonstrating linkage between the new antigen and other

Table 4.1. Lutheran Blood Group Antigens

Known Antithetical Pairs	
Low Frequency	*High Frequency*
Lu^a	Lu^b
Lu9	Lu6
Lu14	Lu8
Au^b	Au^a

High-Incidence Antigens That Genetic (G), Serologic (S), or Biochemical (B) Evidence Suggests Are Encoded by Genes at the Lutheran Locus	
Antigen	*Evidence*
Lu4	S, B
Lu5	S, B
Lu7	S
Lu11	S
Lu13	S, B
Lu16	G, S
Lu17	S

Lutheran antigen polymorphisms. Antigens absent from Lu(a – b –) cells but not unequivocally linked to Lutheran antigens were termed *para-Lutheran antigens*. Some of these para-Lutheran antigens have since been demonstrated to reside on a similar protein as the Lutheran antigens, while at least one antithetical pair of antigens (Au^a/Au^b), previously thought not to be genetically linked to the Lutheran locus, has since been shown also to reside on the Lutheran proteins (Daniels 1990).

The Lu^a antigen, being of moderately low frequency (8 percent of Caucasian populations), not uncommonly induces antibody formation, although the presence of the antibody is often not detected because of the frequent absence of the antigen on cells routinely used to perform antibody screening and because of the often short-lived production of the antibody (Lostumbo et al. 1966). This discrepancy is rarely a problem, however, as anti-Lu^a is often cold-reacting and predominantly IgM. Thus, anti-Lu^a has not been associated with delayed hemolytic transfusion reactions. Likewise, anti-Lu^a only rarely been reported in hemolytic disease of the newborn, perhaps also because of the weakened expression of Lutheran antigens on fetal red cells (Greenwalt et al. 1967).

The Lu^b antigen, present in more than 99.8 percent of persons, is only rarely the target of alloantibody. Unlike anti-Lu^a, however, anti-Lu^b is more often warm-reacting; it has been reported to contain primarily IgG and, at least in some cases, predominantly IgA. Accelerated posttransfusion red cell destruction may occur owing to anti-Lu^b, but this destruction is most often relatively slow, allowing the transfusion of Lu(b +) blood to someone with anti-Lu^b in emergencies. Likewise, hemolytic disease of the newborn does not appear to occur (or occurs in an extremely mild form) owing to anti-Lu^b.

The second most important antithetical pair of Lutheran antigens is Lu6 and Lu9. Lu9 occurs in about 2 percent of donors, while Lu6 occurs in more than 99.9 percent of persons. In studies designed to prove that these antigens are indeed part of the Lutheran system, workers demonstrated strong linkage disequilibrium between Lu^a and Lu9, so Lu(a + b +) cells are much more likely to be Lu:9 than at Lu(a – b +) cells. Antibodies to these antigens, although provoked by red cell transfusions and frequently warm-reacting IgG, have not been implicated in significant red cell destruction.

Finally, Lu14 and Lu8 constitute a third set of antithetical antigens in this system and have negligible clinical impact. Lu8 occurs in 99.9 percent of persons, while Lu14 occurs in only 2.5 percent. In addition, numerous high-frequency antigens are apparently part of the Lutheran system (see below); these include Lu4, Lu5, Lu12, Lu13, and Lu16. The Auberger antigens (Au^a and Au^b), originally thought to be independent from the Lutheran system, now appear to reside on the same protein as Lutheran antigens and are probably part of this system.

BIOCHEMISTRY

Although early work suggested that Lutheran antigens resided on proteins, because proteases and reagents that disrupted disulfide bonds often destroyed antigen activity, identification of the proteins involved was first achieved many years later using a murine monoclonal antibody BRIC108 with anti-Lu^b–like specificity (Parsons et al. 1987). This original work identified two proteins, M_r 85 and 78 kDa, by immunoblotting. That these proteins were actually the targets of human anti-Lu^a and anti-Lu^b was later confirmed by similar methods using human antisera (Fig. 4.1).

Thus far, human antisera to Lu^a, Lu^b, Lu3, Lu4, Lu5, Lu6, Lu8, Lu13,

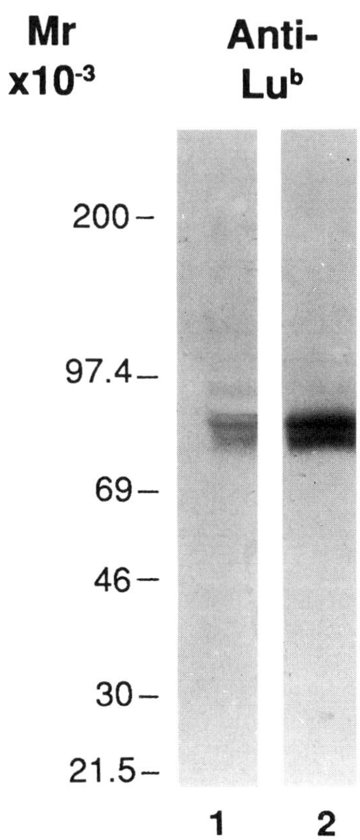

Figure 4.1. Identification of Lutheran proteins by immunoblotting with human anti-Lu^b. Lutheran protein was partially purified by the following technique: Normal Lu(b+) red cells were incubated with ficin to remove proteolytically the N-oligosaccharide-containing portion of glycophorin A. Membranes from these cells were then lysed and passed over a lentil lectin column, and adherent protein was eluted with methyl alpha-D-mannopyranoside. The anti-Lu^b identified reactive protein in membranes pretreated with ficin (lane 1) as well as in the eluate from the lentil lectin column (lane 2).

and Lu14 have all been shown to react with two proteins of molecular weights similar to those originally identified using the monoclonal antibody BRIC108 (Daniels and Khalid 1989), although strict proof that these proteins are the same—that is, that the individual molecule carrying Lu^b simultaneously carries Lu6 and Lu8—is lacking at this time. Furthermore, although all these antigens are absent in Lutheran null phenotypes, no proof of genetic linkage is available for Lu4, Lu5, and Lu13. The possibility remains that the expression of these antigens depends, for example, on posttranslational modification of Lutheran protein by the product of a non-Lutheran gene.

The Lutheran proteins have been characterized only partially. They appear to be of low abundance, as only 2000 to 4000 copies of Lu^b antigen are present per red cell (Merry et al. 1987). Several studies have described Lutheran antigens as being poorly expressed on fetal red cells, although the process whereby Lutheran antigens appear later in development of the newborn remains obscure (Greenwalt et al. 1967; Toivanen and Hirvoven 1973). Work with endoglycosidase F and sialidase has shown that these enzymes changed the migration of Lu protein in SDS-polyacrylamide gels, thus demonstrating the presence of N-linked oligosaccharides (Parsons et al. 1987). Lutheran proteins also appear not to be significantly linked to the red cell cytoskeleton (Judson et al. 1988). However, little else is known about the biochemical nature of these proteins at this time. Work with monoclonal antibodies suggests, however, that the expression of this protein is not limited to erythroid cells; murine monoclonal anti-Lu^b reacts strongly with renal endothelial cells and fetal hepatocytes (Anstee et al. 1988).

NULL PHENOTYPES

Since the discovery of the Lu^a and Lu^b antigens and the determination of their relationship to each other as antithetical, three genetic backgrounds for the Lu(a−b−) phenotype have been described. In a few families, the Lu(a−b−) phenotype has appeared to represent homozygosity for an apparently "amorphic" Lutheran allele (variously called *Lu* or *lu*) that does not encode the production of Lutheran system antigens (Brown et al. 1974). This Lutheran null phenotype is termed autosomal recessive Lu(a−b−). Persons with this phenotype may produce an antibody (called anti-Lu3) that reacts with either Lu(a+) or Lu(b+) red cells but is not separable into anti-Lu^a and anti-Lu^b. Families in which one such amorphic allele is present have also been described (J. L. Crookston and M. Crookston, personal communication, cited in Brown et al. 1974). Unlike the other Lutheran "null" phenotypes, however, recessive Lu(a−b−) red cells have normal expression of all non-Lutheran antigens.

The most common cause of the Lu(a−b−) phenotype appears to be an independently segregating, dominant gene that down-regulates the expression of all Lutheran antigens (Crawford et al. 1961). This gene, traditionally called *In(Lu)* (since it "inhibits Lutheran"), causes extremely weakened expression of inherited Lutheran antigens, so such antigens are not detectable by routine methods (e.g., agglutination assays using human typing sera). At least one study found that the incidence of this gene is as high as 1 in 3000 (Shaw et al. 1984). Also, studies of the strength of expression of Lutheran antigens within and among families suggest that the common variant of this gene [often called *in(Lu)*] regulates the strength of expression of the Lutheran antigens. Thus, within a family, one may correlate the strength of Lu^b expression with homo- or heterozygosity, while such correlations may not be possible from one family to another.

A third Lu(a − b −) phenotype has also been described. This phenotype appears to be due to a second Lutheran regulatory gene, *XS2*, and occurred with an X-linked inheritance pattern (Norman et al. 1986). Like *In(Lu)*, it suppressed but did not abolish expression of all Lutheran system antigens; inherited antigens were still detectable by sensitive means. The effects of the *XS2* gene on non-Lutheran antigens is different, however, from that of the *In(Lu)* gene.

LUTHERAN REGULATORY GENES

THE *IN(LU)* GENE

The *In(Lu)* gene, as stated above, suppresses but does not totally prevent the expression of Lutheran antigens. Although the suppressive effect of the *In(Lu)* gene on Lutheran antigens has not been strictly quantitated, the level of Lutheran antigens expressed by these cells is most likely much less than 50 percent of the normal level. Quantitation of Lu^b antigen as recognized by a monoclonal antibody demonstrated about 500 antigen sites per cell in persons with the *In(Lu)* phenotype. Agglutination techniques using antihuman globulin, which are known to be able to detect 100 to 500 molecules of antibody on a red cell surface, fail to detect Lutheran antigens on *In(Lu)* cells. Given that normal homozygous Lu(b +) cells have 2000 to 4000 copies of the antigen per cell, *In(Lu)* red cells most likely have no more than 500 copies of Lu^b antigen. Furthermore, cells from donors with one copy of an amorphic *Lu* gene have easily detectable Lutheran system antigens, suggesting that a 50 percent reduction of the antigen would not make these cells phenotypically Lu(a − b −).

The true antigen status of *In(Lu)* red cells has been demonstrated by several extremely sensitive tests, such as the absorption and elution of anti-Lu^b and radioimmunoassay. Such procedures have been used to demonstrate low levels of Lutheran antigen expression on *In(Lu)* Lu(a − b −) red cells. The presence of Lutheran antigens on these cells is compatible with the fact that persons with the *In(Lu)* Lu(a − b −) phenotype have never been demonstrated to make antibodies to the Lutheran antigens for which they have genes (such as Lu^b), unlike persons with the recessive Lu(a−b−) phenotype, who may make an antibody (anti-Lu3) that binds to all cells with normal expression of Lu^a or Lu^b antigens.

Perhaps the most fascinating phenomenon associated with the *In(Lu)* gene and the phenotype it produces is that cells of the *In(Lu)* Lu(a−b−) phenotype have depressed expression of a number of apparently unrelated red cell antigens. Early on, workers described the suppression of the P_1, i, and Au antigens by *In(Lu)* (Taliano et al. 1973). Since then, the Auberger antigens have been shown to be borne on Lutheran proteins (Daniels 1990). However, the P_1 and i antigens are known to be primarily glycolipid in nature and dependent on immunodominant oligosaccharide structures.

The first protein shown to be down-regulated by *In(Lu)* was the membrane protein now known as CD44 but originally described as *In(Lu)*-related p80 (Telen et al. 1983, 1984). Following the observation that the In^b antigen was decreased on *In(Lu)* cells (Ferguson and Gaal 1988), the In^a and In^b blood group antigens have both been shown to reside on red cell CD44 (Spring et al. 1988; Telen and Ferguson 1990).

Other proteins have also been shown to be affected by *In(Lu)* (reviewed in Tippett 1990). Lutheran antigens were demonstrated to reside on protein structures, providing evidence for a second protein under *In(Lu)* regulatory control (Parsons et al. 1987; Daniels and Khalid 1989). Although CD44 and Lutheran proteins are of very similar molecular weights, current evidence indicates that they are distinct proteins (Telen et al. 1988). The expression of the red cell receptor for the *Haemophilus influenzae* bacterium and the related AnWj antigen has also been shown to be markedly reduced in the presence of the *In(Lu)* gene (Poole and Giles 1982; Gilsdorf et al. 1989). Expression of the MER2 antigen, a target of murine monoclonal and human antibodies, is also reduced in the presence of the *In(Lu)* gene (Tippett 1986). The red cell antigen produced by the MER2 gene (Daniels et al. 1987), which maps to a part of chromosome 11 separate from the region containing the CD44 gene (Glaser et al. 1989), is incompletely characterized, although it appears likely to be a protein, perhaps of about 70 kDa (Miller et al. 1985). There is also some evidence that several other high-incidence blood group antigens are slightly depressed by the *In(Lu)* gene, although the evidence concerning these antigens is somewhat less definitive (Daniels et al. 1986). These antigens include Kn^a, Sl^a, McC^a, Cs^a, and Yk^a. The antigens of the Kn/McC family, including Sl^a, have recently been shown to reside on the red cell C3b/C4b complement receptor CR1 (Rao et al., 1991).

Thus, the *In(Lu)* gene appears to effect expression of a broad range of antigens, including those on proteins encoded by chromosomes 1 (CR1), 11 (CD44 and MER2), and 19 (Lu antigens). Furthermore, work with the *H. influenzae* receptor and CD44 has demonstrated that the effect of *In(Lu)* is largely limited to erythroid cells, as epithelial cells (in the case of the *H. influenzae* receptor) and lymphocytes (in the case of CD44) appear essentially unaffected. The possibility remains that the *In(Lu)* gene acts by affecting an erythroid-specific DNA-binding protein or is itself differentially expressed in erythroid cells. Exploration of these possibilities is only just beginning and promises to yield interesting data regarding possible mechanisms of action of broad regulatory genes such as *In(Lu)*. No other human regulatory gene has yet been described to have the type of broad but tissue-specific suppressor effects engendered by the *In(Lu)* gene.

In(Lu) Lu(a−b−) red cells have also been seen to have mild morphologic and physiologic abnormalities. Some samples from persons with *In(Lu)* contain significant numbers of acanthocytes and poikilocytes. Numerous workers have noted that these red cells cannot be stored in the usual preservation media, such as acid citrate–dextrose, as well as normal red cells (unpublished observations of this author and others). Udden et al. (1987) documented abnormal K^+-Na^+ balance in *In(Lu)* red cells. However, the molecular mechanism responsible for the cation defect has not been elucidated.

THE *XS2* GENE

The *XS2* gene, which causes an X-linked recessive Lu(a−b−) phenotype, suppresses but does not abolish expression of Lutheran (and Auberger) antigens, similarly to the *In(Lu)* gene. On the other hand, studies of the one family in which this gene has been described showed that it did not suppress the expression of In^b and its protein CD44, nor was the AnWj antigen suppressed (Norman et al. 1986; Telen et al. 1988). Thus, this gene appears to have a unique locus and mechanism of action clearly distinguishable from that of the *In(Lu)* gene. Study of the original extended family with this phenotype has demonstrated the *XS2* gene to lie near the centromere of the X chromosome (Mulley et al. 1988).

Although different from those of *In(Lu)*, the effects of the *XS2* gene may not, however, be limited to Lutheran antigens. Red cells with the X-linked Lu(a−b−) phenotype were noted to have enhanced expression of the i antigen (as opposed to the reduced expression in *In(Lu)* cells) and depression of the I antigen (Norman et al. 1986). The family was not adequately informative for the possible effects of *XS2* on the P_1 antigen, although some weakening of that antigen was suggested. The mechanism of action of the *XS2* gene is thus far completely undefined.

ANTIGENS AFFECTED BY LUTHERAN REGULATORY GENES

As outlined above, numerous red cell antigens appear to be affected by Lutheran regulatory genes. However, this section will deal with only the two well-investigated membrane structures whose expression is down-regulated by the *In(Lu)* gene: *In(Lu)*-related p80 (CD44) and the AnWj *H. influenzae* receptor.

In(Lu)-RELATED p80 (CD44)

The CD44 glycoprotein is widely expressed in many human tissues (Dalchau et al. 1980; Telen et al. 1983; Carter and Wayner 1988). In fact, it was after nearly 10 years of study that numerous independent investigators working in such diverse fields as thymocyte differentiation, red cell antigens, extracellular matrix receptors, and lymphocyte-endothelial binding compared the reactivity of their various monoclonal and polyclonal antibodies and found that they all reacted with the protein designated CD44 by the Third International Workshop on Leukocyte Differentiation Antigens (McKay et al. 1988; Telen et al. 1986; Omary et al. 1988; Picker et al. 1989).

Red cell CD44 was first described in 1983 (Telen et al. 1983) as *In(Lu)*-related p80, the target of a murine monoclonal antibody A3D8. This antibody recognized an antigen expressed by all circulating leukocytes and red cells, including B and T lymphocytes, monocytes, and polymorphonuclear leukocytes. In addition, numerous malignant leukocyte cell lines expressed p80 strongly. Other tissues, including squamous epithelial cells, fibroblasts, and brain, reacted with the A3D8 antibody. In addition, A3D8 antigen activity was found in normal serum and plasma, indicating that the molecule was expressed in both membrane-bound and soluble forms.

Expression of the A3D8 red cell antigen was clearly down-regulated in the presence of the *In(Lu)* gene (Telen et al. 1983, 1987) (see also Fig. 4.2). The red cells of persons with the *In(Lu)* Lu(a−b−) phenotype bound five times less antibody than did cells of normal Lu(b+) or Lu(a+) phenotypes, while cells of other null phenotypes showed no decrease in antibody binding. Interestingly, cord red cells appeared to have normal to increased expression of CD44, as compared with red cells from normal adults. This finding was in contradistinction to data obtained with Lutheran antibodies, which bind only very weakly to cord red cells. Also, despite the marked apparent effect of the *In(Lu)* gene on expression of red cell CD44, the regulatory gene had only modest effect on expression of CD44 by lymphocytes and monocytes (Telen et al. 1983). Serum CD44 expression was also decreased modestly by the *In(Lu)* gene. In total, therefore, *In(Lu)* appeared to have a relatively erythroid-specific effect on CD44 expression.

The initial characterization of the CD44 antigen showed that it was destroyed by a variety of proteases. Using various antibodies and tissues, investigators isolated a protein of 80 to 90 kDa (Haynes et al. 1983; Telen et al. 1984; Letarte et al. 1985). In addition, various workers have described a higher-molecular-weight protein of 170 to 200 kDa. In at least some tissues, this higher-molecular-weight protein appears to contain

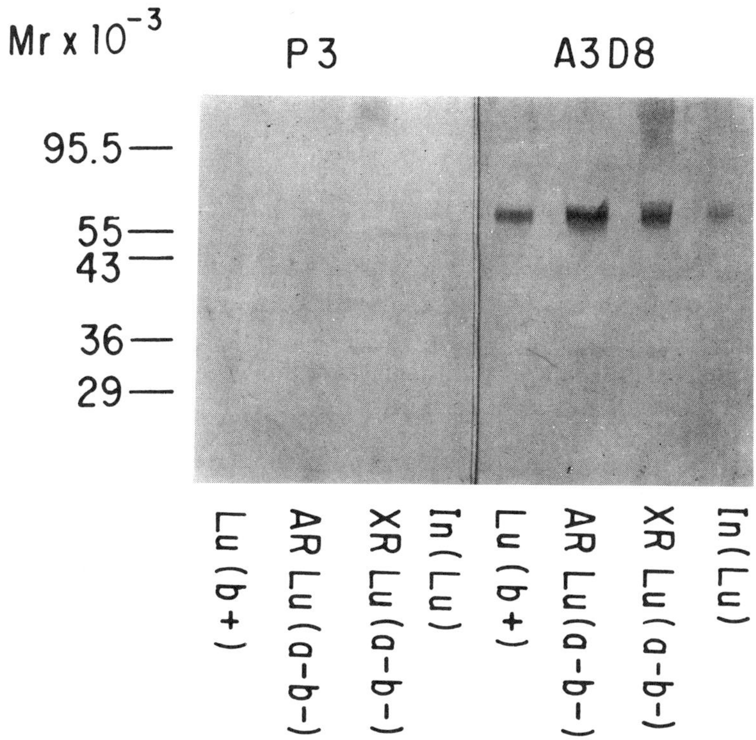

Figure 4.2. Expression of CD44 [*In(Lu)*-related p80] by various Lutheran-null phenotypes. When the A3D8 antibody against CD44 was used to immunoblot membrane proteins from Lu(b+), autosomal recessive (AR) Lu(a−b−), X-linked recessive (XR) Lu(a−b−), and *In(Lu)* Lu(a−b−) red cells, a reduced amount of immunoreactive protein was detectable in the *In(Lu)* membranes, while the recessive Lu(a−b−) red cells had normal to increased amounts of CD44 protein. P3 is a nonreactive murine myeloma protein used as a nonreactive control.

several chondroitin sulfate groups absent from the lower-molecular-weight form (Jalkanen et al. 1988).

Following the initial observation that A3D8 antigen was detectable in plasma and serum, this soluble form of CD44 was isolated and characterized. Serum CD44 appears to be indistinguishable in molecular weight from the red cell form, although there may be subtle antigenic differences (Lucas et al. 1989).

The DNA for CD44 has been cloned, demonstrating that CD44 is a protein of 341 amino acids (Stamenkovic et al. 1989; Goldstein et al. 1989). This work has shown that the CD44 molecule is partly homologous to cartilage link proteins and thus part of a multigene family. The 37-kDa peptide backbone predicted from cDNA sequence appears expressed as a highly N- and O-glycosylated protein of 80 to 90 kDa or linked to multiple chondroitin sulfate moieties to form a protein of 170 to 200 kDa.

In addition, mRNA from epithelial cells, whose CD44 has been described as of slightly higher M_r, is larger than lymphoid CD44 mRNA. Tissue-specific variations of CD44 have yet to be fully characterized.

Numerous investigators have demonstrated that the CD44 molecule has important physiologic roles as a protein affecting cell–cell interaction. The first such role described is that of a ligand important to the homing and adhesion of circulating lymphocytes to the high endothelial cells of venules in lymphatic organs, including lymph nodes and the Peyer's patches of the intestines (Jalkanen et al. 1986; Berg et al. 1988). However, it is not yet known whether CD44 acts to confer organ specificity to the lymphocyte homing process. Such a function would be expected to involve polymorphisms of CD44, either in glycosylation or in primary amino acid sequence. Recently, a variant form of CD44 was described associated with leukocyte uropods; this form appears to contain an additional 134 amino acids and may indicate that function-specific polymorphisms of CD44 do exist (Dougherty et al. 1990). In addition, some evidence suggests that CD44 may act in concert with other molecules to allow lymphocytes to migrate to the appropriate organ.

Nevertheless, several lines of evidence suggest that CD44 is in itself an adhesion molecule. First, work by Aruffo and colleagues (1990) showed that CD44 is a major cell surface receptor for hyaluronate. Second, transfectants containing the baboon CD44 cDNA acquire a new adhesive phenotype (St. John et al. 1990).

There is also good evidence that red cell CD44 is capable of having a regulatory function in cell–cell interaction. Hale and colleagues (1989) demonstrated that antibodies to CD44 inhibit the interaction of the lymphocyte CD2 molecule with red cell LFA-3 during the formation of human lymphocyte-erythrocyte rosettes. Paroxysmal nocturnal hemoglobinuria red cells, which lack the phosphatidylinositol-anchored LFA-3 molecule, do not form such rosettes, indicating the CD44 appears to act via another adhesion protein, presumably LFA-3, which has previously been shown to be a receptor for CD2 (Hale et al. 1990).

The CD44 molecule also appears to have an important role in the activation of both T lymphocytes and monocytes. Antibodies to CD44 up-regulate CD-2– and CD-3–mediated activation of human T cells (Denning et al. 1990). In addition, CD44 antibodies also increase the binding of T lymphocytes to monocytes, again presumably by affecting interactions between other ligands, perhaps again including CD2 and LFA-3 (Denning et al. 1990). This phenomenon, along with the fact that CD44 antibodies also increase monocyte production of interleukin 1 (Denning et al. 1990), suggests that ligand binding to CD44 may serve in vivo to regulate numerous events important in host immunity and inflammation.

Two groups working independently made the connection between the In blood group system and CD44. The impetus for this work was the fact

Table 4.2. The Binding of Human anti-In^b to Purified Red Cell CD44

	Specific cpm Bound	
Target Protein	*anti-In^b #1*	*anti-In^b #2*
Experiment #1		
CD44	1328	2049
CD55	0	4
Experiment #2		
CD44	4699	7003
BSA*	0	0

*BSA = bovine serum albumin.

that In group antibodies did not react or reacted weakly with *In(Lu)* Lu(a−b−) red cells (Ferguson and Gaal 1988). Spring and colleagues demonstrated in 1988 that both In^a and In^b were detectable on CD44 protein purified from red cells of the appropriate phenotypes. Telen and Ferguson in 1990 confirmed this assignment of blood group antigens to CD44 (Table 4.2) and further showed that the In^b antigen was independent of the three epitopes recognized by a large number of murine monoclonal antibodies to CD44 (Fig. 4.3)

AnWj ANTIGEN: THE *HAEMOPHILUS INFLUENZAE* RECEPTOR

The Anton and Wj^a red cell antigens, now determined to be a single antigen designated AnWj, are also affected by the *In(Lu)* gene (Poole and Giles 1982). This antigen appears to be involved in the structure that serves as a receptor for the *H. influenzae* virus. Early evidence of this relationship came from studies which showed that human hemagglutinating strains of *H. influenzae* failed to agglutinate fetal and *In(Lu)* Lu(a−b−) red cells (van Alphen et al. 1986; Gilsdorf et al. 1989). Lack of a relationship to expression of Lutheran antigens was demonstrated by the fact that recessive-type Lu(a−b−) red cells were agglutinated normally. Further research examining the various antigens known to be down-regulated by the *In(Lu)* gene showed that An− red cells were not agglutinated, while variants in the P, Ii, and other systems reacted normally. Also, anti-AnWj antibodies were shown to be capable of blocking the binding of *H. influenzae* to An+ red cells, further supporting the role of the An antigen (van Alphen 1986).

The relationship between the red cell *H. influenzae* receptor and the pathophysiologically important epithelial receptor is not completely clear. Initial studies of persons with An− red cells included infants and persons in whom the An− phenotype was most likely acquired; study of the

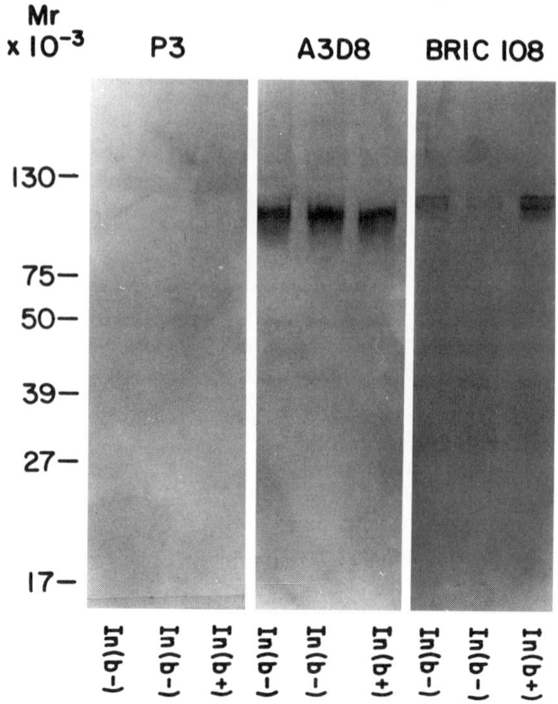

Figure 4.3. The expression of CD44 and Lutheran protein is independent of In phenotype. Immunoblotting demonstrated that CD44 and the Lutheran protein, as detected by murine monoclonal antibodies A3D8 and BRIC108, respectively, were expressed equally by In(a+b–) and In(a–b+) red cells. Polymorphism of the In antigen was not associated with a change in molecular weight of CD44, recognized by antibody A3D8. This immunoblot also illustrates the slightly higher molecular weight of Lutheran protein as compared with CD44.

epithelial cells of infants and An– adults demonstrated presence of the bacterial receptor, showing that the two receptors were independently expressed (van Alphen et al. 1987). In addition, the same investigators were unable to inhibit adherence to epithelial cells with anti-Anton sera, suggesting that the structure of the epithelial receptor was different from that of red cells. However, a more recent study of members of a family with a hereditary form of the An-phenotype showed that *H. influenzae* did not agglutinate red cells from the An– family members and did not adhere to epithelial cells from these same persons (Poole et al. 1989). On the other hand, epithelial cells from persons with the *In(Lu)* gene were able to serve normally as adherence targets for *H. influenzae* species, suggesting again that the effect of the *In(Lu)* gene is tissue-specific.

The biochemical nature of the red cell AnWj structure is largely undetermined. Both the AnWj antigen and the *H. influenzae* receptor are trypsin-resistant, and the AnWj antigen is also resistant to ficin, papain, and sialidase. Efforts to inhibit hemagglutination of red cells by *H. influenzae* with various carbohydrate structures have been unsuccessful (Gilsdorf et al. 1989). Studies of acquisition of the AnWj antigen by the red cells of neonates suggest that the antigen is expressed in a rather sudden fashion, so circulating red cells go from An− to strongly An+ within a few days (Poole and van Alphen 1988). This would seem possible only if the antigen were "manufactured" on the cell surface from a previously existing substrate while cells were in the circulation or if the antigen could be adsorbed from plasma. Although An antigen can be detected in saliva (van Alphen et al. 1989), incubation of AnWj− red cells in plasma from AnWj+ donors does not change AnWj antigen status. Thus, the structure of the AnWj antigen is yet to be elucidated.

FUTURE RESEARCH

Despite the historical importance of the Lutheran blood group system and its regulatory genes, the function of Lutheran protein(s) and the mechanism of action of its regulatory genes remain to be delineated. Especially interesting is the potentially tissue-specific effects of the *In(Lu)* gene. Several groups are currently working to define further the biochemistry of the Lutheran antigens, and it seems reasonable to expect that the structure of the various antigenic polymorphisms designed as blood group antigens will be substantially clarified within the next few years. It is also likely that the structural gene for the Lutheran protein(s) will be identified and sequenced during that time. A number of investigators are also currently looking at the polymorphisms of CD44 to elucidate the nature of the In^a/In^b antigens and the mechanism whereby CD44 may contribute to organ-specific homing of lymphocytes. Likewise, the structures of the AnWj and MER2 antigens are of continued interest and will most likely be clarified in the coming few years.

However, perhaps most exciting is that the mechanism of action of the *In(Lu)* and *XS2* genes will be defined in the near future. The broad but relatively tissue-specific effects of the *In(Lu)* gene make it especially interesting as an object of investigation, as this gene may be an example of a heretofore undescribed class of regulatory genes. Although early speculation raised the possibility that the *In(Lu)* gene encoded a glycosyltransferase, our current knowledge of its target antigens makes it perhaps more likely that *In(Lu)* encodes a DNA-binding protein or a product that targets such a binding protein. Since a number of such proteins are erythroid-specific, such a mechanism would provide built-in tissue specificity. Although current data allow only speculation, the next few years should provide more concrete information on which to base our understanding of the *In(Lu)* gene.

ACKNOWLEDGMENTS

This work has been funded in part by grants RO1 HL35572 and RO1 HL44042 from the National Heart, Lung, and Blood Institute, National Institutes of Health. M. J. Telen is the recipient of Research Career Development Award KO4 HL02233 (NHLBI, NIH).

REFERENCES

Anstee, D. J., G. Mallinson, J. E. Yendle, C. Holmes, and M. J. A. Tanner. 1988. Evidence for the occurrence of Lu^b-active glycoproteins in human erythrocytes, kidney and liver. Proceedings of the Twentieth Congress of the International Society for Blood Transfusion, Manchester, British Blood Transfusion Society, p. 263 (abstract).

Aruffo, A., I. Stamenkovic, M. Melnick, C. B. Underhill, and B. Seed. 1990. CD44 is the principal cell surface receptor for hyaluronate. *Cell* 61:1303–13.

Berg, E. L., L. A. Goldstein, M. A. Jutila, M. Nakache, L. J. Picker, P. R. Sheeter, N. W. Wu, D. Zhou, and E. C. Butcher. 1988. Homing receptors and vascular addressins: Cell adhesion molecules that direct lymphocyte traffic. *Immunol. Rev.* 108:5–18.

Brown, F., S. Simpson, S. Cornwall, B. P. L. Moore, R. Oyen, and W. L. Marsh. 1974. The recessive Lu(a−b−) phenotype: A family study. *Vox Sang.* 26:259–64.

Callender, S. T., and R. R. Race. 1946. Serological and genetical study of multiple antibodies formed in response to blood transfusions by a patient with lupus erythematosus diffusus. *Ann. Eugen.* 13:102–17.

Carter, W. G., and E. A. Wayner. 1988. Characterization of the class III collagen receptor, a phosphorylated transmembrane glycoprotein expressed in human nucleated cells. *J. Biol. Chem.* 263:4193–4201.

Cook, P. J. L. 1965. The Lutheran-Secretor recombination fraction in man: A possible sex difference. *Ann. Hum. Genet.* 28:393–401.

Crawford, M. N., T. G. Greenwalt, T. Sasaki, P. Tippett, R. Sanger, and R. R. Race. 1961. The phenotype Lu(a−b−) together with unconventional Kidd groups in one family. *Transfusion* 1:228–32.

Cutbush, M., and I. Chanarin. 1956. The expected blood-group antibody, anti-Lu^b. *Nature* 178:855–56.

Dalchau, R., J. Kirkley, and J. W. Fabre. 1980. Monoclonal antibody to a human brain–granulocyte–T lymphocyte antigen probably homologous to the W3/13 antigen of the rat. *Eur. J. Immunol.* 10:745–49.

Daniels, G. 1990. Evidence that the Auberger blood group antigens are located on the Lutheran glycoproteins. *Vox Sang.* 58:56–60.

Daniels, G., and G. Khalid. 1989. Identification, by immunoblotting, of the structures carrying Lutheran and para-Lutheran blood group antigens. *Vox Sang.* 57:137–41.

Daniels, G. L., M. A. Shaw, C. G. Lomas, M. R. Leak, and P. Tippett. 1986. The effect of *In(Lu)* on some high-incidence antigens. *Transfusion* 26:171–72.

Daniels, G. L., P. Tippett, D. K. Palmer, Y. E. Miller, D. Geyer, and C. Jones. 1987. MER2, a red cell polymorphism defined by monoclonal antibodies. *Vox Sang.* 52:107–10.

Denning, S. M., P. T. Le, K. H. Singer, and B. F. Haynes. 1990. Antibody against the CD44 p80 lymphocyte homing receptor molecule augments human peripheral blood T cell activation. *J. Immunol.* 144:7–15.

Dougherty, G. J., P. Lansdorp, and R. K. Humphries. 1990. Molecular cloning of CD44R, a novel uropod-associated form of the CD44 homing receptor. *Exp. Hematol.* 18:585 (abstract).

Eiberg, H., J. Mohr, L. Staub Neilsen, and N. Simsonsen. 1983. Genetics and linkage relationships of the C3 polymorphism: Discovery of *C3-Se* linkage and assignment of *LES-C3-DM-Se-PEPD-Lu* synteny to chromosome 19. *Clin. Genet.* 24:159–70.

Ferguson, D. J., and H. D. Gaal. 1988. Some observations on the In^b antigen and evidence that anti-In^b causes accelerated destruction of radiolabeled red cells. *Transfusion* 28:479–82.

Gilsdorf, J. R., W. J. Judd, and M. Cinat. 1989. Relationship of *Haemophilus influenzae* type b pilus structure and adherence to human erythrocytes. *Infect. Immun.* 57:3259–60.

Glaser, T., D. Housman, W. H. Lewis, D. Gerhard, and C. Jones. 1989. A fine-structure deletion map of human chromosome 11p: Analysis of J1 series hybrids. *Somat. Cell Mol. Genet.* 15:477–501.

Goldstein, L. A., D. F. Zhou, L. J. Picker, C. N. Minty, R. F. Bargatze, J. F. Ding, and E. C. Butcher. 1989. A human lymphocyte homing receptor, the Hermes antigen, is related to cartilage proteoglycan core and link proteins. *Cell* 56:1063–72.

Greenwalt, T. J., T. T. Sasaki, and E. A. Steane. 1967. The Lutheran blood groups: A progress report with observations on the development of the antigens and characteristics of the antibodies. *Transfusion* 7:189–200.

Hale, L. P., K. H. Singer, and B. F. Haynes. 1989. CD44 antibody against *In(Lu)*-related p80, lymphocyte-homing receptor molecule inhibits the binding of human erythrocytes to T cells. *J. Immunol.* 143:3944–48.

Haynes, B. F., E. A. Harden, M. J. Telen, M. E. Hemler, J. L. Strominger, T. J. Palker, R. M. Scearce, and G. S. Eisenbarth. 1983. Differentiation of human T lymphocytes I: Acquisition of a novel human cell surface protein (p80) during normal intrathymic T cell maturation. *J. Immunol.* 131:1195–1200.

Haynes, B. F., M. J. Telen, L. P. Hale, and S. M. Denning. 1989. CD44—A molecule involved in leukocyte adherence and T-cell activation. *Immunol. Today* 10:423–28.

Jalkanen, S. T., R. F. Bargatze, L. R. Herron, and E. C. Butcher. 1986. A lymphoid cell surface glycoprotein involved in endothelial cell recognition and lymphocyte homing in man. *Eur. J. Immunol.* 15:1195–1202.

Jalkanen, S. T., M. Jalkanen, R. Bargatze, M. Tammi, and E. C. Butcher. 1988. Biochemical properties of glycoproteins involved in lymphocyte recognition of high endothelial venules in man. *J. Immunol.* 141:1615–23.

Judson, P. A., F. A. Spring, S. F. Parsons, D. J. Anstee, and G. Mallinson. 1988. Report on group 8 (Lutheran) antibodies. *Rev. Fr. Transfus. Immuno-hematol.* 31:433–40.

Letarte, M., S. Iturbe, and E. J. Quackenbush. 1985. A glycoprotein of molecular weight 85,000 on human cells of B-lineage: Detection with a family of monoclonal antibodies. *Mol. Immunol.* 22:113–19.

Lewis, M., H. Kaita, G. Coghlan, S. Philipps, E. Belcher, P. J. McAlpine, G. R. Coopland, and R. A. Woods. 1988. The chromosome 19 linkage group *LDLR. C3, LW, APOC2, Lu, Se* in man. *Ann. Hum. Genet.* 52:137–44.

Lostumbo, M. M., P. V. Holland, and P. J. Schmidt. 1966. Isoimmunization after multiple transfusions. *N. Engl. J. Med.* 275:141–44.

Lucas, M. G., A. M. Green, and M. J. Telen. 1989. Characterization of the serum *In(Lu)*-related antigen: Identification of a serum protein related to erythrocyte p80. *Blood* 73:596–600.

Marsh, W. L., P. J. Brown, J. DiNapoli, M. L. Beck, M. Wood, R. Wojcicki, and C. de al Camara. 1983. Anti-Wj: an antibody that defines a high-incidence antigen modified by the *In(Lu)* gene. *Transfusion* 23:128–30.

McKay, C. R., J. F. Maddox, and G. L. Wijffels. 1988. Characterization of a 95,000 molecule on sheep leucocytes homologous to murine Pgp-1 and human CD44. *Immunology* 65:93–99.

Merry, A. H., B. Gardner, S. F. Parsons, and D. J. Anstee. 1987. Estimation of the number of binding sites with murine monoclonal anti-Lu^b on human erythrocytes. *Vox Sang.* 53:57–60.

Miller, Y. E., N. Sullivan, J. Bill, D. Geyer, and C. Jones. 1985. Monoclonal antibodies to two tightly linked distinct chromosome 11 encoded cell surface antigens. *Am J Hum Genet* 37:A233.

Mohr, J. 1954. *A Study of linkage in man.* Copenhagen: Munksgaard.

Mulley, J. C., P. C. Norman, P. Tippett, and R. W. Beal. 1988. A regional localization for an X-linked suppressor gene (XS) for the Lutheran blood group. *Hum. Genet.* 78:127–29.

Norman, P. C., P. Tippett, and R. W. Beal. 1986. An Lu(a – b –) phenotype caused by an X-linked recessive gene. *Vox Sang.* 51:49–52.

Omary, M. B., I. S. Trowbridge, M. Letarte, M. F. Kagnoff, and C. M. Isacke. 1988. Structural heterogeneity of human Pgp-1 and its relationship with p85. *Immunogenetics* 27:460–64.

Parsons, S. F., G. Mallinson, P. A. Judson, D. J. Anstee, M. J. A. Tanner, and G. L. Daniels. 1987. Evidence that the Lu^b blood group antigen is located on red cell membrane glycoproteins of 85 and 78 kd. *Transfusion* 27:61–63.

Picker, L. J., J. de los Toyos, M. J. Telen, B. F. Haynes, and E. C. Butcher. 1989. Monoclonal antibodies against CD44 [*In(Lu)*-related p80], Pgp-1, and the Hermes class of lymphocyte receptors bind to the same molecule. *J. Immunol.* 142:2046–51.

Poole, J., and C. M. Giles, 1982. Observations on the Anton antigen and antibody. *Vox Sang.* 43:220–22.

Poole, J., C. Levene, L. van Alphen, R. Sela, M. Bennett, and P. Spruell. 1989. Serological and microbiological studies in a family showing inheritance of AnWj antigen. *Transfusion* 29S:34.

Poole, J., and L. van Alphen. 1988. *Haemophilus influenzae* receptor and the AnWj antigen. *Transfusion* 28:289.

Rao, N., D. J. Ferguson, S. F. Lee, and M. J. Telen. 1991. Identification of human erythrocyte blood group antigens on the C3b/C4b receptor (CR1). *J. Immunology* 146:3502–07.

Renwick, J. H., S. E. Bundey, M. A. Ferguson-Smith, and M. M. Izatt. 1971. Confirmation of linkage of the loci for myotonic dystrophy and ABH secretion. *J. Med. Genet.* 8:407–16.

Shaw, M. A., M. R. Leak, G. L. Daniels, and P. Tippett. 1984. The rare Lutheran blood group phenotype Lu(a – b –): A genetic study. *Ann. Hum. Genet.* 48:229–37.

Spring, F. A., R. Dalchau, G. L. Daniels, G. Mallinson, P. A. Judson, S. F. Parsons, J. W. Fabre, and D. J. Anstee. 1988. The In^a and In^b blood group antigens are located on a glycoprotein of 80,000 MW (the CDw44 glycoprotein) whose expression is influenced by the *In(Lu)* gene. *Immunology* 64:37–43.

Stamenkovic, I., M. Amiot, J. M. Pesandro, and B. Seed. 1989. A lymphocyte molecule implicated in lymphocyte homing is a member of the cartilage link protein family. *Cell* 56:1057–62.

Taliano, V., R.-M. Guevin, and P. Tippett. 1973. The genetics of a dominant inhibitor of the Lutheran antigens. *Vox Sang.* 24:42–47.

Telen, M. J., G. S. Eisenbarth, and B. F. Haynes. 1983. Human erythrocyte

antigens: Regulation of a novel red cell surface antigen by the inhibitor Lutheran *In(Lu)* gene. *J. Clin. Invest.* 71:1878–86.
Telen, M. J., and D. J. Ferguson. 1990. Relationship of In^b antigen to other antigens on *In(Lu)*-related p80. *Vox Sang.* 58:118–21.
Telen, M. J., A. M. Green, and T. Young. 1988. Serological and biochemical characterization of monoclonal antibodies against red cell markers related to expression of Lutheran blood group antigens. *Rev. Fr. Transfus. Immunohematol.* 31:421–28.
Telen, M. J., T. J. Palker, and B. F. Haynes. 1984. Human erythrocyte antigens II: The *In(Lu)* gene regulates expression of an antigen residing on an 80-kilodalton protein of human erythrocytes. *Blood* 64:599–606.
Telen, M. J., I. Rogers, and M. Letarte. 1987. Further characterization of erythrocyte p80 and the membrane protein defect of *In(Lu)* Lu(a – b –) erythrocytes. *Blood* 70:1475–81.
Telen, M. J., H. Shehata, and B. F. Haynes. 1986. Human medullary thymocyte p80 antigen and *In(Lu)*-related p80 antigen reside on the same protein. *Hum. Immunol.* 17:311–24.
Tippett, P. 1986. Contributions of monoclonal antibodies to understanding one new and some old blood group systems. *In Red cell antigens and antibodies*, ed. G. Garratty. 83–98. Arlington, VA: American Association of Blood Banks.
——— 1990. Regulator genes affecting red cell antigens. *Trans.Med. Rev.* 4:56–68.
Toivanen, P., and T. Hirvonen. 1973. Antigens Duffy, Kell, Kidd, Lutheran and Xg^a on fetal red cells. *Vox Sang.* 24:372–76.
Udden, M. M., M. Umeda, Y. Hirano, and D. M. Marcus. 1987. New abnormalities in the morphology, cell surface receptors, and electrolyte metabolism of *In(Lu)* erythrocytes. *Blood* 69:52–57.
van Alphen, L., J. Poole, L. Geelen, and H. C. Zanen. 1987. The erythrocyte and epithelial cell receptors for *Haemophilus influenzae* are expressed independently. *Infect. and Immunity* 55:2355–58.
van Alphen, L., J. Poole, and M. Overbeeke. 1986. The Anton blood group antigen is the erythrocyte receptor for *Haemophilus influenzae*. *FEMS Microbiol. Lett.* 37:69–71.
van Alphen, L., M. van Ham, L. Geelen-van den Broek, and T. Pieters. 1989. Relationship between secretion of the Anton blood group antigen in saliva and adherence of *Haemophilus influenzae* to oropharynx epithelial cells. *FEMS Microbiol. Immunol.* 47:357–62.

5

THE KIDD ANTIGENS AND UREA TRANSPORT

Robert B. Gunn, M.D.,
J. Jay Gargus, M.D., Ph.D.,
and Otto Fröhlich, Ph.D.

The Kidd blood group antigen was discovered by Drs. Allen, Diamond, and Niedziela in 1951 at Children's Hospital in Boston. They detected a new antibody in the serum of Mrs. Kidd, the mother of a child with hemolytic disease of the newborn. The corresponding antigen is now called Jk^a. The antibody to the other allele, Jk^b, was discovered by Plaut and colleagues in 1953. Finally, in 1959, the rare phenotype Jk(a−b−) was described in a Filipino family of Chinese ancestry (Pinkerton et al. 1959). In 1982 Heaton and McLoughlin reported that the red cells from these rare individuals with the Jk(a−b−) phenotype had a much slower lysis in 2 M urea than Jk-positive cells.

Red cells are nearly perfect osmometers: they swell and shrink by net water movements, so the internal and external osmolarities become equal. Urea, which rapidly permeates normal red cell membranes, equilibrates and thus cannot balance the normal impermeant osmolytes within red cells. As the urea enters the cell, water follows, the cell swells, and lysis occurs. The much slower lysis of Jk(a−b−) cells might be due to very slow urea entry into the cells.

The transport of urea in red cells has been known since the 1930s to vary greatly between species. The hemolysis times in urea solutions are much shorter for red cells from mammals compared with those from fish, amphibians, reptiles, or birds, implying that the urea permeability is higher in mammalian than in nonmammalian red cells. This increased permeability of mammalian red cells cannot be explained by nonfacilitated linear diffusion of urea across the lipid bilayer of these cells but may be due to the presence of a specific urea transport pathway. In 1970 two lines of evidence suggested that much of the mammalian urea transport might be mediated. First, Hunter (1970) showed that swelling rates of red cells in urea solutions exhibited saturation kinetics; thus, urea was not transported by simple diffusion. Second, Macey and Farmer (1970) showed that phloretin, the aglycone of the sugar transport inhibitor phloridzin, inhibited urea transport without having an effect on water transport. Thus, water and urea appeared to travel by separate pathways. Wieth and colleagues (1974) first reported ^{14}C-urea and ^{14}C-thiourea fluxes that showed saturation kinetics in human red cells. In contrast, they found that in chicken erythrocytes the urea flux was proportional to the urea concentration; was slow, with a rate coefficient of 0.0008 s^{-1}; and was not inhibited by phloretin. Thiourea fluxes also showed no evidence for a specific pathway in chickens and were 1.8 times faster than urea fluxes under comparable conditions, probably reflecting the higher partition of thiourea into the lipid phase of the cell membrane. In contrast to chicken red cells, human red cells were found to be highly permeable to urea with a rate coefficient of 6.6 s^{-1} at 25°C and 1 mM extracellular urea. They confirmed the finding that phloretin strongly inhibited the urea flux but also showed that thiourea was a competitive inhibitor of ^{14}C-urea fluxes. Furthermore, the thiourea flux in human cells had two components: a phloretin-insensitive linear component and a phloretin-sensitive saturating component with K_m = 15 to 20 mM for thiourea that was competitively inhibited by urea. Thus, chicken red cells have no mediated urea or thiourea transport while human red cells have a mediated transport mechanism shared by urea and thiourea. The slow nonmediated pathway in both cell types is consistent with lipid bilayer permeability. Further detailed kinetic studies by Brahm (1983) and by Mayrand and Levitt (1983) have confirmed and extended these findings and identified a large number of compounds that inhibit the mediated pathway.

The physiologic function of mediated urea transport in red cells has been considered by Macey and Yousef (1988). They modeled the transit of red cells through the renal vasa recta where the blood, which is isoosmotic in the rest of the circulation (300 mOsm total), becomes hyperosmotic in both salt (600 mOsm) and urea (600 mOsm). Since red cells behave as nearly perfect osmometers they would be expected to lose about 75 percent of their water if both salt and urea were impermeant. The rapid mediated transport of urea allows it to equilibrate across the red cell membrane and thus reduce water loss to only 50 percent. In addition to avoiding a rheologic disaster in the renal papilla, a more important function of the mediated mechanism may be to allow the rapid removal of urea from the red cells as they ascend the vasa recta from the papilla to the isoosmotic renal cortex. The kinetics of urea transport are such that net efflux is more enhanced than net influx under equal but opposite gradients (Fröhlich, unpublished observations). This allows the red cells to shed their internal urea and avoid swelling and lysis as they emerge into the cortex where the urea concentration is nominal. In their modeling, Macey and Yousef (1988) showed a range of nonmediated and mediated flux rates at which red cell transit is safe, without lysis. Not only does the rapid equilibration of urea across the red cell prevent red cell shrinkage and later lysis, but it also reduces the amount of urea washed out of the papilla by a given degree of vasa recta blood flow and thus tends to preserve renal concentrating ability.

Mediated urea transport occurs in the most distal portions of the renal collecting duct. Passive urea transport in the kidney has been known to be important for many years (Berliner et al. 1958; Kokko and Rector 1972; Stevenson 1972). Recently, Knepper and co-workers (Sands et al. 1987; Chou and Knepper 1989; Chou et al. 1990), using isolated segments of the medullary collecting duct, have demonstrated urea fluxes that show saturation, specific inhibition, and competition with urea analogues. The ability of the kidney to concentrate urea in the renal medulla is due in part to the rapid equilibration of the final concentrated urine urea with the medullary interstitium.

Selective salt and water transport result in a concentrated urea in the tubular fluid. The presence of a urea transporter in the terminal portion of the inner medullary collecting duct then allows the equilibration of the high tubular urea concentration with the interstitium of the tip of the papilla and thus regenerates and increases the medullary interstitial urea concentration.

CHARACTERISTICS OF THE UREA TRANSPORTER

It is not known whether erythrocytes and renal cells share the same urea transport mechanism, though the two transport systems share several characteristics. Both are inhibited reversibly by phloretin, irreversibly by pCMBS (p-chloromercuribenzenesulfonate), and inhibited by the much more slowly transported urea congener thiourea. The apparent substrate affinities of both tissues are in the range of several hundred millimolar for urea. One might therefore suspect that the two transport mechanisms are the same or at least similar. However, since kinetic studies are very difficult with the renal tubule preparations, most of the kinetic studies on urea transport have been performed on erythrocytes.

THE UREA TRANSPORTER BEHAVES LIKE A CHANNEL

The kinetics of red cell urea transport suggest that the urea transport protein is most likely a channel since the flux rate is so great and the number of transporter proteins is probably low. Channel-type transporters typically have higher turnover rates than carriers and thus a high flux requires fewer transporter units per cell. A typical value for urea equilibrium exchange transport near substrate saturation ($>$ 2 M on both sides of the membrane) is about 50 mol (kg Hb $\times$ min)$^{-1}$ at 0°C. This corresponds to a transport rate of 1.8×10^{10} urea molecules per second per cell. The fastest known carrier-type transport protein, the erythrocyte anion exchanger, has a turnover rate of about 300 s^{-1} or a transport rate of 3×10^8 molecules s^{-1} cell^{-1} at 0°C. This means that if the urea transporter were a carrier, it would have to exist at a density at least comparable to that of the erythrocyte anion carrier (band 3), which at 10^6 copies per cell is the most abundant of the intrinsic membrane proteins. However, essentially all major proteins in the erythrocyte membrane have been identified, leaving only minor components as candidates for the transporter protein.

If the urea transporter is the Jk antigen–bearing protein (see below), one has an independent determination of the number of transport sites. There are only about 14,000 copies of the Jk antigen per red cell (Masouredis et al. 1980). With this small number of transporters, one calculates a turnover rate of $1.3 \times 10^6\ s^{-1}$ at 0°C. This is too rapid for a carrier-type mechanism and suggests that the urea transporter functions as a channel.

The notion that the urea transporter is a nonelectrolyte channel is further supported by the experiments of Yousef and Macey (1989). In stopped-flow experiments they measured urea permeability as a function of the urea concentration. They could fit these data to a model of a simple channel but not of a simple carrier. In preliminary observations Fröhlich and Trammel (1987) found that the unidirectional efflux of urea as well as that of the more slowly transported analogue thiourea was inhibited by extracellular urea and thiourea, respectively. Such trans-inhibition could be exhibited by both a channel and a carrier mechanism. In the case of a channel mechanism, it could be due to blockage of outward-moving substrate by extracellular binding of unlabeled substrate. In the case of a carrier mechanism, it would be expected if the translocation rate in the unloaded state is much more rapid than the translocation rate in the substrate-loaded state, a possibility that was not excluded by the kinetic analysis of Yousef and Macey.

However, two other observations argue against a carrier mechanism altogether. First, thiourea transport exhibits no transinhibition by intracellular thiourea, in contrast to the strong transinhibition by extracellular thiourea (Fröhlich and Trammel 1987; Brahm, personal communication). This observation rules out a symmetric carrier, but does not exclude the possibility of an asymmetric carrier mechanism in which the outward translocation rate constant is greater than the inward translocation rate constant, for both the slowly translocated loaded forms and the rapidly translocated unloaded forms of the hypothetical carrier. Second, thiourea tracer efflux is transinhibited by both extracellular thiourea *and* extracellular urea (Fröhlich, unpublished observations). Since urea equilibrium exchange is at least two orders of magnitude faster than thiourea equilibrium exchange, one would expect that a carrier mechanism would demonstrate urea transstimulation of unidirectional thiourea efflux at least relative to extracellular thiourea. Instead, urea transinhibited to about the same extent as thiourea. Thus the possibility of a carrier mechanism for urea transport is essentially eliminated. However, these observations also indicate that the urea transport pathway is considerably more complex than a simple channel since substrates differentially block the channel mouths at the inside and the outside of the cell.

THE UREA TRANSPORTER IS SPECIFIC FOR UREA

It has been suggested that the transport pathway that mediates urea transport is also the main transport pathway for other substrates for which the red cell membrane possesses a high permeability. The list of such substrates includes water, ethylene glycol, and even chloride (Solomon et al. 1983). The evidence for this notion was derived from measurements of phenomenologic reflection coefficients, as calculated from volume-related changes in light scattering that occur when cells are mixed with solutions of the different nonelectrolytes. However, compelling evidence argues in favor of the competing notion that urea, water, ethylene glycol, and chloride are each transported by a separate and substrate-specific pathway. This evidence includes inhibitors that are specific for only one substrate class. Three examples: first, the stilbene disulfonates inhibit only anion transport and leave nonelectrolyte movements unaltered (Fröhlich and Jones 1988); second, the sulfhydryl reagent pCMBS reacts with urea and water transport with greatly differing affinities (Toon and Solomon 1986); and third, phloretin does not affect water permeability (Macey and Farmer 1970) while it noncompetitively inhibits anion transport (Fröhlich and Gunn 1987) and competitively inhibits urea transport (Fröhlich, unpublished observations). Also, as mentioned above, the erythrocytes of some animals lack one of the transport pathways: the urea permeability of chicken red cells is so low that it corresponds to that of a lipid bilayer, but their water and anion transport rates are comparable to those found in mammalian cells (Wieth et al. 1974). Further, the flow-tube experiments of Brahm and Galey (1987) demonstrated essentially no effect of osmotic gradients (i.e., net water movements) on urea transport, even though one would expect such flux coupling if urea and water moved along the same pathway. The conclusion from the kinetic and inhibitor studies mentioned above is that while it is possible that the urea channel permits the occasional entry of water molecules along with the primary substrate urea, it is clear that the primary pathways for water and anions (and probably also ethylene glycol) occur elsewhere on separate transport units/proteins, not on the urea transporter.

The best evidence in favor of the notion of separate transport proteins comes from recent studies with human erythrocytes of a rare blood type. Blood type Jk(a − b −) cells lack mediated urea transport (Fröhlich et al. 1991). Several observations led us to this conclusion: The permeability of Jk(a − b −) cells for urea is very low; it corresponds to that found in chicken erythrocytes (Wieth et al. 1974) and the cholesterol-containing

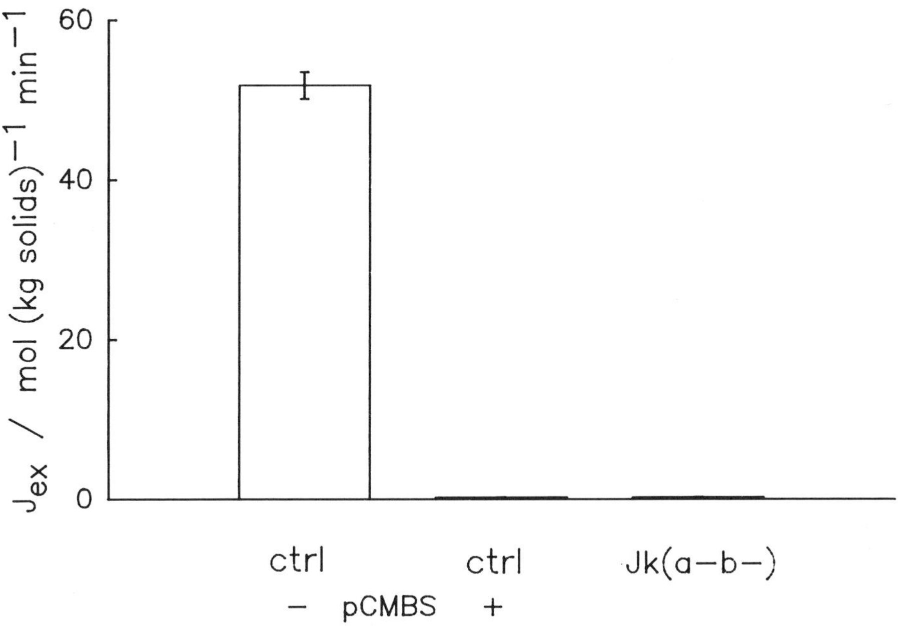

Figure 5.1. A comparison of the urea (U) fluxes from normal cells (control), inhibitor-treated normal cells, and Jk(a − b −) cells. The fluxes are equilibrium exchange fluxes at $U_i = U_o = 2$ M, at 0°C. The inhibitor treatment consisted of exposing the Jk-positive cells to 100 μm p-chloromercuribenzene (pCMBS) for 30 minutes at 22°C, followed by washes to remove unreacted pCMBS. Note that pCMBS reduced the control urea flux in control cells to nearly the level found in Jk(a − b −) cells. (*Source:* From Fröhlich et al. 1991.)

lipid bilayer (Finkelstein 1976), or to the permeability of inhibitor-treated control cells (Fig. 5.1). Also, inhibitors of urea transport reduce thiourea fluxes in control cells to the rates found in Jk(a − b −) cells, while the thiourea fluxes in Jk(a − b −) cells are not affected by these inhibitors. Furthermore, the rate of the small unidirectional thiourea efflux across the membrane of Jk(a − b −) cells is not transinhibited by extracellular thiourea (Fig. 5.2). These results are consistent with a passive diffusion process through the lipid bilayer of the Jk(a − b −) cell. Finally, the Jk(a − b −) cells, with their compromised urea permeability, exhibit the *same* rates of water, ethylene glycol, and chloride transport as control cells (Fröhlich et al. 1991). The most parsimonious explanation by far is that Jk(a − b −) cells lack only one protein found in control cells, and that this protein possesses both Jk antigenic determinants and urea transport function (see below). The other proteins, which are responsible for transporting other nonelectrolytes and anions, are the same in Jk(a − b −) and Jk-positive cells.

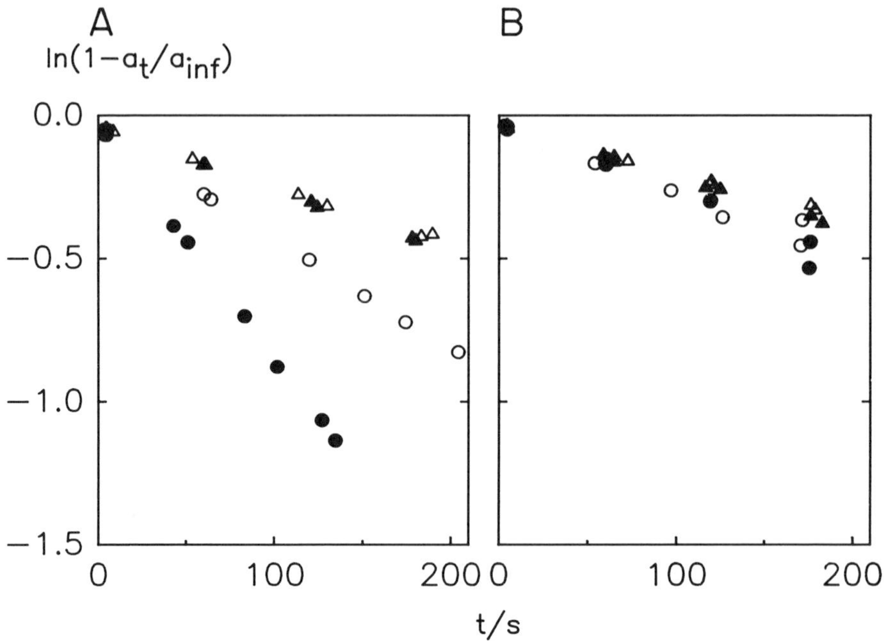

Figure 5.2. A comparison of thiourea (TU) fluxes from normal cells (A) and Jk(a−b−) cells (B). The fluxes are unidirectional fluxes with TU_i = 70 μM and TU_o = 0 (solid symbols) or 70 mM (open symbols). Also included are data obtained in the presence of the competitive inhibitor thionicotinamide (TN = 4 mM; triangles). The ordinate is a logarithmic measure of the extent of loss of tracer from the cell (or appearance in the medium); the slope is proportional to the flux rate. Note that in Jk(a−b−) cells there is no inhibition by extracellular TU or TN and that in the presence of TN both cell types exhibit the same flux rates. (*Source:* From Fröhlich et al. 1991.)

THE Jk(A−B−) MUTATION

For many years it has been suggested that red cell urea transport is a good model for that in the kidney, where it has a key role in the concentrating mechanism. But even this central aspect of urea transport remains controversial. Models of the nephron suggest that eliminating urea permeability would reduce maximally concentrated urine (U_{osm} max) from a standard of 1200 mOsm to about 900 mOsm. In work with Jeff Sands and Juha Kokko in the renal division at Emory University, we brought two unrelated Jk(a−b−) patients and one obligate heterozygote into our Clinical Research Center to define their U_{osm} max by dehydrating them and administering antidiuretic hormone (ADH). In both homozygotes U_{osm} max was 800 mOsm, indicating a marked concentrating defect (Sands et al. 1990). Most simply, this finding suggests that the same locus defined by their mutation encodes both the kidney and red blood cell transporter, and that urea transporter function is completely absent in both tissues. Thus, as far as transport is concerned, the mutation looks like a "knockout" or "null," not a more subtle structural mutation.

The salient features of the Kidd antigen system would arise if the Kidd locus encoded a membrane protein and the Jk^a and Jk^b alleles represented alternative sequences in one region of the gene which, through selection, have become polymorphic in the population. This implies that the two alleles hold the majority of their sequences, and therefore the epitopes they likely define, in common. The strongest argument for this model is the nature of the rare Jk^{ab} antibody (also referred to as Jk3). Multiparous or transfused null homozygotes frequently produce the unique Jk^{ab} antibody. It recognizes determinants of the Kidd antigen protein distinct from the antithetical Jk^a or Jk^b epitopes (Woodfield et al. 1982). These Jk^{ab} determinants are absent from all Jk(a−b−) red cells but are found on all Kidd-positive cells (Jk^a and/or Jk^b). Red cells with the Jk^{ab} antigen, but neither the Jk^a nor the Jk^b antigen, have yet to be found (although a family with weakly antigenic determinants has been reported [Okubo et al. 1986] that could be interpreted to show the negative interallelic complementation [Fincham 1983] of a novel transdominant, functionally altered Kidd allele). These findings fit with the notion that Jk(a−b−) cells are homozygous null for one protein; the null mutants, lacking the entire protein, would lack the Jk^{ab} as well as Jk^a and Jk^b determinants.

Again, like transport, the antigen phenotype of Jk(a−b−) cells is a null. Null phenotypes are important in translating genotype to phenotype because there is only one way to lack a protein but many ways to alter it, some of which can produce complex phenotypes. It is essential to understand the null phenotype to understand the physiologic role played by the protein (Fincham 1983).

The observation of two rare phenotypes covarying in families or in a population can either suggest that both phenotypes are different functional manifestations of the same single causal gene or may simply be a reflection of the close proximity in the genome of two different genetic loci (Gargus and Mitas 1988). Given a large population survey, one would expect to be able to distinguish these two possibilities through the discovery of an individual in whom the linkage phase, and hence established concordance, was broken through meiotic synapsis and recombination. Such a nonconcordant individual has not been found in the Kidd/urea lysis system.

The association established in the literature between the Jk(a−b−) phenotype and the urea lysis-resistant phenotype is remarkable. A chi-square analysis of the data taken from three large published population surveys (Heaton and McLoughlin 1982; Woodfield et al. 1982; Okubo et al. 1983) yields an aggregate χ^2 value that is astronomical, 3.78×10^5. (With one degree of freedom a χ^2 value of 15 has a $p < .0001$.) Clearly chance alone is not responsible for the observed covariance in populations.

What is observed is not a simple genetic linkage between two adjacent chromosomal loci, which each by chance happens to encode one of the few red blood cell membrane proteins. If there are two distinct loci then there must be a complete *linkage disequilibrium.* This is because the association observed is not between the rare phenotype of lysis resistance and the Kidd *locus,* but rather between the lysis resistance and a very rare *allele* at the Kidd locus, the null allele. Such disequilibria have been reported in regions very close to a number of loci—for example, the cystic fibrosis locus (Estivill et al. 1988). A number of explanations for this type of disequilibrium can be advanced (Fincham 1983), but the simplest would be the following event: the rare mutation that causes resistance to urea lysis occurred *by chance* in a chromosome that happened to possess the $Jk(a-b-)$ allele. This event would have needed to occur so recently, and the two loci be so close, that sufficient time had yet to pass to allow recombinational events to randomize this region of the chromosome. The implication, of course, would be that all individuals with these two phenotypes inherited a chromosomal segment *directly descended* from the progenitor in whom the recent mutation occurred. However, this mechanism would be very unlikely to explain the association of the mutations now found in distinct isolated populations (Haribi 1984; Salmon et al. 1984).

Finding the covarying phenotypes to be both *null* suggests two possible mechanisms for the observed concordance. First, it is most likely that both phenotypes result from the lack of one gene product. Second, it remains a formal possibility that one small chromosomal deletion has eliminated *two* tightly linked loci. In a given population over time, a deletion chromosome could have spread, such that all individuals receiving the chromosome would be null hemizygotes at all loci spanned. (The Asian malaria belt distribution of the common $\alpha°$-thalassemia alleles follows this model [Levitan, 1988].) However, one would expect that in each isolated ethnic background the primary mutation was different, or that sporadic new mutations would be different, with some failing to span both loci (as is seen in α-thalassemia). Hence it would be surprising that in all genetic backgrounds studied thus far, the null transport phenotype predicts the null antigen phenotype, and vice versa. Under the first mechanism, the single-gene model, concordance would be guaranteed since any and all null mutations would produce both null phenotypes whether the mutation was inherited or new.

Recently a different type of information about the Kidd locus has become available through pedigree analysis and genetic linkage studies. The Kidd locus has been mapped to human chromosome 18 by linkage to a DNA restriction fragment length polymorphism (RFLP) disclosed by anonymous probe L2.7 (Geitvik et al. 1987). Although the probe and antigen loci are statistically quite close in the genome, separated by only a recombination fraction of 3 percent in family studies, it is likely they are physically separated by a distance of over three million nucleotide base pairs (standardly one finds roughly a million base pairs per percent recombination), a very large distance to traverse with molecular techniques, making a "reverse genetics" locus-based cloning strategy unattractive.

Characterization of the Kidd antigen suggests its molecular weight is about 45 kDa (Sinor et al. 1987). However, the Kidd antigen protein has not been isolated or purified. Therefore, standard protein-based approaches to this gene, either through microsequencing and screening a cDNA library with an oligonucleotide probe, or the production of a heterologous antibody for immunoscreening an expression cDNA library, are also frustrated (Gargus and Mitas 1988). However, highly specific *homologous* antisera are available for the two allelic forms of the Jk antigen as a result of isoimmunization (via transfusion or pregnancy). This homologous isoantibody allowed a novel approach to gene isolation (Gargus et al. 1988). Since an isoantigen is one that genetically varies between individuals of a species (members of which share in common nearly all antigenic determinants), the antisera produced in isoimmunization are highly specific, the specificity of such antisera being the basis of blood and tissue typing. In other red cell antigen systems (Salmon et al. 1984), isoantibody specificity has been shown to reflect an antiserum's ability to discriminate a change in one amino acid in allelic forms of glycophorin B (the Ss antigen system) or two amino acids in allelic forms of glycophorin A (the MN antigen system).

The specificity of the Kidd antiserum suggested it would be a useful reagent in expression library screening. For this reason it was elected to screen a human reticulocyte cDNA expression library (Gargus et al. 1988). Using dilutions of pooled anti-Jk^a and anti-Jk^b antisera, five independent recombinant λgtll clones were identified by their production of immunoreactive protein. This reflected a frequency of detection of 1.5×10^{-5} per recombinant clone. Two independent clones from separate screenings of the library, λpp10 and λpp11, were plaque-purified to homogeneity, and both were found to react with anti-Jk^{a-}, but not with anti-Jk^{b-}, antiserum, showing the allelic specificity of the isolation. This isolation also proves that the Jk^a epitope is protein, not carbohydrate, since the expressing bacteria do not glycosylate proteins.

Both λpp10 and λpp11 contain a 2.3-kb cDNA insert in the EcoRI cloning site of the vector (Gargus et al. 1988). These cDNA inserts were then excised from a preparative gel and subcloned into the EcoRI site of the Bluescript plasmid vector for further characterization. Digestion of these plasmid constructs with a variety of restriction enzymes allowed the generation of a restriction map of the two cDNA inserts, which were superimposable (Allen et al. 1988). Finding a single restriction map in two independent immunoreactive cDNA isolates argues strongly for the specificity of the isolation.

The Bluescript clones were sequenced by dideoxy termination (Allen et al. 1988). The deduced sequence yielded an open-reading frame (ORF) that was appropriately positioned to produce the antibody-detected fusion protein. Translation of the ORF revealed a sequence with no homology in the protein database. By two different algorithms (Eisenberg and Kyte-Doolittle), its predicted structure is consistent with a transmembrane orientation. It has a globular N-terminal domain (which is probably cytosolic) followed by six long α helical runs of 20 to 25 amino acids each, all highly hydrophobic except the fifth helix, which is neither hydrophobic nor clearly amphipathic. The disposition of this fifth helix is unclear, and so, therefore, is that of the C-terminus (Gargus et al. 1991). There are no consensus N-glycosylation sites to help orient this region. Algorithms that identify antigenic determinants, however, predict strongly antigenic domains between helix three and four and between helix five and six. Perhaps together these regions form the labile Jk^a epitope on the external face of the membrane. The cysteine-rich nature of the extreme C-terminus (four of the last 12 amino acids) might provide another hint to orientation. The inhibitory effect of extracellular disulfide reagents on urea transport suggests some functionally important extracellular cysteines.

To prove conclusively that this cDNA encodes the transporter or the antigen would require the identification of a known amino acid sequence from the isolated protein. However, no amino acid sequence is known. This leaves functional expression as the only possible strong proof of identity available. There is no established functional definition of the Jk^a antigen other than that it reacts with the anti-Jk^a antibody. But since this antibody was used in the cloning, this argument is reduced to a tautology. There is, on the other hand, an established physiologic and functional definition of the urea transporter. For this reason eukaryotic expression constructs of the cDNA were made (Gargus et al. 1991). Preliminary data on constructs transfected into $LMTK^-$ fibroblasts suggest the presence of a new, very fast component of urea transport that is both phloretin and thionicotinamide inhibitable and is not present in the untransformed cells (Gargus et al. 1991).

REFERENCES

Allen, F. H., L. K. Diamond, and B. Niedziela. 1951. A new blood-group antigen. *Nature* 167:482.

Allen, J. R., M. Mitas, L. Malone, B. Brunner-Jackson, D. S. Wimalasena, and J. J. Gargus. 1988. Inborn error in human urea transport: Analysis of the cDNA encoding the putative transporter. *Am. J. Hum. Genet.* 43:A1.

Berliner, R. W., N. G. Levinsky, D. G. Davidson, and M. Eden. 1958. Dilution and concentration of the urine and the action of antidiuretic hormones. *Am. J. Med.* 27:730–44.

Brahm, J. 1983. Urea permeability of human red cells. *J. Gen. Physiol.* 82:1–24.

Brahm, J., and W. R. Galey. 1987. Diffusional solute flux during osmotic water flow across the human red cell membrane. *J. Gen. Physiol.* 89:703–16.

Chou, C.-L., and M. A. Knepper. 1989. Inhibition of urea transport in inner medullary collecting duct by phloretin and urea analogues. *Am. J. Physiol.* 257:F359–65.

Chou, C.-L., J. M. Sands, H. Nonoguchi, and M. A. Knepper. 1990. Concentration dependence of urea and thiourea transport in rat inner medullary collecting duct. *Am. J. Physiol.* 258:F486–94.

Estivill, X., M. Farrall, R. Williamson, M. Ferrari, M. Seia, A. M. Giunta, G. Novelli, L. Potenza, B. Dallapicolla, G. Borgo, P. Gasparini, P. F. Pignatti, L. De Benedetti, E. Vitale, M. Devoto, and G. Romeo. 1988. Linkage disequilibrium between cystic fibrosis and linked DNA polymorphisms in Italian families: A collaborative study. *Am. J. Hum. Genet.* 43:23–28.

Fincham, J. R. S. 1983. *Genetics*. 315–84, 522. Boston, Jones & Bartlett.

Finkelstein, A. 1976. Water and nonelectrolyte permeability of lipid bilayer membranes. *J. Gen. Physiol.* 68:127–35.

Fröhlich, O., and R. B. Gunn. 1987. Interactions of inhibitors on the anion transporter of the human erythrocyte. *Am. J. Physiol.* 252:C153–62.

Fröhlich, O., and S. C. Jones. 1988. Kinetic independence between red cell anion exchange and urea transport. *Biochim. Biophys. Acta* 943:531–34.

Fröhlich, O., R. I. Macey, J. Edwards-Moulds, J. J. Gargus, and R. B. Gunn. 1991. Urea transport deficiency in Jk(a − b −) erythrocytes. *Am. J. Physiol.* 260:C778–83.

Fröhlich, O., and D. Trammell. 1987. Is the red cell urea transporter a carrier or a channel? *Biophys. J.* 51:514a.

Gargus, J. J., B. Brunner-Jackson, and L. Malone. 1988. Cloning the human gene encoding a putative urea transport mechanism. *FASEB J.* 2:A300.

Gargus, J. J., and M. Mitas. 1988. Physiological processes revealed through an analysis of inborn errors. *Am. J. Physiol.* 255:F1047–58.

Gargus, J. J., E. Steele, Y. Feng, W. L. Whaley, and L. Malone. 1991. Expression studies of human urea transporter cDNA. *Biophys. J.* 59:330a.

Geitvik, G. A., Hoyheim, T. Gedde-Dahl, K. H. Grzeschik, R. Lothe, H. Tomter, and B. Olaisen. 1987. The Kidd (Jk) blood group locus assigned to chromosome 18 by close linkage to a DNA-RFLP. *Hum. Genet.* 77:205–209.

Haribi, B. 1984. Jk(a − b −) phenotype does exist in Caucasians. *Transfusion* 24:184.

Heaton, D. C., and K. McLoughlin. 1982. Jk(a − b −) red blood cells resist urea lysis. *Transfusion* 22:70–71.

Hunter, F. R. 1970. Facilitated diffusion in human erythrocytes. *Biochim. Biophys. Acta* 211:216–22.

Karan, D., and R. I. Macey. 1990. Temperature- and concentration-dependence of urea permeability of human erythrocytes determined by NMR. *Biochim. Biophys. Acta* 1024:271–77.

Kokko, J. P., and F. C. Rector. 1982. Countercurrent multiplication system without active transport in inner medulla. *Kidney Int.* 2:214–23.

Levitan, M. 1988. *Textbook of Human Genetics*. 325–28.New York, Oxford University Press.

Levitt, D. G., and H. J. Mlekoday. 1982. Reflection coefficient and permeability of urea and ethyleneglycol in the human red cell membrane. *J. Gen. Physiol.* 81:239–54.

Macey, R. I., and R. E. L. Farmer. 1970. Inhibition of water and solute permeability in human red cells. *Biochim. Biophys. Acta* 211:104–106.

Macey, R. I., and L. W. Yousef. 1988. Osmotic stability of red cells in renal circulation requires rapid urea transport. *Am. J. Physiol.* 254:C669–74.

Masouredis, S. P., E. Sudora, L. Mahan, and E. J. Victoria. 1980. Quantitative immunoferritin microscopy of Fy^a, Fy^b, Jk^a, U and Di^b antigenic site numbers on human red cells. *Blood* 56:969–77.

Mayrand, R. R., and D. G. Levitt. 1983. Urea and ethylene glycol-facilitated transport systems in the human red cell membrane: Saturation, competition and asymmetry. *J. Gen. Physiol.* 81:221–37.

Okubo, Y., T. Tomita, N. Nagao, H. Yamaguchi, and M. Tanaka. 1983. Mass screening donors for —D— and Jk(a – b –) using the Groupamatic-360. *Transfusion* 23:362.

Okubo, Y., H. Yamaguchi, N. Nagao, T. Tomita, T. Seno, and M. Tanaka. 1986. Heterogeneity of the phenotype Jk(a – b –) found in Japanese. *Transfusion* 26:237–39.

Pinkerton, F. J., L. E. Mermod, B. A. Liles, J. A. Jack, and J. Noades. 1959. The phenotype Jk(a – b –) in the Kidd blood group system. *Vox Sang.* 4:155–60.

Plaut, G., E. W. Ikin, A. E. Mourant, R. Sanger, and R. R. Race. 1953. A new blood-group antibody, anti-Jk^b. *Nature* 171:431.

Salmon, C., J.-P. Cartron, and P. Rouger. 1984. *The human blood groups.* 257–87. Chicago, Year Book.

Sands, J. M., J. J. Gargus, O. Fröhlich, R. B. Gunn, and J. P. Kokko. 1990. Importance of carrier-mediated urea transport to urine concentrating ability in patients with Jk(a – b –) blood type. *J. Am. Soc. Nephrol.* 1:678.

Sands, J. M., H. Nonoguchi, and M. A. Knepper. 1987. Vasopressin effects on urea and H_2O transport in inner medullary collecting duct subsegments. *Am. J. Physiol.* 253:F823–32.

Sinor, L. T., K. L. Eastwood, and F. V. Plapp. 1987. Dot-blot purification of the Kidd blood group antigen. *Med. Lab. Sci.* 44:294–96.

Solomon, A. K., B. Chasan, J. A. Dix, M. F. Lukacovic, M. R. Toon, and A. S. Verkman. 1983. The aqueous pore in the red cell membrane: Band 3 as a channel for anions, cations, nonelectrolytes and water. *Ann. N.Y. Acad. Sci.* 414:97–124.

Stevenson, J. L. 1972. Concentration of urine in a central core model of the renal counterflow system. *Kidney Int.* 2:85–94.

Toon, M. R., and A. K. Solomon. 1986. Control of red cell urea and water permeability by sulfhydryl reagents. *Biochim. Biophys. Acta* 860:361–75.

Walter, A., J. Gutknecht. 1986. Permeability of small nonelectrolytes through lipid bilayer membranes. *J. Membr. Biol.* 90:207–17.

Wieth, J. O., J. Funder, R. B. Gunn, and J. Brahm. 1974. Passive transport pathways for chloride and urea through the red cell membrane. In L. Bolis, K. Bloch, S. E. Luria, and F. Lynen, eds. 317–37. *Comparative biochemistry and physiology of transport.* Amsterdam, Elsevier North-Holland.

Woodfield, D. G., R. Douglas, J. Smith, A. Simpson, L. Pinder, and J. M. Stavely. 1982. The Jk(a – b –) phenotype in New Zealand Polynesians. *Transfusion* 22:276–78.

Yousef, L. W., and R. I. Macey. 1989. A method to distinguish between pore and carrier kinetics applied to urea transport across the erythrocyte membrane. *Biochim. Biophys. Acta* 984:281–88.

6

THE PROTEIN AND GENE STRUCTURE OF RED CELL GLYCOPHORINS

Jean-Pierre Cartron, Ph.D.
and Jacqueline London, Ph.D.

Of the many proteins that compose the red cell membrane, the group of glycoproteins collectively designated "glycophorins," owing to their high carbohydrate content (Marchesi et al. 1972), are singularly important. Glycophorins are a model of membrane proteins used to probe questions of structure and function and as specific markers of erythroid differentiation (see reviews by Bretscher 1973; Marchesi et al. 1976; Wise 1984). A large body of information on these proteins has accumulated, mainly on the major member, glycophorin A. Despite this interest, the function of these proteins remains elusive. They might play a structural role in the preservation of the red cell shape. It has also been suggested that the large amount of sialic acids carried by these glycoproteins confers to the red cells a strong negative charge that keeps erythrocytes apart from each other (Bretscher 1973). They may also serve as ligands for viruses, bacteria, and parasites (for reviews, see Burness 1981; Hadley et al. 1986; Gahmberg et al. 1988).

Four main glycophorins, which can be specifically detected by periodic acid–Schiff (PAS) staining after the separation of red cell membranes by sodium dodecyl sulfate–polyacrylamide gel electrophoresis (SDS-PAGE) (Laemmli 1970; Fairbanks et al. 1971), have been identified and are known under different nomenclatures (Table 6.1). We use the designations glycophorins A (GPA), B (GPB), C (GPC) (Furthmayr 1978a, 1978b) and D (GPD) (Dahr 1986). A new member, glycophorin E (GPE) has been identified in the course of molecular genetic studies (Kudo and Fukuda 1990; Vignal et al. 1990b).

These proteins represent about 2 percent of the total erythrocyte membrane proteins; their main properties are summarized in Table 6.1. Glycophorins A and B represent 85 and 10 percent, respectively, of the PAS-positive material of the erythrocyte membrane, whereas glycophorins C and D represent only 4 and 1 percent, respectively. Glycophorin E is undetectable by this staining. These data correlate grossly with the

Table 6.1. Nomenclature and Properties of the Major Red Cell Membrane Glycoproteins

Properties	Red Cell Membrane Glycophorins				
	GPA	*GPB*	*GPC*	*GPD*	*GPE*
Synonyms	PAS-1 MN SGP GP α	PAS-3 Ss SGP GP δ	PAS-2 Comp D GP β	Comp E GP γ	
Blood group antigens	MN	Ss	Ge:3,4	Ge:2,3,4	M
PAS-positive material (%)	85	10	4	1	undetected
Apparent molecular mass (kDa)	36	20	32	23	17
Copies cell ($\times 10^{-3}$)	500–900	100–300	50–100	20	?
Polypeptide chain (residues)	131	72	128	107	59
O-linked sugar chains	15	11	12	6	?
N-linked sugar chains	1	0	1	0	0
Percent solubilized by 5% (w/v) Triton X-100	89	92	20	30	?

number of copies of each glycoprotein, which ranges from approximately 10^6 per cell for GPA, 1 to 3 $\times$ 10^5 per cell for GPB, 0.5 to 1.0 $\times$ 10^5 per cell for GPC, and 2 $\times$ 10^4/cell for GPD. This may be compared to 10^6 copies per cell for the band 3 (anion transporter) and to the 5 $\times$ 10^5, 4 $\times$ 10^5, 1 $\times$ 10^5, and 2 $\times$ 10^5 copies per cell of the skeletal proteins actin, spectrin (α and β), ankyrin, and protein 4.1, respectively. The membrane glycophorins also differ by their apparent molecular mass (estimated on SDS gels), by the composition of their carbohydrate chains, and by their extractibility with a nonionic detergent like Triton X-100 (see Table 6.1). Importantly, these molecules are the carriers of blood group antigens: MN on GPA, Ss on GPB, and Gerbich (Ge) on GPC and GPD. Many variants of these antigens are known, which may be of significance in transfusion medicine (Race and Sanger 1975; Mollison et al. 1987).

The purpose of this chapter is to summarize the current literature on the molecular characterization of the genes encoding these proteins and their variants, with the aim of better understanding their polymorphisms, evolution, and mode of regulation. Whether or not these genes define a new family will also be addressed. The structure and antigenic properties of the erythrocyte membrane glycoproteins will be discussed only briefly, since they have been reviewed extensively (Anstee 1980, 1981; Dahr 1986; Lisowska 1989; Blanchard 1990). Similarly, the isolation and structural analysis of the cDNA and genes encoding GPA and GPB will not be discussed in detail, since this has been the subject of a recent review (Cartron et al. 1990).

GLYCOPHORINS A, B, AND E AND THE BLOOD GROUP MNSs LOCUS

MNSs BLOOD GROUPS AND GLYCOPHORINS A AND B

The Basic Nomenclature of MNSs Antigens. The M and N antigens were discovered by Landsteiner and Levine (1927) following the deliberate immunization of rabbits with human red cells, but the S and s antigens defined by human antisera were described later (Sanger and Race 1947; Sanger et al. 1948; Levine et al. 1951). Serologic and family studies reviewed in great detail by Race and Sanger (1975) and Issitt (1981, 1985) summarized the complexity of this blood group system; therefore, most of the information needed for an understanding of those antigens will be found under those references.

After the recognition that M and N as well as S and s were the products of allelic genes, respectively, it was shown that the genes encoding MN and Ss antigens are closely linked on chromosome 4q28-q31 (Cook et al. 1981), and that recombination between the two loci could occur, albeit rarely (Gedde-Dahl et al. 1967). Current genetic studies have recognized four common gene complexes (haplotypes) inherited "en bloc" from one generation to another. In the North European population the frequency of these haplotypes is approximately 0.24 for *MS,* 0.30 for *Ms,* 0.07 for *NS,* and 0.38 for *Ns.* The combination of these common haplotypes produce ten genotypes and nine phenotypes that are easily detected by the M-, N-, S-, and s-specific antisera.

In 1953, Wiener and colleagues identified the U antigen, which is common in Caucasians but absent from approximately 1 percent of blacks. It was found later that the U-negative red cells are also S-negative and s-negative (S−s−U− phenotype) but that among S−s− blacks, about 16 percent are weakly U-positive. These findings strongly suggested that the U antigen was encoded by an allele (S^u or *u*) at the *Ss* locus. Two other high-frequency antigens in the Caucasian population, En^a and Wr^b, deserve to be mentioned. Darnborough and colleagues (1969) described an unusual phenotype called En(a−) in a young English woman (MEP) whose red cells exhibited a marked sialic acid deficiency and absence of MN antigens. The serum of Mrs. MEP contained a new antibody reacting with all human red cells except her own. The term "En" was proposed to indicate that En(a−) individuals have an abnormal red cell *en*velope owing to the lack of a common En^a antigen, serologically defined by the serum MEP. The Wr^b antigen is also a high-frequency red cell antigen, which is defined by an antibody present in the serum of a rare (and still unique) individual (Mrs. Fr.) (Adams et al. 1971) assumed to be homozygous for the rare Wr^a antigen first identified by Holman (1953). Rare individuals that lack M and N antigens are all Wr(a−b−) and frequently develop anti-Wr^b in their serum. Also of interest, anti-Wr^b is a common autoantibody present in the sera of patients suffering from autoimmune hemolytic anemia (see Petz and Garraty, 1980). Whereas the En^a antigen is clearly encoded by an allele at the *MN* locus, the genetic inheritance of Wr^b is still a matter of speculation (see below).

A large number of antigens encoded by alleles at the *MN* and *Ss* loci have been described, and many others are still candidates. These variants are currently identified either by the absence of expression of one of the common antigens M, N, S, s, U, En^a, and Wr^b, or by new antigenic properties revealed in most instances by antibodies produced by alloimmunization during transfusion or pregnancy. The description of these variants is beyond the scope of this chapter but can be found in the reviews mentioned above. Only those antigens that have been investigated at the protein and/or DNA level will be briefly mentioned, like the low-frequency antigens M^g or M^c and He (Henshaw) or M^v, which are encoded by alleles at the *MN* and *Ss* locus, respectively (Table 6.2). Another category of low-incidence antigens that have been extensively investigated are those of the Miltenberger (Mi) series, which are serologically distinguished into eight subclasses (Mi.I to Mi.VIII) by a panel of human antibodies (see Giles et al. 1982). Immunochemical as well as biochemical investigations at the protein and DNA level, reported below, have clearly established that some of these antigens are encoded by alleles of the *MN* locus (Mi.I, Mi.II, Mi.VII, and Mi.VIII), whereas others are encoded by hybrid gene fusion products of the *MN* and *Ss* loci (Mi.V) or are the result of gene conversion at the *Ss* locus (Mi.III and Mi.VI).

GPA and GPB Are the Carriers of MNSs Blood Group Antigens. The demonstration that the MN antigens are carried by red cell membrane sialoglycoproteins emerged more than 30 years ago with the finding that these antigens are inactivated by treatment with neuraminidases from influenza viruses and *Vibrio cholerae* (for review see Springer and Huprikar, 1972). Since these pioneer investigations, many studies have been performed to characterize and purify the red cell membrane glycoproteins. One of the major advances in that field was the electrophoretic separation of SDS–solubilized cell membranes in SDS-PAGE, either in a continuous (Fairbanks et al. 1971) or more reliably in the discontinuous buffer system of Laemmli (1970). Other important steps were the development of purification methods that permitted isolation of the red cell membrane components in a water-soluble form (for reviews see Steck 1974; Marchesi et al. 1976). Using a combination of these methods, Hamaguchi and Cleve (1972) assigned the MN and Ss antigens to a major and a minor red cell sialoglycoprotein now called *glycophorin A* (GPA) and *glycophorin B* (GPB), respectively. These findings were largely confirmed by the discovery and biochemical characterization of genetic variants lacking red cell expression of MN antigens [En(a−) phenotype], Ss antigens (S−s−U− phenotype), or even all MNSs antigens (Mk phenotype) that were found

Table 6.2. Some Well-Characterized Variants of Glycophorins A and B

Variant	Protein*: *Residues (kDa)*	Protein*: *Alteration*	Gene Structure†	Associated Antigens‡	Comments
Normal glycophorins					
GPA (MN)	131 (36)	^{1}(S/L)-S-T-T-^{5}(G/E)	7 exons (> 30 kb)		^{49}R-T-V-Y-P (see Mi.VII and VIII)
GPB (Ss, 'N')	72 (20)	^{29}(M/T)	5 exons (> 30 kb)		
GPA and/or B Deficiency					
En(a−) Fin		GPA absent	Deletion (S)		GPB and GPE genes present
S−s−U−		GPB absent	Deletion or mutation (S)		GPA and GPE genes present
Mk		GPA and B absent	Deletion (S)		GPE gene present
GPA and B Variants					
GPA mutants					
M^g	131 (34)	^{1}L-S-T-N-E		M^g	Not N-glycosylated at position 2,3
M^c	131 (36)	^{1}S-S-T-T-E			Evolutionary link M→N
Mi.I/Mi.II	131 (32)	^{28}(T→M/L)		Mi^a, V^w/Hut	Absence of N-glycan
MiVII/Mi.VIII	131 (36)	^{49}T-T-V-^{52}(S/Y)-P		Nob/Nob, Hop	Evolutionary link GPA→Mi.VII
GPB mutants					
He	72 (20)	^{1}W-S-T-S-G		He	No 'N' reactivity
M^v	72 (20)	Abnormal N-ter		M^v	
Hybrid Glycoproteins					
A-B hybrids					
En(a−) UK	72? (20)	$(A\text{-}B)^{MEP}$	Hybrid gene (S)	(M)	Cross-over within N-terminus
Mi.V	104 (30)	(1–58A/27–72B)	6 exons	Hil	
B-A hybrids					
St^a	99 (24)	(1–26B/59–131A)	6 exons	Stones	Protease-resistant antigen
Dantu	99 (24)	(1–39B/71–131A)	6 exons	Dantu	Protease-resistant antigen
B-A-B hybrids					
Mi.III/Mi.VI	103 (28)	(1–26B/31 new res/27–72B) ^{48}(R/T)	6 exons	Mi^a, Mur, Hil (Mi.III) Mi^a, Mur, Hil, Hop (Mi.VI)	Enhanced 'N' reactivity

*Protein sequences given in the one-letter amino acid code.
†Gene structures characterized by Southern blot hybridization only are indicated by (S).
‡Low-frequency antigens associated with protein variants.

deficient for GPA, GPB, or both GPA and GPB proteins, respectively (see reviews by Anstee 1980, 1981; Dahr 1986).

PROTEIN STRUCTURE OF GLYCOPHORINS

Molecular Analysis of GPA, GPB, and GPE. The primary structure of the GPA and GPB proteins was deduced from protein sequencing and nucleotide sequencing of the cDNAs (reviewed by Dahr 1986; Blanchard 1990; Cartron et al. 1990), whereas the structure of the GPE protein was derived from cDNA sequence exclusively (Kudo and Fukuda 1990; Vignal et al. 1990b). A schematic representation of the three proteins structure is given in Figure 6.1, showing how the protein segments are encoded by the different exons of each gene (see below). All proteins are synthesized with a cleavable leader peptide sequence of 19 residues and all are similarly organized in three distinct domains, including an extracellular

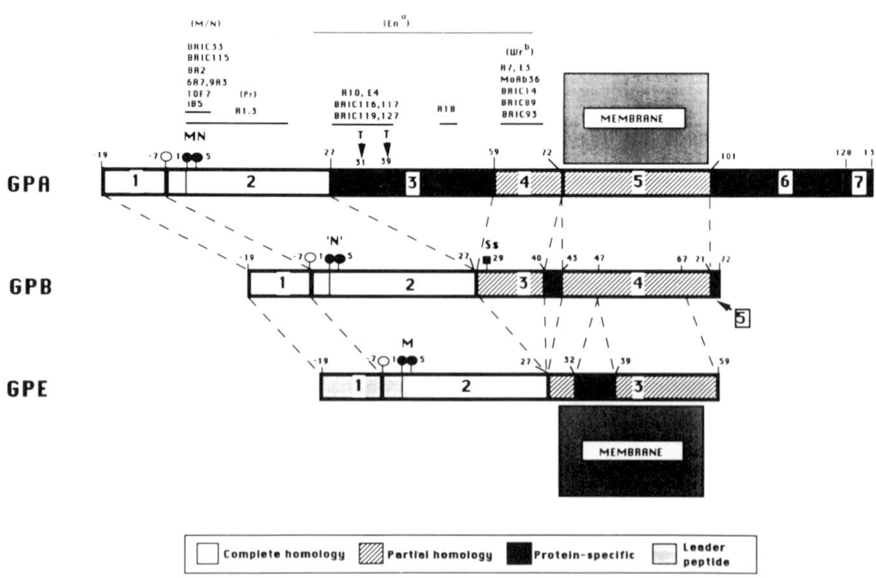

Figure 6.1. Protein structure from human glycophorins A, B, and E. GPA, GPB and GPE proteins are represented with their cleavable signal peptide of 19 residues, denoted by negative numbers. Position +1 above protein diagrams refers to the first amino acid of the mature protein. The picture delineates the protein segment homology between the three glycophorins and their general organization in terms of amino acids encoded by exons 1 to 7 of the GPA gene, 1 to 5 of the GPB gene, and 1 to 3 of the GPE gene (see also Fig. 6.2). Polymorphic positions on the leader peptide (−7) and on the mature proteins (MN, 'N' and Ss) are indicated by open and black circles and a black square, respectively. T arrows denote trypsin cleavage sites of GPA on intact red cells. A proposed map of the epitopes recognized by murine monoclonal antibodies against GPA (horizontal bars) is represented above the GPA structure (see text).

region that carry glycans chains and blood group antigenic determinants, a single hydrophobic domain that spans the phospholipid bilayer, and a more or less extended intracellular domain that may interact with membrane as well as with cytosolic protein components. Remarkably, GPA, B, and E are homologous both at the protein and the DNA level, and thus define a new family of gene-related molecules derived from a common ancestral gene during evolution, as discussed below. The highest protein homology sequence occurs at the first 26 amino acid residues of the mature proteins, which are entirely identical, except for the MN polymorphisms present at positions 1 and 5. Glycophorin A is extensively characterized and was the first membrane protein to be fully sequenced (Tomita and Marchesi 1975; Tomita et al. 1978). The mature glycoprotein consists of 131 amino acids and has a molecular weight of 31 kDa. The overall content of carbohydrate is approximately 60 percent of the protein mass, of which about half are N-acetyl neuraminic acids (sialic acids). Glycophorin A carries 16 oligosaccharide chains, including a single N-glycan chain attached at ^{26}Asn (Yoshima et al. 1980; Irimura et al. 1981) and 15 sialotetrasaccharide chains O-glycosidically linked to Ser and Thr residues (Thomas and Winzler 1969) clustered in the extracellular domain. Although MN antigens are specified by amino acid polymorphisms at positions 1 and 5 (M = ^{1}Ser/^{5}Gly; N = ^{1}Leu/^{5}Glu) of GPA (Dahr et al. 1977; Wasniovska et al. 1977; Furthmayr 1978a), some anti-M and anti-N antibodies are carbohydrate-dependent (Judd et al. 1979).

Many murine monoclonal antibodies directed against human glycophorins have been produced and characterized (for review see Lisowska 1989). Most react specifically with GPA, and the epitopes they recognize have been mapped on this protein mainly by agglutination (and its inhibition), competitive binding assay, immunofluorescence, and Western blot analysis using either intact red cells or membranes from normal or variant cells carrying well-characterized glycophorin species (see Lisowska 1989; Gardner et al. 1989). Some of these epitopes are shown in Figure 6.1. Certain antibodies directed against the N-terminal region of GPA are M-specific (6A7, 9A3, E3) or N-specific (iB5, 8A2), whereas others that do not discriminate between M and N blood groups have specificities equivalent to those defined by human antibodies like anti-Pr (R1.3), anti-En^{a} (R10, R18, 10F7), or anti-Wr^{b} (R7, MoAb36, BRIC14), although the fine properties between these antibodies (protease and glycosylation dependence) may slightly differ (for discussion see Lisowska 1989). This is obvious for En^{a} antigens, which represent heterogeneous structures spreading over residues 27 to 72 of GPA (see Fig. 6.1). The Wr^{a}/Wr^{b} specificity is not so clear-cut, however, since it is not simply a polymorphism of GPA. Indeed, Dahr and colleagues (1986) could not demonstrate any amino acid sequence difference in GPA from Wr(b−) and Wrb(+) red cells and found that Wr^{b} was a labile structure located within 62 to 72 of GPA that requires lipids for antigenic activity. They suggested

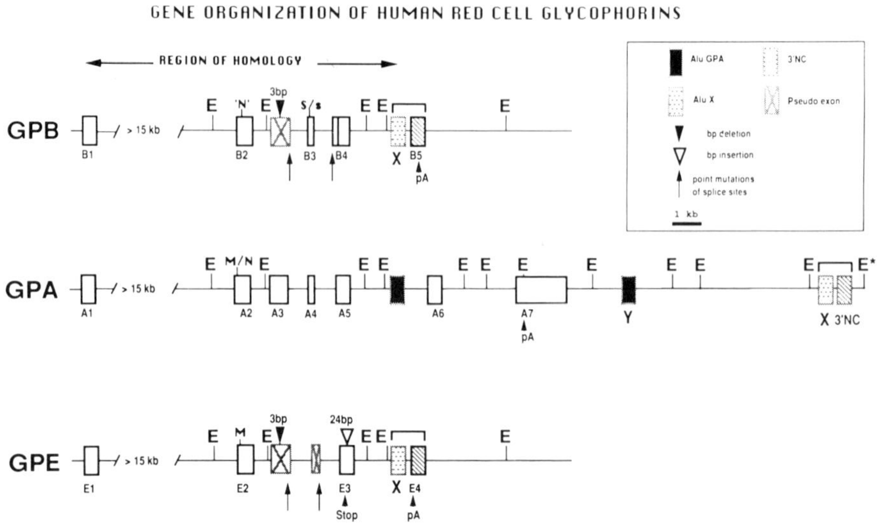

Figure 6.2. Genomic organization of human red cell glycophorins. The diagram shows an *Eco*R1 (E) restriction map of the glycophorin genes. Solid squares refer to exons and pA to a polyadenylation site. Other symbols are given in the top right insert. The sequence homology between the three genes extends from the 5′ region down to the Alu repeats located in the intron 5 of GPA gene or the equivalent positions in the intron 4 and intron 3 of the GPB and GPE genes, respectively. Downstream of this position the nucleotide sequences of GPB and GPE are still similar but differ completely from those of the 3′ region of GPA. The nucleotide sequence 3′NC downstream the Alu element, denoted X in the GPA gene (horizontal bar), is identical to those of exon B5 and E4 of the GPB and GPE gene, respectively, suggesting that these genes acquired their 3′ regions by unequal crossing-over between the Alu repeats located inside and outside the GPA gene (see also Fig. 6.3).

further that a complex between GPA and band 3 might be important for Wr^b expression. This hypothesis has been recently confirmed by elegant immunoprecipitation studies carried out with murine monoclonal anti-Wr^b antibodies (Telen and Chasis 1990). Whether a polymorphism of band 3 is responsible for Wr^b antigen remains unresolved.

Glycophorin B consists of 72 amino acids, among which only six are exposed on the cytoplasmic side, including three basic amino acids. This glycoprotein does not carry an N-linked carbohydrate chain since the consensus sequence Asn-Asp-*Thr* (amino acid residues 26 to 28) present on GPA protein is modified into Asn-Gly-*Glu* on GPB, but carries approximately 11 O-linked oligosaccharide chains. Like GPA, the carbohydrate content of GPB is close to 50 percent of the protein mass. Glycophorin B also expresses an unusual form of blood group N antigen (noted ‘N’) due to a ^{1}Leu/^{5}Glu polymorphism, which, unlike the N antigen of GPA, is resistant to trypsin hydrolysis on native red cells (Dahr et al. 1975a). The blood group Ss polymorphism is determined by a Met/Thr exchange at position 29 defining the S and s antigens, respectively (Dahr et al. 1980). Residues 27 to 58 and 101 to 131 of GPA (encoded by exons A-3, A-6, and A-7; see below) are not represented in GPB but a new sequence (residues 40 to 42) is absent from GPA (see Fig. 6.1). Glycophorin B carries a cysteine at position 50 and an alanine at the carboxy end of the protein, which are absent in GPA and were detected only by cDNA nucleotide sequencing (Siebert and Fukuda 1987). Monoclonal antibodies that react with the N-terminal region of the blood type GPA, except those that are M-specific, react also with GPB (see Fig. 6.1). However, GPB-specific or S/s-specific monoclonal antibodies have not been reported, although a murine monoclonal anti-S might have been produced recently (Anstee and Lisowska 1990). Like Wr^b, the antigenic reactivity of U is apparently lipid-dependent, and residues 33 to 40 of GPB represent the essential part of this antigen (Dahr and Moulds 1987).

The predicted mature GPE protein consists of 59 amino acids (see Fig. 6.1) and should express the blood group M antigen as amino acids 1 and 5 are Ser and Gly, respectively. As the consensus N-glycosylation sequence (^{26}Asn-X-Ser/Thr) is not present no N-glycan is attached to ^{26}Asn, but the protein may carry O-linked oligosaccharides such as those present on the NH_2-terminal region of GPA and GPB. Since residues 27 to 39 of GPB (encoded by exon B-3) are absent from GPE, the protein should not express Ss blood group antigens. From amino residue 27 up to the carboxy end, GPE is similar to GPB but with distinct features: (1) both polypeptides contain a cysteine residue but not at a conserved position (residues 50 and 57, respectively); (2) GPE contains an insertion of eight amino acids (positions 32 to 39), including two tryptophans that are present neither in GPB nor GPA proteins, and the putative transmembrane domain has an overall reduced hydrophobicity and is separated into two hydrophobic subregions; and (3) a premature stop codon interrupts the GPE protein sequence at position 59. Until recently, a glycoprotein with the properties expected for GPE had not been identified on control or variant human erythrocytes, including homozygous Mk erythrocytes, which lack both GPA and GPB and are unreactive with anti-M/N or anti-S/s reagents (see below). Glycophorin E might be expressed at a low copy number or at a certain stage of differentiation or ontogenesis and, therefore, may be difficult to detect by conventional methods for glycoprotein identification. In addition, like GPB, the GPE protein has a very short C-terminal domain and might be inefficiently inserted into the membrane (see Fig. 6.1). Preliminary evidence suggests, however, that a murine anti-M monoclonal antibody is able to detect the GPE gene product as a 20-kDa component on immunoblots irrespective of the MN status of the red cell membrane proteins (Anstee 1990). Whether GPE carries as yet unidentified blood group antigens encoded by the new eight amino acid sequence is unknown. Similarly, whether a blood group N-like GPE protein (N-ter amino acids ^{1}Leu/^{5}Glu) may exist remains undetermined. This is not unlikely since evolutionary considerations suggest that the GPE gene derived from a duplication of the GPB gene. However, it might have arisen from microconversion events such as those found in Mi.III and Mi.VI genes (see below).

Molecular Analysis of Glycophorins in Selected Variants. Red cell glycophorins from several MNSs variants have been characterized, mainly by SDS-PAGE, and occasionally purified and partially sequenced in order to provide a molecular basis to the antigenic diversity of these proteins. Some of the results are summarized in Table 6.2 but will not be discussed here as a full description can be found in extensive reviews (Anstee 1980, 1981; Dahr 1986; Blanchard, 1990). Several variants of the O-glycans attached to human glycophorins A and B are known to result from either inherited (Cad) or acquired (T and Tn) conditions. These variants will not be discussed in the present review, but it is interesting to note that the cells carrying certain of these determinants resist the *in vitro* invasion by laboratory strains of *Plasmodium falciparum* merozoites (Cartron et al. 1983).

Nonhuman Homologs of Glycophorins. Glycophorin-like molecules have been detected on red cells of several animal species, but only those from pig, horse, and dog have been purified and completely sequenced (for review see Krotkiewski 1988), including the monkey glycophorin MK from *Macaca fuscata* (Murayama et al. 1989). All these molecules are carbohydrate-rich (25 to 70%), and the apparent molecular weight of the monomers ranged from 20 to 50 kDa between species. Notably, the neuraminic (sialic) acids carried by glycophorins are exclusively of the N-acetyl type in humans and of the N-glycolyl type in other species, except in rodents, which exhibit both the N-acetyl and O-acetyl types. There is a significant sequence homology between the hydrophobic transmembrane domains of all animal glycophorins and human GPA (and GPB), but not of GPC. This was confirmed by molecular cloning of a mouse glycophorin (Matsui et al. 1989). Only the monkey glycophorin MK exhibited a striking homology with the extracellular and intracellular domain of GPA and demonstrated MN blood activity, as did other higher primates (Wiener et al. 1972). Immunostaining analysis confirmed that red cells from nonhuman primates carry glycoproteins related to human GPA, but a GPB-like protein was detected only in chimpanzees (Lu et al. 1987a). These findings suggested that the genes encoding the glycophorins derived from a common ancestor, and this was further investigated at the DNA level to delineate the evolutionary relationship between these genes (see below). This is consistent with the identification of an M^c-specific sequence considered as the evolutionary link between M and N (see Table 6.2) at the N-terminus of the red cell glycoprotein from M blood-type chimpanzee (Blumenfeld et al. 1983).

PUTATIVE FUNCTION OF GLYCOPHORINS A AND B

The discovery that red cells deficient in GPA, GPB or both proteins [En(a−), S−s−U, and Mk variants, respectively] have no detectable anomaly of morphology, function, and survival provided a strong indication that these proteins had no vital functions (reviewed by Furthmayr 1978a; Anstee 1980, 1981), even at an early stage of erythroid differentiation, since the absence of cell surface expression has been recently correlated with large gene deletions (see below).

Another property of the red cell glycophorins is related to their elevated sialic acid content, resulting in their ability to bind viruses, bacteria, and parasites. For instance, purified glycophorins and red cells from genetic variants deficient for these proteins inhibit or resist, respectively, invasion by certain strains of *Plasmodium falciparum* parasites (for review see Chapter 12; Mitchell and Bannister 1988). Other strains of parasites, however, are not dependent on sialic acids for invasion and may efficiently penetrate into Tn as well as homozygous Mk red cells (Mitchell et al. 1986; Hadley et al. 1987), but the ligand(s) used by these parasites have not been identified yet. Interestingly, parasites that exhibited low invasion of sialic acid–deficient red cells maintained after several cycles their ability to invade untreated and neuraminidase-treated erythrocytes at equivalent rates, suggesting an adaptative capacity to switch from a sialic acid–dependent to a sialic acid–independent mode of invasion (Dolan et al. 1990).

In the course of these studies, it was found that murine monoclonal antibodies against red cell glycophorin determinants, particularly Wr^b, were potent inhibitors of invasion (Pasvol et al. 1982; Facer 1984), although Wrb(−) red cells were normally invaded (Hermentin et al. 1984; Cartron et al. 1984). As an explanation, it was proposed that anti-GPA antibodies inhibited invasion by reducing membrane deformability and not by using the Wr^b antigen as receptor (Pasvol et al. 1989). This is consistent with previously established findings indicating that binding of antibody to GPA reduced membrane deformability, presumably by inducing an interaction between GPA and the skeletal proteins (Chasis et al. 1985, 1988; Chapter 7) that are known to regulate the mechanical properties of red cells (see Bennett 1985, 1990). It is suspected, however, that a membrane defect rather than rigidity of red cells by itself specifically inhibited invasion (Nagel 1990).

As noted above, GPA associates with skeletal proteins only after ligand binding, and its C-terminal domain is crucial in this process. At variance, GPC and GPD apparently bind permanently to the skeletal proteins. The glycophorin–skeletal proteins interaction probably occurs via protein 4.1 and is mediated by phosphoinositides (for review see Anderson 1989), but as only GPC and GPD deficient red cells exhibit morphologic abnormalities (see below) it is likely that only the interactions involving these proteins are of physiologic importance (see Chapter 7).

GENE STRUCTURE OF GPA, GPB, AND GPE

Gene Organization. The GPA, GPB, and GPE genes have been fully characterized (Kudo and Fukuda 1989, 1990; Vignal et al. 1989, 1990b). A simplified representation of the three genes structure is given in Figure 6.2. The GPA and GPB genes extend over 30 kb of DNA and comprise seven exons (A-1 to A-7) and five exons (B-1 to B-5), respectively. Their detailed structure has been reviewed recently (Carton et al. 1990). The GPE gene has a genomic structure similar to the GPB gene and is composed of four exons (E-1 to E-4). The difference in exon numbering between each gene arises because exon A-3 and A-3 plus A-4 of the GPA gene are pseudoexon structures in the GPB and GPE genes, respectively (see Fig. 6.2 and below). Typically, the three genes are extensively homologous in their 5′ region (> 95% identity) up to Alu repeated sequences present in introns 5, 4, and 3 of the GPA, GPB, and GPE genes, respectively (see Fig. 6.2 and below).

Exons 1 and 2 of each gene are identical, except for nucleotide exchanges responsible for a polymorphism of amino acids −7 (signal peptide) and +1 and +5 (MN), and are separated by a large intron (> 15 kb). So far, no overlapping clone has been identified.

Exons A-2 to A-4 encode the extracellular domain of mature GPA, whereas these domains are encoded by exons B-2 plus B-3 and exon E-2, respectively, of the GPB and GPE genes. The transmembrane domain of the GPA, GPB, and GPE proteins is encoded by exons A-5, B-4, and E-3, respectively. Because of splice-site mutations, exon sequences A-3 and A-3 plus A-4 of the GPA gene are spliced out from the GPB and GPE mRNAs, and the encoded protein segments (amino acids 27 to 58 and 27 to 71, respectively) are not expressed in the GPB and GPE proteins, respectively (see Fig. 6.2). Moreover, a nucleotide substitution atct → ag/CT in the third intron of the GPB gene creates a new 5′ splice site and therefore exon B-4 contains three additional codons encoding amino acids 40 to 42 that are not present in the GPA protein (see Figs. 6.1 and 6.2). The nucleotide sequence encoded by exon E-3 differs significantly from those encoded by its counterparts A-5 and B-4 in the GPA and GPB genes, respectively. Indeed, in addition to frequent point mutations (leading to amino acid substitutions) there is an in frame insertion of 24 bp encoding eight amino acids found neither in GPA nor in GPB and a premature stop codon (due to a C → T nucleotide exchange in the CGA codon 68 of GPB) shortening the reading frame by five codons as compared with GPB. The origin of the 24-bp insertion is unknown, but this sequence is present with a partial homology not only in a GPE downstream sequence (58% homology) but also in GPA and GPB at corresponding positions and even with a higher degree of homology (83% and 67% respectively).

DNA sequences encoding the 3′ region of GPA differ completely from those encoding the 3′ sequences of GPB and GPE. The transition point is defined by intronic Alu sequence repeats (see Fig. 6.2). The C-terminal region of GPA (30 amino acids) is encoded by exons A-6 and A-7, whereas the short C-terminal region of GPB is encoded by exon B-4 (homologous to exon A-5) and exon B-5, which has no equivalent in the GPA gene. The GPE protein is virtually devoid of cytoplasmic segment, and exon E-4 corresponds only to 3′ untranslated sequences.

Evolution of the Glycophorin Gene Family. The transition site from the homologous to nonhomologous regions in the GPA and GPB genes was positioned at a sequence of an Alu family (Kudo and Fukuda 1989), and the same transition site separated homologous and nonhomologous regions within the GPE gene (Kudo and Fukuda 1990; Vignal et al., 1990b).

Alu elements are genomic sequences of about 300 bp interspersed every 3 to 5 kb in the human genome and most are flanked on both sides by short direct repeats (seven to 20 bp) which represent a duplication of the random genomic target site where the Alu sequence is integrated (Van Arsdell et al. 1981; Daniels and Deininger 1985). Six different classes, all derived from a common ancestor, have been identified (Ullu et al. 1982). Comparison of the nucleotide sequences surrounding Alu sequences and their direct flanking repeats in the three glycophorin genes clearly suggested that two sequential duplications through unequal crossing-over occurred during evolution, as shown from Figure 6.3. Accordingly, GPA probably arose from a first duplication of an ancestral gene. The GPB and GPE genes evolved later from duplication of one of the duplicated genes, which acquired 3′ sequences different from those of GPA following homologous recombination at Alu sequences (Kudo and Fukuda 1989, 1990).

Based on intron sequence divergence of the GPA and GPB genes and on sequence divergence of the 3′ regions of the GPB and GPE genes, it was estimated that the first gene duplication of the ancestral GPA gene occurred nine to 35 million years ago, whereas the second duplication generating GPB and GPE took place five to 21 million years ago (Kudo and Fukuda 1989, 1990).

Preliminary results obtained in the authors' laboratory (Vignal et al., unpublished data) strongly suggest that the right side of the Alu sequence and the 3′ untranslated sequences found in GPB and GPE originate from a genomic sequence located within a *Eco*RI fragment positioned between the GPA and GPB genes on chromosome 4. Sequencing of this fragment indicated that it includes an Alu element (named X in Fig. 6.2) followed by a nucleotide sequence (named 3′NC in Fig. 6.2) identical to that which is present at the 3′ end of the GPB and GPE genes. Presumably, the 3′ regions of the GPB and GPE genes were generated by homologous recombination between the X (Alu) sequence and the second Alu se-

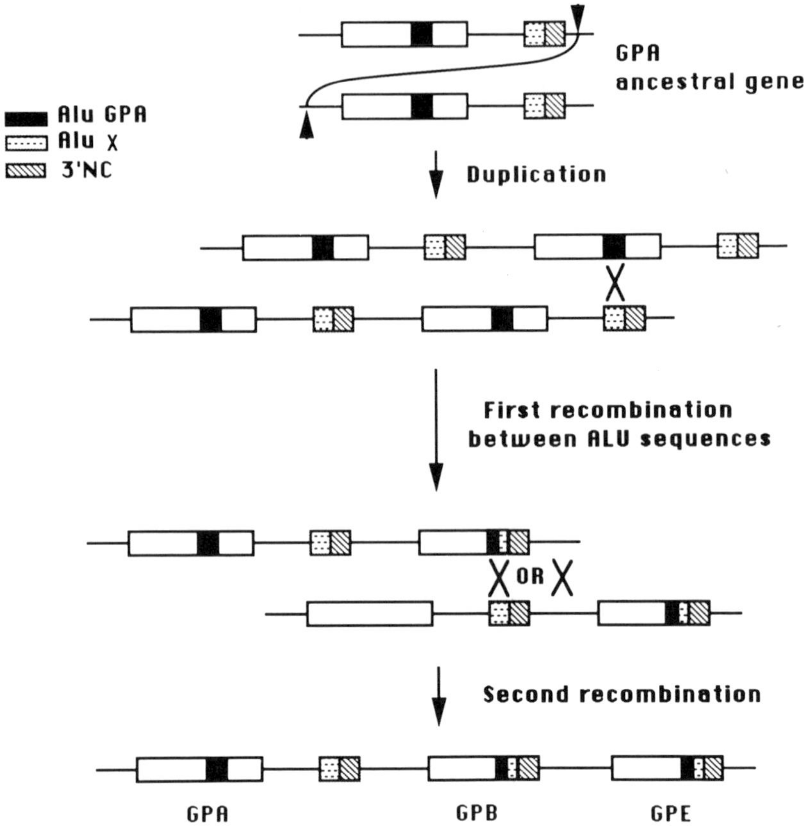

Figure 6.3. Evolution of the glycophorin gene family. The glycophorin genes presumably evolved from a common ancestral gene by duplication during evolution, and the GPB and GPE genes acquired their 3′ region by recombination at Alu repeats (Kudo and Fukuda 1990). Recent evidence (see text) suggests that this recombination event involved Alu elements, denoted Alu GPA and Alu X (see also Fig. 6.2) located inside and outside the GPA gene.

quence within intron 5 of the GPA gene, as proposed in Figure 6.3. Another Alu element (named Y in Fig. 6.2) is present within a 2.9-kb *Eco*RI fragment downstream from exon A-7 of the GPA gene, but it is not followed by sequences related to the GPB or GPE genes (Vignal et al., unpublished data).

All these findings indicate clearly that the three closely related glycophorin genes define a new gene family. Phylogenetic studies carried out by restriction DNA analysis on Southern blot from humans, chimpanzees, gibbons, and gorillas are consistent with this concept and provide further information on the evolution of this gene family. Indeed, the GPA-related gene was identified in all primates, whereas the GPB gene was detected only in humans, chimpanzees, and gorillas, thus suggesting that the GPB gene appeared later than GPA in an ancestor common to humans, chimpanzees, and gorillas (Rearden et al. 1990b). This is consistent with the early detection of GPA only in Capuchin monkeys (Créau-Goldberg et al. 1989). Similar investigations indicated that the chimpanzee genome contains at least three related genes closely homologous to the human GPA, GPB, and GPE genes, which most likely share a similar gross structural organization (Lu et al. 1990).

Chromosome Assignment and Gene Cluster Organization. The blood group *MNSs* locus has been assigned by linkage analysis to chromosome 4q28-q31 (Cook et al. 1981). This was confirmed by direct assignment by in situ hybridization of a GPA cDNA probe to human metaphasic chromosomes (Rahuel et al. 1988a). From the identification of hybrid glycophorin variants generated by unequal crossing-over, it was postulated that GPA and GPB are adjacent genes in that order downstream in the direction of transcription (Anstee 1980, 1981). This is consistent with the linkage disequilibrium between a *Stu*I restriction-fragment–length polymorphism (RFLP) for GPA and the blood groups MN and Ss in Caucasians (Murray et al. 1988). The GPE gene has been assigned to chromosome 4 by Southern blot hybridization to DNA from a human hybrid 9TK cell line retaining only chromosome 4 as the residual human chromosome (Vignal et al. 1990b) and by *in situ* hybridization (Kudo and Fukuda, 1990). Moreover, studies of the deletion occurring in different glycophorin variants (see below) strongly suggests that the three genes are in the order GPA-GPB-GPE on chromosome 4 (Vignal et al. 1990b). This alignment is consistent with the presumption that the three genes evolved from a common ancestor to form a small gene cluster by duplication and diversification (Fig. 6.3).

GENOMIC STRUCTURE OF GLYCOPHORIN VARIANTS

A large number of glycophorin variants have been extensively characterized by immunochemical studies (reviewed by Furthmayr 1978a; Anstee et al. 1980, 1981; Dahr 1986; Blanchard 1990) but as yet relatively few have been investigated at the genomic level. This section will focus on the recent advances in this area that have led to the description of the glycophorin gene family and to general models of the organization and rearrangements of these genes in normal individuals and their variants.

Variants Lacking GPA and/or GPB. These variants have been explored only by Southern blot hybridization.

En(a−) variant. This rare phenotype was discovered in 1969 simultaneously in England and in Finland (Darnborough et al. 1969; Furuhjelm et al. 1969) and later in Canada (Taliano et al. 1980). Serologic and immunochemical studies of the variant's families have shown that the *En(Fin)* gene complex is a silent gene producing no GPA and thus no MN antigens except for the typical trypsin-resistant 'N' reactivity carried by GPB (Dahr et al. 1975a). The cells are deficient in sialic acids but the Ss antigens are normal. Genomic analysis of the En(a−) Finnish DNA by Southern blot hybridization with GPA and GPB cDNA probes after cleavage by several restriction enzymes indicated that all restriction fragments from the GPA gene were absent whereas those from the GPB and GPC genes were normally present (Rahuel et al. 1988b). Thus the absence of the GPA protein in this variant originates from a large GPA gene deletion.

The English En(a−) variant was more complex since it arose from the uncommon genotype *En(UK)/Mk,* in which *Mk* indicated heterozygosity for a silent gene that suppressed the expression of both MN and Ss antigens (see below). Genomic studies described below have shown this gene to be an A-B hybrid gene producing a glycoprotein composed of the N-terminus of GPA linked to the C-terminus of GPB.

S−s−U− variant. Red cells that are deficient for the S, s and U (and 'N') antigens define the phenotype S−s−U− and were discovered by Greenwalt and colleagues (1954). This phenotype is prevalent among selected populations, in particular among blacks in which the incidence varies from 1 to 37 percent in certain regions in Africa, as compared with an incidence of < 0.001 percent among whites (Lowe and Moores 1972). The phenotype is heterogeneous since about 16 percent of S−s− individuals are U-positive. Biochemical investigations have shown that S−s−U− red cells either lack GPB (Dahr et al. 1975b) or carry a defective molecule that is not glycosylated (Tanner et al. 1977).

The genomic DNA from several unrelated S−s−U− individuals has been examined by Southern hybridization in several laboratories (Huang et al. 1987; Tate et al. 1989; Rahuel et al. 1991). In most instances, the lack of cell surface expression of GPB was correlated with a large deletion of the GPB gene (exons B-2 to B-5), whereas the GPA and GPC genes were normally present.

Few other individuals exhibit apparently partial deletions (Huang et al. 1989b), whereas still another (Del.) has normal GPB restriction fragments and so far a normal promoter structure region (Rahuel et al. 1991). These findings are consistent with the heterogeneity of the S−s−U− phenotypes and indicate that distinct gene alterations (deletions, alteration of either transcription and translation, or both) may generate the S−s−U− condition.

Mk variant. Metaxas and Metaxas-Bühler (1964) first described red cells from Mk heterozygous individuals that express only 50 percent of MN and Ss antigens, suggesting the presence of a silent allele at the *MN* and *Ss* loci. This silent haplotype has since been found in rare heterozygous variants such as *Mi.V/Mk* and *En/Mk*. Two exceptional Mk homozygous individuals have been discovered in a Japanese family (Tokunaga et al. 1979). Homozygous Mk red cells lack GPA and GPB and all MN and Ss antigens, including the associated antigens such as U, En^a, and Wr^b (see Race and Sanger 1975; Issitt 1981, 1985). These cells are sialic acid–deficient but exhibit a hyperglycosylation of protein band 3 similar to that observed in En(a−) variants, whereas GPC and GPD are normally expressed.

Southern blot hybridization clearly established that both the GPA and GPB genes were absent in the DNA from one of the original homozygous Mk donors (R.S.) (Tate et al. 1989; Vignal et al. 1990b), thus indicating that *Mk* is a silent gene complex caused by a very large deletion of the *MN* and *Ss* loci that produces neither GPA nor GPB proteins.

Hybrid Glycoproteins. It is well known from the study of hemoglobin and haptoglobin gene families (Bunn and Forget 1986; Maeda and Smithies 1986) that homologous DNA sequences of adjacent genes may recombine by unequal crossing-over following misalignment of the homologous chromosomes during meiosis. For instance, the unequal crossing-over between the δ and β globin genes results in the production of a first chromosome lacking the normal δ and β genes but carrying a δ-β fusion product (Lepore hybrid) and of a second chromosome carrying the normal δ and β genes and a β-δ gene fusion product (anti-Lepore hybrid). The δ-β fusion product encodes a globin variant made of the N-terminus of the δ chain linked to the C-terminus of the β chain, whereas the β-δ gene product encodes a reciprocal protein made of the N-terminus of the β chain linked to the C-terminus of the δ chain.

Segregation analysis has established that the MN and Ss antigens carried by GPA and GPB proteins, respectively, are defined as the products of two closely linked (adjacent) genes on chromosome 4 (Race and Sanger 1975; Issitt 1985). Moreover, amino acid sequencing of GPA and GPB proteins as well as nucleic acid analysis of the glycophorin A and B genes themselves have conclusively demonstrated that these genes are highly homologous and were derived from each other by duplication of an ancestral gene (see above). This suggests, therefore, that unequal crossing-over may also occur between the GPA (A) and GPB (B) genes to produce Lepore (A-B) as well as anti-Lepore (B-A) hybrid gene fusion products. Indeed, both types of hybrids have been observed and characterized at the protein and DNA level. Some properties of selected hybrids are summarized in Table 6.2, and a schematic representation of their gene structure is shown in Figure 6.4.

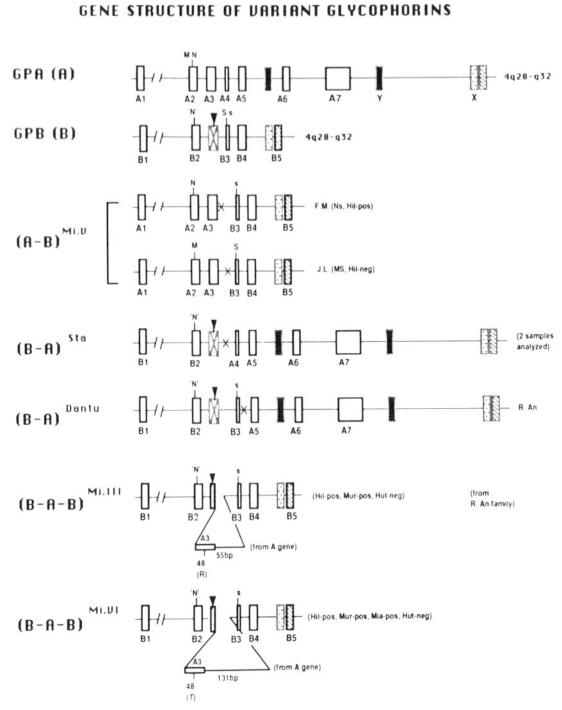

Figure 6.4. Gene structure of variant glycophorins. A schematic representation of the genomic structure from glycophorin variants based on the genomic organization of the GPA (A) and GPB (B) genes (see text). Symbols as in Fig. 6.2. The 3′ region downstream from exon A-7 in the $(B-A)^{Sta}$ and $(B-A)^{Dantu}$ hybrid genes is postulated from the structure of the GPA gene.

A-B Hybrids. The best A-B hybrid glycoproteins of the Lepore type characterized so far are the En(UK) and the Mi.V variants.

The *En(UK)* gene complex was the first reported example of a gene presumably encoding a hybrid red cell glycoprotein (Dahr et al. 1978). As noted above, the English type of En(a−) phenotype arose from the uncommon genotype *En(UK)/Mk;* which produced neither GPA nor GPB proteins. Curiously, however, the *En(UK)* complex produced a small amount of trypsin-resistant ‘M’ antigen (not found on normal cells) carried by a glycoprotein possessing a serine residue at its N-terminus and migrating as GPB on SDS gels. It was postulated that this unusual glycoprotein is a hybrid polypeptide chain having at least the N-terminal serine of a M-specific GPA and the C-terminal part of a S-specific GPB (Dahr et al. 1978). Additional studies with murine monoclonal antibodies against human glycophorins have confirmed this prediction (Bigbee et al. 1984).

More recently, genomic studies with glycophorin cDNA probes confirmed that the En(UK) complex is a hybrid gene comprising the 5′ region of the GPA gene linked to the 3′ region of the GPB gene (Rahuel et al. 1988b). However, because of the very high homology between exons A-2 and B-2 it was not possible to identify the crossing-over point. Unfortunately, this variant was not available for further analysis by genomic sequencing.

Homozygous Mi.V red cells (F.M. donor, typed as NNss, Hil+) lack GPA and GPB proteins but carry a glycoprotein of approximately 30 kDa (see Table 6.2) migrating at an intermediate position between GPA and GPB on SDS gels (Vengelen-Tyler et al. 1981). The Mi.V gene from this donor is a hybrid gene composed of exons A-1 to A-3 linked to exons B-3 to B-5 (Vignal et al. 1989). The structure of the hybrid protein was deduced from PCR amplification of the A-3/B-3 junction and nucleic acid sequencing. The Mi.V protein (F.M.) is made of 104 residues composed of amino acid residues 1 to 59 of GPA fused to amino acid residues 27 to 72 of GPB (Fig. 6.4). As expected, this hybrid protein carries the N and s antigens determined by the N-terminus of GPA (^{1}Leu/^{5}Glu) and by the C-terminus of GPB (^{61}Thr, equivalent to ^{29}Thr on normal GPB).

Another Mi.V-like sample (J.L. donor, typed as MNSs, Hil−), noted Mi.V*, was analyzed both at the protein and genomic levels (Johe et al. 1989; Kudo et al. 1990). The glycoprotein pattern after SDS-PAGE was similar to other Mi.V variants (Lu et al. 1987b) but Mi.V* red cells do not present the blood group Hil reactivity of this class of Miltenberger variants (Giles 1982). The amino acid sequence of the Mi.V* protein was similar to the F.M. protein, except for the polymorphisms at positions 1 and 5 (Ser/Gly) and 61 (Met), responsible for the blood groups M and S, respectively (Johe et al. 1989). Genomic analysis confirmed these findings and revealed that Mi.V* is encoded by a hybrid gene fusion product composed of exons A-1 to A-3 from the GPA gene and B-3 to B-5 of GPB gene, as was shown for Mi.V (F.M.). Further investigations have shown that both Mi.V variants originate from an unequal crossing-over occurring in the homologous intron separating exons A-3/A-4 and B-2/B-3 of the original genes (see Fig. 6.4). The breakpoints, however, were different, as determined by PCR amplification and sequence analysis (Kudo et al. 1990; Vignal et al., unpublished data). In Mi.V* the putative crossing-over sequence (5′-CTTTA-3′) is located around the 3′ end of intron 3 of the GPA gene, while in Mi.V (F.M.) it takes place close to the 5′ end. It is noteworthy that in the region of the Mi.V crossing-over a sequence ATTTACA similar to that found in Mi.V* is also present. It was reported by Rearden and associates (1990a) that the crossing-over sequence found in Mi.V* and in the St^{a} variant (see below) is homologous to that found in the haptoglobin-related genes (Maeda and Smithies 1986). Presumably, the homologous recombination through unequal crossing-over in St[a], Mi.V, Mi.V*, and haptoglobin-related genes can be facilitated by the sequence 5′-(C/A)TTTA(A/T/C)A-3′ present in different positions or even in the reverse orientation close to the cross-over point in these genes.

B-A Hybrids. The St[a] (Stones) and Dantu gene complexes produce GPA, GPB (except in some Dantu variants of black origin lacking GPB; see below), and a hybrid protein of approximately 24 kDa that migrates between GPA and GPB on SDS-PAGE gel electrophoresis (Tanner et al. 1980; Anstee et al. 1982; Blanchard et al. 1982; Unger et al. 1987; Contreras et al. 1984). The St[a] and Dantu proteins (PJ and NE samples, respectively) were the first anti-Lepore type hybrid red cell membrane glycoproteins to be fully sequenced (Blanchard et al. 1987a; Dahr et al. 1987). Both proteins contain 99 amino acid residues but they differ by several characteristics: (1) the St[a] protein contains residues 1 to 26 of GPB and 59 to 131 of GPA, whereas Dantu protein is composed of residues 1 to 39 of GPB and 71 to 131 of GPA; (2) the St[a] antigen is located within residues 25 to 30 (T N G E R V Q), whereas the Dantu antigen is located within residues 28 to 40 (E T G Q L V H R F Y V P E I), presumably at the junctions between the GPB and GPA protein sequences; and (3) the Dantu protein exhibits a blood group s reactivity whereas the St[a] protein exhibits neither S nor s reactivity.

Analysis of St[a] (Japanese family O.S.) and Dantu (black family R.An.) genomes by Southern blot hybridization confirms that both contain a B-A hybrid gene composed of six exons that differ in their structure (see Fig. 6.4). The St[a] gene comprises exons B-1 to B-2 linked to exons A-4 to A-7, whereas the Dantu gene includes exons B-1 to B-3 linked to exons A-5 to A-7 (Huang and Blumenfeld 1988; Huang et al. 1989a; Rearden et al. 1990a).

The crossing-over point of the St[a] hybrid gene obtained by PCR amplification on genomic DNA was proposed to be located 220 bp upstream of the first nucleotide of exon A-4 within the 5′-TTAAAAGT-3′ sequence, which was shown to be homologous in the reverse orientation to that found in haptoglobin-related hybrid genes (Maeda and Smithies 1986). This sequence is related to the consensus 5′-(C/T)TTTA(A/T/C)A-3′ already mentioned in the crossing-over required for generating MiV, MiV*, and haptoglobin-related genes. The crossing-over point of the Dantu hybrid gene (R. An.) is located within the homologous intronic regions separating exons B-3/B-4 and A-4/A-5 (see Fig. 6.4), but its exact position has not been determined. The Dantu chromosome R.An. is peculiar since it contains a duplication of the hybrid gene and a deletion of the GPB gene. The origin of such a haplotype would require two unequal homologous crossing-overs giving rise to the duplication of the Dantu gene *cis* to the GPB gene deletion (Huang and Blumenfeld,

1988). Whether a similar duplication occurs in other Dantu samples is unknown.

A comparison of junction sequence in the St^a and Mi.V glycoproteins indicates an exact reciprocal arrangement (see above), strongly suggesting that a reciprocal recombination event gave rise to these hybrid proteins (Tate and Tanner 1988). Genomic studies have confirmed this presumption by showing that the unequal crossing-over occurs in intron 3 of the GPA gene, which does not contain Alu repeats, as diagramatically depicted in Figure 6.4. The putative cross-over points in this intron, however, were not identical in each instance (Rearden et al. 1990a; Kudo et al. 1990).

Other examples of Dantu and St^a chromosomes giving rise to different proteins have been reported but were not investigated at the DNA level. Among the Dantu variants, some that do not produce GPB (Tanner et al. 1980; Dahr and Moulds 1987) occur in blacks (Ph, NE donors), whereas the first reported case of Dantu in a Caucasian donor (MD) produces GPA, GPB, and the Dantu hybrid protein (Dahr et al. 1989b). As the GPA level was low in Dantu^{NE} red cells, it was postulated that the GPA and the hybrid proteins might compete to bind the band 3 necessary for GPA incorporation in the membrane, thus lowering the number of GPA molecules that can be detected in these variants (Unger et al. 1987; Dahr et al. 1989a). A second variety of St^a gene (M^Z complex) that differs from common St^a (M^r complex) by producing weak M and N antigens has been purified and partially sequenced (Dahr et al. 1990). Although the M^r protein is a hybrid molecule, as described above, the M^z molecule (E.Z. donor) seems likely to be a variant of GPA lacking residues 27 to 58 encoded by exon A-3.

B-A-B Hybrids. Previous investigations of Mi.III, Mi.IV, and Mi.VI erythrocytes, which are common among Orientals, suggested that these cells carry an abnormal form of GPB that migrates on SDS-PAGE with an apparent size of approximately 28 kDa (for review see Anstee 1980). It has been postulated that these gene complexes are generated by insertion of a fragment of the GPA gene into the GPB gene (Laird-Fryer et al. 1986). Genomic DNAs from individuals exhibiting Mi.III and Mi.VI phenotypes were recently investigated by Southern blot hybridization and nucleotide sequencing after allele-specific PCR amplification between exons 2 and 4 of each gene (Huang and Blumenfeld 1991). The Mi.III and Mi.VI genes were found to be identical to the GPB gene except that in both an internal segment of GPB (pseudoexon region) has been replaced by its exonic counterpart of the GPA gene, thus resulting in very peculiar B-A-B hybrid gene structures (see Fig. 6.4). This replacement creates a composite exon flanked by functional 3′ and 5′ splicing sites derived from the GPB intron 2 (pseudoexon region) and the portion of

A-3 exon and intron 3 of the GPA gene that is inserted, respectively. This composite sequence in the Mi.III protein has been confirmed by peptide sequencing (Huang and Blumenfeld 1991), and these findings correlate well with previous hybrid gene structure predictions (Laird-Fryer et al. 1986) and with immunochemical analysis carried out with Mi.III, Mi.IV, and Mi.VI (King et al. 1989). Nucleotide sequencing also predicts that Mi.III and Mi.VI proteins differ from each other by one amino acid residue at position 48 (Arg/Thr) due to a single nucleotide G/C exchange. Moreover, the Mi.III and Mi.VI genes differ further in the location of upstream (B-A) and downstream (A-B) breakpoints and the length of GPA sequence replaced (55 to 131 bp, respectively). The B-A rearranged region of the two genes contains a sequence of 35 bp rich in A and T residues and multiple inverted repeats, which might serve as a recombinational hot spot. This sequence contains the CTTTAAA, motif previously mentioned for recombination in Mi.V, Mi.V*, and haptoglobin genes. It is suggested that gene conversion rather than double crossing-over might account for the origin of both variants (Huang and Blumenfeld 1991).

These results identified a new class of hybrid glycophorin genes in which unexpressed intronic sequences can be used to generate composite exons presumably responsible for antigenic diversity. Further investigation should reveal whether other Miltenberger variants that share antigenic epitopes with Mi.III and Mi.VI are also formed by microconversion events.

REARRANGEMENTS OF GLYCOPHORIN GENES IN VARIANTS

Current models of evolution (see Fig. 6.3) and of the structure of gene fusions generated by unequal crossing-over (see Fig. 6.4) suggest that the GPA and GPB genes are adjacent in this order, in the direction of transcription on chromosome 4. The position of the GPE gene, discovered more recently, was deduced from the rearrangements of the glycophorin genes occurring in GPA and GPB deletion variants, which all contain a copy of the GPE gene (Vignal et al. 1990a, 1990b). Surprisingly, the absence of a given protein(s) could be correlated with the absence of the corresponding gene, but careful nucleotide analysis of exons 1 and their 5′ flanking sequences revealed that only the bulk of the gene was missing (Fig. 6.5). For instance, in the Finnish type of En(a−) variant, exons A-2 to A-7 were absent but exon A-1 and its 5′ flanking region were still present. Similarly, in the S−s−U− genome, exons B-2 to B-5 were missing but exon B-1 and upstream sequences were still present. In the homozygous Mk variant, the large deletion (> 100 kb) could be accounted for by the lack of the entire GPB gene (exons B-1 to B-5) and of exons A-2 to A-7 of the GPA gene, but exon A-1 was still present (see Fig. 6.5). Moreover, exon E-1 of the GPE gene was also missing, suggesting that exon A-1 was presumably linked to exons E-2 to E-4 of the GPE gene.

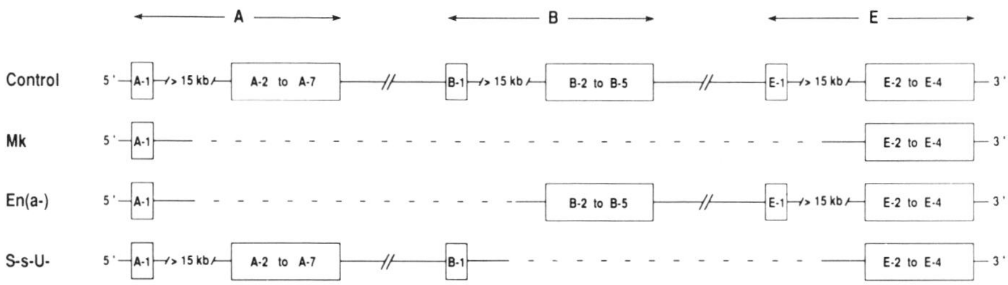

Figure 6.5. Rearrangement of the glycophorin genes in deletion variants. The postulated deletions occurring in the En(a−), S−s−U−, and Mk variants are indicated in dotted lines. For each gene, exon 1 is represented separately, as it is located at least 15 kb upstream from the bulk of the gene. The distance separating each gene is unknown (vertical bars). (*Source:* From Vignal et al. 1990.)

From these findings a model of gene rearrangements occurring in the deletion variants has been proposed. Accordingly, all variants appear as hybrid gene structure (Lepore type) resulting from unequal crossing-over within the large first intron of the three genes. At the protein level, these hybrid structures are undetectable, since the exon 1 of each gene encodes a similar amino acid segment of the signal peptide, which is removed from the mature protein. SDS-PAGE studies of red cell membranes from the deletion variants do not indicate any significant alteration of the level of membrane glycophorins other than the affected one(s) (for reviews see Anstee 1980, 1981; Dahr 1986). This suggests first that regulatory sequences for accurate transcription and translation are preserved in the hybrid structures shown in Figure 6.5, and second that the bulk of the GPB gene under the control of exon A-1 and upstream sequences (GPA promoter) is transcribed and/or translated at the same level as it is under the control of its own promoter. Since the GPA protein level is much higher than the GPB level on normal red cells (see Table 6.1), and since the GPE protein is probably expressed at a low yield in erythrocyte membranes, it may be postulated that the rearrangements occurring in En(a−), S−s−U−, and Mk variants remove regulatory sequences necessary for efficient transcription of GPA and GPB genes. It may also be possible that the absence of regulation takes place at the translation level, but the demonstration of this assumption requires the availability of mRNA samples from these individuals.

Obviously, unequal crossing-over between homologous regions of the glycophorin genes is a basic mechanism that explains the generation of hybrid as well as deletion variants. Different homologous regions are used that are located either in introns 1 for the deletion variants (see Fig. 6.5) or in introns 3 and 4 of GPA gene and their homologous positions in the GPB gene for the other hybrid variants investigated so far (see Fig. 6.4). Moreover, microconversion events also occur, as found in Mi.III and Mi.VI variants, therefore still increasing the high degree of the glycophorin genes and gene products. These variations might even be more important than presently recognized since only rearrangements associated with a functional abnormality or with new antigenic properties would be easily detected.

Although the glycophorin gene cluster contains several Alu elements, which are presumably involved in evolution (see Figs. 6.2 and 6.3), so far these sequences have not been used to generate the gene diversity that naturally occurs in the glycophorin variants described above, in contrast to what is observed for genes such as the low-density lipoprotein receptor (Lehrman et al. 1987), the adenosine deaminase (Markert et al. 1988), the human growth hormone (Vnencak-Jones et al. 1988), and the human complement C1 inhibitor (Stoppa-Lyonnet et al. 1990). Obviously, other sequences having a greater length of homology might preferentially participate in the recombinational events as suggested by the rather homologous sequences found in the Mi.V, Mi.III/Mi.VI, and Dantu variants (see above).

It has also been reported that the glycophorin gene cluster is relatively more prone to mutation by radiation, as a high incidence of somatic mutations was detected in atomic bomb survivors (Langlois et al. 1987; Kyoizumi et al. 1989a). Similarly, this mutation rate is increased in patients with Bloom's syndrome (Kyoizumi et al. 1989b), suggesting that propensity to the development of malignancies results from increased frequency of spontaneous mutations and somatic recombinations. A better characterization of the glycophorin gene cluster in these pathological situations might help us understand the mechanisms of the somatic mutations.

EXPRESSION AND TISSUE SPECIFICITY OF GLYCOPHORINS A, B, AND E

The expression of glycophorin genes has been explored by direct analysis of membrane proteins by SDS-PAGE and by cell surface analysis with immunofluorescent probes. With the availability of cDNA probes, the mRNA level of a variety of cell lines and tissues has also been explored. More recently, the structural and functional analysis of glycophorin gene transcription was documented.

Cell Expression of GPA and GPB. During normal erythroid development, GPA is expressed rather late on morphologically recognizable precursors but is not detectable on the progenitors BFU-E (burst forming unit–erythroid) or CFU-E (colony forming unit–erythroid) as deduced from indirect immunofluorescence and biochemical analysis (Gahmberg et al. 1978; Robinson et al. 1981; Fukuda and Fukuda 1984; Fukuda 1985). Glycoprotein A (the most extensively studied) was also found to be restricted to the erythroid cell lineage in the hematopoietic tissue. Both GPA and GPB reached the maximum expression at the basophilic normoblast stage and remained at a constant amount per cell through further maturation (Loken et al. 1987), in contrast to previous findings suggesting an increased O-glycosylation and the late development of MN antigens with erythroid differentiation (for review see Gahmberg et al. 1988).

Because of its erythroid specificity, GPA was used as a specific marker to characterize and identify malignant hematopoietic cells expressing antigenic markers of erythroid differentiation (Greaves et al. 1983; Villeval et al. 1986). Glycophorin expression in various cell types was also studied by Northern blot analysis, and the results confirmed that GPA and GPB were restricted to erythroid cell lineage (Villeval et al. 1989; Le Van Kim et al. 1989).

A few reports based on indirect studies suggest that molecules immunologically related to glycophorins might be present on nonerythroid tissues. This has been clearly established for GPC by Northern blot analysis, PCR amplification of mRNA, and cell surface characterization (see below), but still remains indirect evidence for GPA and GPB expression (Le Van Kim et al. 1989). For instance, glycophorin-like molecules have been detected at the surface of rat thymocytes (Brown et al. 1981) and more recently in human kidney endothelium (Harvey et al. 1988) and at the surface of bovine and rat cultured endothelial cells (Schnitzer et al. 1990). Although there is no GPA-specific mRNA in human kidney extracts (Cartron, unpublished data), it is possible that Northern blot analysis is not sensitive enough to detect such a message if present at a low concentration. Since glycophorins are heavily glycosylated molecules that carry oligosaccharide chains shared by other membrane proteins (like the sialylated O-glycans), any possible cross-reaction has to be ruled out before any definitive conclusion can be made. All these findings, however, clearly need further investigations to characterize the putative glycophorin homologues of these tissues and to understand their function, if any.

Transcription of Glycophorin Genes. Four mRNA species of 2.8, 1.7, 1.0, and 0.6 kb were detected in K562 cells and human fetal liver and spleen erythroblasts with a full-length cDNA probe. The 2.8, 1.7, and 1.0 species originate from the GPA gene, whereas the 0.6 kb derived from the GPB gene (Siebert and Fukuda; 1986a, 1987; Tate and Tanner 1988; Rahuel et al. 1989). Nucleotide sequencing of several human fetal liver cDNA clones and transcription start point (cap site) determination by primer extension analysis conclusively demonstrated that the production of the multiple GPA mRNAs is governed by poly(A) site choice generating 3′ regions of different length but not by 5′ region heterogeneity since all GPA mRNAs exhibit the same cap site located 56 nucleotides upstream of the A of the initiating methionine codon (Rahuel et al. 1989;

Hamid et al. 1990). As the 1.7-kb species is always predominant over the 1.0- and 2.8-kb species, the three mRNAs may not be processed with the same efficiency. In addition, the 3′ UT regions may have some role in the three mRNAs' stability (see Bernstein and Ross 1988). More recent studies have indicated that GPB and GPE mRNAs exhibit the same cap site as GPA (Vignal et al. 1990a).

The GPA, GPB, and GPE messages were remarkably decreased in the RNA preparations from phorbol esters (TPA)–treated K562 cells, indicating that the transcription of these genes is coordinately down-regulated by TPA treatment (Siebert and Fukuda 1986b; Kudo and Fukuda 1990). This correlates well with the similarity of the promoter regions presently characterized.

Promoters of GPA, GPB and GPE. There is a significant difference in the cell surface expression of GPA, GPB, and GPE. The factor(s) that control the quantitative level of these protein is unknown, but may involve regulatory sequences in the promoter region of the genes. The 5′ flanking regions (about 300 bp) of the three glycophorin genes that exhibit a promoter activity are > 98 percent homologous and differ only by a few point mutations (Vignal et al. 1990a). The structure is rather simple and lacks TATA and CAAT consensus sequences often found in eukaryotic genes (Breathnach and Chambon 1981). Like other erythroid genes they contain a CACCC box and several GATA-1 motifs (synonyms NF-E1, GF-1, Eryf-1) that are important for accurate erythroid transcription (see Yamamoto et al. 1990 and a review by Orkin 1990). The importance of zinc-finger transcription factor GATA-1 was highlighted by the recent demonstration that in chimeric mice, cells carrying a null mutation in the GATA-1 gene lacked erythroid development (Pevny et al. 1991). The promoter elements characterized thus far in the glycophorin genes are consistent with the findings that glycophorin mRNAs are found only in cells or tissues of erythroid lineage. As none of the point mutations identified in these promoters affect any of the potential regulatory elements (CACC or GATA-1 motifs), such differences should not account significantly for the differential transcription levels observed between the three genes. Nevertheless, it is possible that unknown enhancers or silencers might be present in other regions of the three genes that have a critical role in regulating transcription levels, as was shown for the globin genes (reviewed by Evans et al. 1990).

GLYCOPHORINS C AND D AND THE BLOOD GROUP GERBICH LOCUS

Glycophorins C and D are quantitatively minor sialoglycoproteins of the red cell membrane contributing 4 and 1 percent to the PAS-positive material, and their apparent molecular mass estimated by SDS-PAGE is

32,000 and 23,000, respectively. Recent evidence indicates that these glycoproteins carry the blood group Gerbich antigens and are involved in the mechanical properties of the erythrocyte membrane.

GERBICH ANTIGENS AND GLYCOPHORINS C AND D

The Nomenclature of Gerbich Antigens. The Gerbich antigens (Ge) were discovered by Rosenfield and associates in 1960 and found present on the majority of human red cells (> 99%) except those from some ethnic groups within the Melanesian population. Three high-incidence antigens, Ge:1, 2, and 3, serologically defined by three human antisera were first described and shown to identify four phenotypes (Booth and McLoughlin 1972) that include the normal Ge-positive type designated Ge:1,2,3 and three rare variant types lacking one or several of these antigens, which are respectively known as the Melanesian type (Ge: −1,2,3), the Yussef (Yus) type (Ge: −1, −2,3), and the Gerbich (Ge) type (Ge: −1, −2, −3). However, since anti-Ge:1 (made by Melanesians Ge: −1,2,3) antisera and Melanesian red cells are generally not available, the Ge:1 terminology is often omitted.

Recently, a new category of Ge-negative red cells lacking GPC and GPD and exhibiting a marked degree of elliptocytosis but clinically no significant hemolysis has been described. This new phenotype, called "Leach," can be distinguished from the other Ge-negative variants (Ge: −2, −3), since it is not reactive with Ge-related murine monoclonal antibodies that bind to GPC on immunoblots (Anstee et al. 1984a, 1984b). More recently, a human antibody with a similar specificity was found in the serum from another Leach donor (McShane and Chung 1989) and proposed to define the Ge:4 antigen that is common to all red cells (including the Yus- and Ge-types) except those from the Leach individuals (Table 6.3). Presumably, the antibody developed by a nontransfused patient who develops anemia following gold therapy for rheumatoid arthritis has a similar specificity (Beattie and Sigmund 1987; Daniels et al. 1988). Presently, except for the original Leach phenotypes described (P.L. and K.W.), only three families (Cud., MWB, and LN) in which this phenotype is inherited have been published. All Leach individuals have elliptocytic red cells that are deficient in GPC and GPD (Daniels et al. 1986; Rountree et al. 1989; McShane and Chung 1989).

The high incidence of Ge-negative phenotypes in Melanesians was thought to be related to the high prevalence of malaria on the northeast coast of New Guinea, suggesting that this phenotype may confer a selective advantage against the disease (Dahr et al. 1985). This is in good correlation with the reduced invasion of Leach erythrocytes by *Plasmodium falciparum* parasites, although Ge: −2,3 and Ge: −2, −3 red cells are normally invaded (Pasvol et al. 1984). Red cells from Melanesians with hereditary ovalocytosis also are resistant to invasion by *P. falciparum* parasites, but this is not related to the Gerbich status of the red cells

Table 6.3. Genetic Conditions Associated with Membrane Defects of GPC, GPD, and Ge Blood Group Antigens

Genetic Condition	Red Cell Morphology	Sialoglycoproteins			Protein Band 4.1	Gerbich Antigens	Frequency
		GPA and B	*GPC and D*	*Abnormal Component**			
Gerbich Deficiency: Leach	Elliptocytosis (20–50%)	Present	Absent	No	Present	Ge: −2, −3, −4	Very rare
Gerbich Deficiency: Ge-Type	Normal	Present	Absent	Yes	Present	Ge: −2, −3, +4	Rare
Gerbich Deficiency: Yus-Type	Normal	Present	Absent	Yes	Present	Ge: −2, +3, +4	Rare
4.1 Deficiency	Elliptocytosis (100%)	Present	Decreased (by 70%)	No	Absent	Decreased	Very rare

*Glycoproteins of electrophoretic mobility intermediate between those of GPC and GPD. Identified as truncated GPC proteins (see text).

(Kidson et al. 1981). Rather, recent evidence suggests that ovalocytic red cells carry a structurally and functionally abnormal band 3 protein that contains an eight–amino acid deletion presumably responsible for the increased binding of band 3 to the membrane skeleton (Liu et al. 1990; Jones et al. 1991; Jarolim et al. 1991). This molecular lesion might explain the increased rigidity of ovalocytes and their resistance to invasion by malaria parasites.

GPC and GPD Are the Carriers of Gerbich Antigens. The discovery of the Leach phenotype strongly suggested that the Ge antigens were carried by GPC and/or GPD. Moreover, the Ge:2 and Ge:3 determinants were found to be neuraminidase-sensitive and located on trypsin-sensitive structures, indicating that these antigens could be carried by red cell membrane sialoglycoproteins (Dahr et al. 1985). This was further confirmed by immunoblotting analysis with human antisera showing that the Ge:3 antigen is present on both GPC and GPD, whereas Ge:2 is present only on GPD (Dahr et al. 1987; Reid et al. 1987a). The Ge:2 epitope is sialic acid–dependent and is located on the N-terminal tryptic glycopeptide from GPD comprising 20 to 30 amino acids. On GPC, the Ge:3 epitope is located in proximity to a tryptic cleavage site at position 48, within residues 40 to 55, and probably includes the O-glycosylated chain attached on Ser^{42} (Dahr et al. 1987). The location of the Ge:1 and Ge:4 epitopes is still unknown.

The Ge-type (Ge: −2, −3) and Yus-type (Ge: −2,3) of Ge-deficient red cells also lack GPC and GPD, but SDS-PAGE analysis revealed that these cells carry instead different glycoprotein components migrating as diffuse bands of 24 to 26 and 25 to 28 kDa, respectively, which are not present in Leach erythrocytes (Anstee et al. 1984b; Dahr et al. 1985). The diffuse migration pattern was related to the presence of N-linked oligosaccharide chains containing repeating units of N-acetyllactosamine that are endo-β-galactosidase-sensitive (Reid et al. 1987a). Further investigations demonstrated that polyclonal antibodies raised against purified GPC or GPD react with antigenic determinants common to the C-terminal domain of both glycoproteins as well as with epitopes present on the abnormal glycoproteins of the Ge-type and Yus-type of erythrocytes, suggesting that all these glycoproteins are immunologically related (Reid et al. 1987a; El-Maliki et al. 1989). It was postulated that the abnormal glycoproteins of Ge: −2, −3 and Ge: −2,3 cells are the result of an unequal crossing-over between the genes encoding GPC and GPD (Anstee et al. 1984b; Dahr et al. 1985), but this assumption was not correct since later studies have demonstrated that GPC and GPD are encoded by a single gene (see below). Remarkably, Ge-negative erythrocytes (except Ge: −2,3) exhibit a reduced expression of Kell antigens, particularly of K:11(Coté), but the molecular basis of this phenotypic association is not known (Race and Sanger 1975; Anstee et al. 1984b), although the region encoding the Ge:3 antigens might be critical for such postulated protein-protein interaction.

STRUCTURAL CHARACTERIZATION OF GPC AND GPD

Primary Sequence of GPC. The complete amino acid sequence of GPC was deduced by cloning the cDNA from a human reticulocyte library (Colin et al. 1986) using partial protein sequence information (Furthmayr 1978b; Dahr et al. 1982; Blanchard et al. 1987b). Glycophorin C is a single polypeptide chain of 128 residues (Fig. 6.6), synthesized without a signal peptide, and has a calculated M_r of 14,000, indicating that the mature glycoprotein of apparent M_r 32,000 on SDS gels contains approximately 50 percent sugars (Colin et al. 1986; High and Tanner 1987).

```
GPC                          ●
Met Trp Ser Thr Arg Ser Pro Asn Ser Thr Ala Trp Pro Leu Ser    15
ATG TGG TCG ACG AGA AGC CCC AAC AGC ACG GCG TGG CCT CTC AGC    45
                            GPD
Leu Glu Pro Asp Pro Gly Met Ala Ser Ala Ser Thr Thr Met His    30
CTC GAG CCT GAT CCG GGG ATG GCC TCT GCC TCC ACC ACA ATG CAT    90
   i1
Thr Thr Thr Ile Ala Glu Pro Asp Pro Gly Met Ser Gly Trp Pro    45
ACT ACC ACC ATT GCA GAG CCT GAT CCA GGG ATG TCT GGA TGG CCG   136
                    i2                                 △
Asp Gly Arg Met Glu Thr Ser Thr Pro Thr Ile Met Asp Ile Val    60
GAT GGC AGA ATG GAG ACC TCC ACC CCC ACC ATA ATG GAC ATT GTC   180

Val Ile Ala Gly Val Ile Ala Ala Val Ala Ile Val Leu Val Ser    75
GTC ATT GCA GGT GTG ATT GCT GCT GTG GCC ATC GTC CTA GTC TCC   225
            i3
Leu Leu Phe Val Met Leu Arg Tyr Met Tyr Arg His Lys Gly Thr    90
CTC CTC TTC GTC ATG CTG CGC TAC ATG TAC CGG CAC AAG GGC ACG   270

Tyr His Thr Asn Glu Ala Lys Gly Thr Glu Phe Ala Glu Ser Ala   105
TAC CAC ACC AAT GAG GCC AAG GGC ACG GAG TTT GCT GAG AGT GCA   315

Asp Ala Ala Leu Gln Gly Asp Pro Ala Leu Gln Asp Ala Gly Asp   120
GAT GCA GCC CTG CAG GGA GAC CCT GCC CTC CAA GAT GCT GGT GAT   360
                      G
Ser Ser Arg Lys Glu Tyr Phe Ile                               128
AGC AGC AGA AAG GAG TAC TTT ATT                               384
```

Figure 6.6. Nucleotide sequence and deduced protein structure of GPC. Glycophorin C is a single-chain polypeptide of 128 amino acids containing one N-glycan chain attached to [8]Asn (black circle). Sequences boxed refer to the hydrophobic protein domain that spans the phospholipid bilayer, and i_1, i_2, and i_3 to intronic sequences interrupting the GPC gene. The broken arrow GPD indicates the N-terminal origin of GPD that is presumably generated by leaky translation of the GPC mRNA at [22]Met (see text). The open triangle indicates the nucleotide deletion (position 134) occurring in a Leach variant (LN) that lacks cell-surface expression of GPC and GPD (McShane and Chung 1989). This single point mutation results in a premature stop codon TAA at position 167 to 169 (underlined by a double bar) and to a truncated protein that is most likely secreted and degraded (Telen et al. 1991).

Glycophorin C shares no structural homology with GPA and GPB. Typically for integral membrane proteins, it is organized in three distinct domains. The extracellular NH_2 terminal domain comprises 57 amino acids and includes a single N-glycosylation site on ^{8}Asn, several potential O-glycosylation sites on Ser and Thr residues (approximately 12 chains), as well as the Ge:3 determinant located around residue 48. This region is followed by a stretch of 24 nonpolar amino acids (residues 58 to 81) corresponding to the intramembranous domain spanning the phospholipid bilayer and by the third protein domain (residues 82 to 128), which is intracytoplasmic and contains the COOH-terminal end of the molecule (see Fig. 6.6).

Murine monoclonal antibodies directed against Ge-related antigens have been useful to characterize Ge-deficient red cells as well as to distinguish GPC, GPD, and their variants. The epitopes recognized by these antibodies that react with GPC but not with GPD have been characterized (Dahr et al. 1989a). They were all specific for the NH_2-terminal region of GPC (residues 1 to 22) not found in GPD, and all except one (APO-3) require sialic acids for binding (Fig. 6.7).

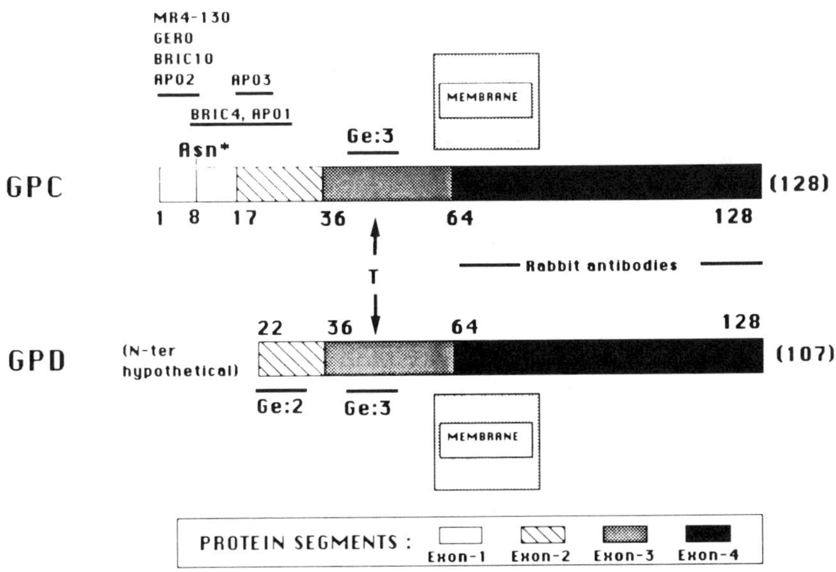

Figure 6.7. Protein structure of human glycophorins C and D. General organization of the GPC and GPD proteins (128 and presumably 107 residues, respectively) showing the protein segments encoded by the four exons of the GPC gene. Numbers denote amino acid residues and T a trypsin cleavage site on intact red cells. The map of epitopes recognized by murine monoclonal antibodies anti-GPC and by polyclonal human (Ge:2, Ge:3) and rabbit antibodies is indicated by horizontal bars.

Primary Sequence of GPD. Several lines of evidence suggest that GPD is a truncated form of GPC: (1) the C-terminal domain of GPD is immunologically related to GPC (see above and Fig. 6.7); (2) partial protein sequencing indicates that GPD is identical to residues 22 to 128 of GPC (El-Maliki et al. 1989); (3) murine monoclonal antibodies reacting with the N-terminal region of GPC (see above) do not recognize GPD, either by agglutination or by immunoblotting or immunoprecipitation (Dahr et al. 1989a); (4) the apparent molecular weight of GPD is 23 kDa, approximately 9kDa less than GPC; (5) GPD does not bind the *Lens culinaris* lectin that reacts with the N-glycan chain present on GPC (Le Van Kim et al. 1987); and (6) GPC and GPD are encoded by the same gene (see below).

These findings indicate that GPC and GPD have an identical carboxy terminal sequence but differ in the N-terminal region. It is assumed that GPD lacks the first 21 amino acids of GPC, but the complete protein sequence of this glycoprotein has not yet been determined, presumably because the N-terminus is blocked (El-Maliki et al. 1989). Currently, the most likely explanations to account for this hypothesis are either a post-translational processing of GPC, alternative initiation of the mRNA at the AUGs at positions 1 and 22, or both. Indeed, examination of the GPC cDNA sequence indicates that the nucleotides surrounding the ATG codon for ^{1}Met (5′-CA GGA *ATG* T-3′) does not fit properly with the consensus translation initiation sequence (5′-CCA GCC *ATG* G-3′) found in viral and eukaryotic mRNAs (Kozak 1984). However, the ATG codon for ^{22}Met is present in the optimal context for binding of ribosomes, with a purine at position −3 from the initiator ATG and a guanine at position +4 (see Fig. 6.6). Since both AUGs are in the same reading frame, GPC and GPD might be produced by the alternative use of these translation initiation sites from a unique mRNA, according to the leaky scanning mechanism permitting the ribosome to initiate either at the first or at the second internal AUG, as described for some viral mRNAs (Kozak 1986, 1989). The use of the second AUG would result in the translation of a polypeptide chain of 107 amino acid residues having the expected size for GPD, assuming the presence of only six O-glycosidically linked tetrasaccharide chains. Such a mechanism has been described for the invariant chain associated with the human HLA-DR antigens (Strubin et al. 1986) and more recently for the rat *Pit*-1 transcription factor (Voss et al. 1991).

Preliminary experiments with recombinant expression vectors carrying either the intact GPC cDNA or variants mutated on codons for ^{1}Met and ^{22}Met support the reinitiation of translation mechanism (Le Van Kim et al., unpublished data).

THE PUTATIVE FUNCTION OF GPC AND GPD

That Leach erythrocytes are partly elliptocytic is reminiscent of a previous observation by Müeller and Morrison (1981) indicating that elliptocytic red cells from a child whose clinical and genetic background could not be documented lack protein 4.1 and GPC (see Table 6.3). In addition, it was shown that GPC and GPD were linked to the membrane skeleton, as these glycoproteins remained firmly associated with the skeletal proteins spectrin, ankyrin, actin, and protein 4.1 following extraction of red cell membranes with a nonionic detergent (Müeller and Morrison 1981; Anstee et al. 1984b). All these findings suggested that GPC and GPD may represent, in addition to band 3 and ankyrin (reviewed by Bennett 1990), another membrane attachment site, via protein 4.1, for the erythrocyte skeletal proteins and that presumably these glycoproteins have some functional role maintaining the normal shape and deformability of the red cell (Chasis and Mohandas 1986; Reid et al. 1987b; Chapter 7).

Investigations of patients homozygous and heterozygous for protein 4.1 deficiency confirmed these preliminary observations and demonstrated that the content of GPC and GPD as well as the Ge blood group antigens are reduced by about 70 percent in homozygous patients, whereas the content of GPA and GPB is normal (Alloisio et al. 1985; Sondag et al. 1987). These findings, therefore, suggest that protein 4.1 might be critical for the correct insertion or transport of GPC and GPD to the red cell surface. A confirmation of these conclusions has been provided recently (Reid et al. 1990).

Since the membrane level of GPC in obligate heterozygotes from a Leach family was found normal by flow cytometry analysis with a murine monoclonal anti-GPC antibody (BRIC10), it was suggested that GPC might be synthetized in excess (Reid et al. 1990). However, carbohydrate staining after SDS-PAGE and agglutination studies with another monoclonal antibody (MR4-130) indicated an expected reduction of approximately 40 to 50 percent of GPC and GPD in heterozygotes from other Ge-deficient red cells (Le Van Kim et al. 1987).

The functional importance of GPC and GPD has been deduced from ektacytometry analysis under constant and variable shear stress, respectively, showing that ghosts from Leach erythrocytes have a reduced mechanical stability and membrane deformability, whereas other Ge-deficient red cell ghosts (Ge-type and Yus-type) exhibited normal properties, as GPA- and GPB-deficient membrane did (Reid et al. 1987b). Since Leach erythrocytes apparently have a normal complement of the other skeletal proteins, the morphologic abnormalities are presumably due to the glycoprotein deficiency. However, a careful examination of two unrelated Leach red cell samples carried out recently indicated a quantitative reduction by 10 to 20 percent of the protein 4.1 content, which may account for the elliptocytosis associated with this phenotype (Cartron and Delaunay, unpublished data).

Very recently, the rigidity and microviscosity of individual Leach red cells measured by the micropipette technique were found to be normal, although the cells were mechanically unstable (Nash et al. 1990). These contradictory results were explained by considering that the results from the ektacytometer are influenced by red cell shape rather than membrane properties. In addition, elliptocytes from Leach cells were found to be denser and smaller and to have less surface area than the discocytes from the same donor. It was suggested, therefore, that elliptocytes are formed from red cells initially released into the circulation with a normal shape. The membrane instability resulting from the defective interaction between GPC and protein 4.1 in these cells caused the progressive distortion of shape as red cells are exposed to shear stress and elongation in the circulation (Nash et al. 1990).

Ge-type and Yus-type erythrocytes are deficient in GPC and GPD but are not elliptocytic (see Table 6.3). As discussed below, these cells carry an abnormal glycoprotein component and it is assumed that this new glycoprotein is able, as are GPC and GPD normally, to interact with membrane skeletal proteins, thereby preserving the cells with a normal shape.

STRUCTURAL ORGANIZATION OF THE GERBICH GENE

The GPC gene is organized into four exons distributed over 13.5 kb of DNA (Colin et al. 1989; High et al. 1989); the complete structure has been reviewed recently (Cartron et al. 1990). Briefly, exons 1 and 2 and most of exon 3 encode the extracellular domain of the GPC protein, whereas exon 4 encodes both the hydrophobic membrane spanning domain and the COOH terminal domain of the protein. Remarkably, exons 2 and 3, which are homologous, are carried by two 3.4-kb direct repeats located in tandem that are themselves highly homologous (< 5% divergence). These two domains, which do not include Alu elements, very likely arose from a rather recent duplication of the unique domain of an ancestral gene (Fig. 6.8). Because of these repeats, genomic clones of GPC inserted in lambda phages and propagated in *Escherichia coli* rearranged spontaneously at high frequency by a deletion of 3.4 kb. The same deletion is responsible for the DNA genomic structure of Ge-type and Yus-type variant individuals whose red cells lack GPC and GPD (Colin et al. 1989; High et al. 1989), as shown below.

Several lines of evidence indicate that the same gene encodes GPC and GPD: (1) there is a single copy of the GPC gene by haploid genome and no GPC-related gene potentially encoding the GPD protein (Le Van Kim et al. 1987); (2) Northern blot hybridization demonstrates a single mRNA species of 1.1 kb in erythroid tissues (Colin et al. 1986); and (3) Southern blot analysis of the DNA from Ge:−2,3 and Ge:−2,−3 individuals indicates that these conditions are associated with a constant deletion of 3.4 kb within the GPC gene (Le Van Kim et al. 1987). Since GPC and GPD are the carriers of Gerbich antigens, this unique gene encoding GPC and GPD has been called *Gerbich (Ge),* and the structural locus has been localized on chromosome 2q14-q21 by in situ hybridization

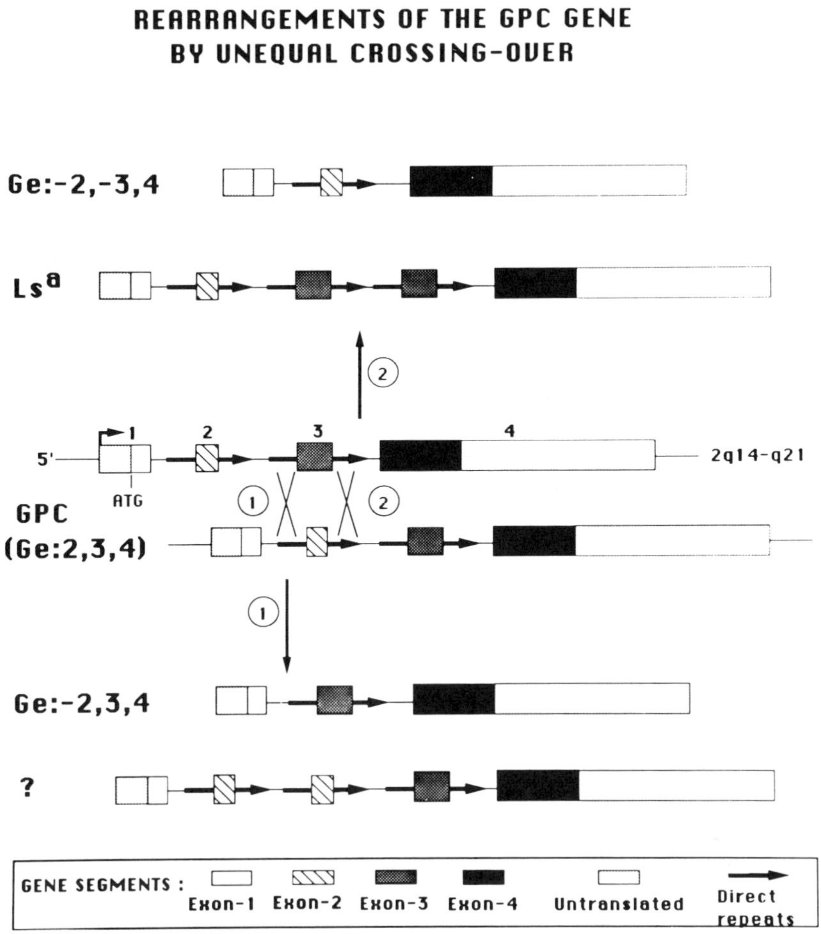

Figure 6.8. Rearrangement of the Gerbich gene in GPC variants. The exon structure (solid boxes) of the Gerbich gene encoding GPC and GPD on chromosome 2q14-q21 is indicated. This gene contains two homologous direct repeats of 3.4 kb (arrows) that encompass exon 2 and 3, respectively. Exon 3 encodes the amino acid sequence that includes the Ge:3 epitope. Unequal crossing-over between these repeats 5′ to exons 2 and 3 (pathway 1) generates two gene fusion products, one lacking exon 2 that encodes the truncated GPC protein with Ge: −2,3,4 specificity (Yus-type variant), and a second characterized by a duplication of exon 2 that may encode a new protein not yet identified (question mark). Unequal crossing-over 3′ of exons 2 and 3 (pathway 2) also generates two gene fusion products, one lacking exon 3 that encodes the truncated GPC protein with Ge: −2, −3,4 specificity (Ge-type variant) and a second characterized by a duplication of exon 3 that encodes the Ls^a variant of GPC protein.

to human metaphasic chromosomes (Le Van Kim et al. 1987; Mattei et al. 1986).

GENE STRUCTURE OF GE VARIANTS

Leach-Type (Ge: −2, −3, −4). The Leach-type of red cells are partially elliptocytic and lack GPC and GPD as well as any GPC- or GPD-related sialoglycoproteins. Four unrelated individuals with this phenotype have recently been analyzed by Southern blot analysis. Three of them (Cud, MWB, and PL) exhibited a 7-kb deletion encompassing exons 3 and 4, whereas exons 1 and 2 were normally present, but it was not clarified whether these deleted genes were transcribed (Tanner et al. 1988, High et al. 1989; Telen et al. 1991a). If so, they would be translated into an abnormal GPC molecule lacking the transmembrane and cytoplasmic domains that could be secreted and/or degraded, thus providing a good explanation for the absence of GPC and GPD on Leach red cells. Preliminary studies, however, indicate that no mRNA could be detected on Northern blots from the MWB Leach variant leukocytes (Colin et al., unpublished data).

A fourth Leach-type individual (LN donor) was shown to be quite different. First, the restriction pattern of the genomic DNA was surprisingly normal and a GPC mRNA of normal size was detected on Northern blots prepared from the donor lymphocytes (Telen et al. 1991a). Polymerase chain reaction amplification and sequencing of LN leukocyte RNAs revealed two alterations within codons 44 to 45: first, a G→T transition changed ^{44}Trp to ^{44}Leu, and second, a deletion of one nucleotide altered the reading frame, resulting in a premature stop codon at the fifty-sixth triplet. The resulting predicted 55 amino acids protein should be devoid of a transmembrane and C-terminal region as compared with GPC and should carry a new short C-terminal end. Presumably this protein is either secreted or degraded and not expressed at the cell surface. These investigations demonstrate that the Leach phenotypes (GPC and GPD "null" erythrocytes) arise by distinct mechanisms, as already found for S−s−U− variants that lack cell-surface expression of GPB.

Yus-Type (Ge: −2,3,4) and Ge-Type (Ge: −2, −3,4). These variants lack GPC and GPD but carry an GPC/D-related glycoprotein of molecular weight intermediate between GPC and GPD (see Table 6.3). In both variants, the genomic DNA is characterized by a deletion of 3.4 kb within the GPC gene (Le Van Kim et al. 1987; Tanner et al. 1988). This deletion eliminates exons 2 and 3 in Ge: −2,3,4 and Ge: −2, −3,4 variants, respectively. Analysis of the deletion breakpoints revealed that distinct unequal crossing-overs between the two homologous repeated domains of the GPC gene are responsible for generating these defective genes, as shown in Fig. 6.8. Recombination between the repeats occurring 5′ of exons 2 and 3 gives rise to one chromosome deleted of exon 3 (Ge: −2,3,4 gene of Yus-type) and to another chromosome carrying a duplication of exon 2, which potentially may encode a new Ge variant (see Fig. 6.8). Recombination between the repeats occurring 3′ of exons 2 and 3 gives rise to one chromosome deleted of exon 3 (Ge: −2, −3,4 of Ge-type) and to another chromosome carrying a duplication of exon 3 (Colin et al. 1989), which has been identified in the genome of individuals carrying the Ls[a] antigen as a DNA insertion of 3.3 kb (High et al. 1989).

The defective gene of Ge: −2,3,4 individuals (Yus-type) is transcribed into a message that links exons 1 and 3 with a conserved reading frame and is translated into a protein of 109 amino acids lacking the 19 amino acids encoded by exon 2 (amino acids 17 to 35). This protein carries the amino acid region 40 to 55 encoded by exon 3 (amino acids 36 to 63), which contains the Ge:3 antigen. Conversely, the defective gene of Ge: −2, −3,4 individuals (Ge-type) is transcribed into a message that links exons 2 and 4 with a conserved reading frame and is translated into a protein of 100 amino acids lacking the 28 amino acids encoded by exon 3 (amino acids 36 to 63). This protein, therefore, lacks amino acids encoding the Ge:3 antigen. These results were recently confirmed by reticulocyte RNA amplification indicating that as compared with the normal GPC mRNA of Ge:2,3,4 individuals, Yus-type variants exhibit a 57-bp deletion corresponding to exon 2, whereas Ge-type variants exhibit an 84-bp deletion corresponding to exon 3 (Chang et al. 1991). Both defective genes have an identical 3′ region that includes exon 4 of the GPC gene (amino acids 64 to 128), which encodes the transmembrane and the C-terminal end of the protein, and therefore the truncated forms of GPC present on these cells are potentially able, like GPC, to interact with the skeletal membrane proteins. This would prevent the cells from becoming elliptocytic in the absence of the normal GPC and GPD counterparts. The truncated forms of the GPC proteins encoded by these abnormal genes have all the properties expected for the unusual glycoproteins characterized by SDS-PAGE on Ge-type and Yus-type erythrocytes. Interestingly, a CPC mRNA isoform produced by alternative splicing of exon 2 that is translated as a truncated protein identical to that which accumulates in Ge: −2,3,4 variants (Yus-type) has been identified in normal tissues (Le Van Kim et al. 1990).

It is expected that Ge: −2, −3,4 red cells should carry also a 79-amino-acid protein that represents a shortened form of the 100-amino-acid protein deleted of its first 21 residues, according to the same mechanism that generates GPD from GPC (leaky translation). Similarly, the chromosome with a duplication of exon 3 (see Fig. 6.8) should encode two Ls[a] proteins of 156 and 135 residues, and the chromosome with a duplication of exon 2 should encode for two new protein variants of 147 and 126 residues. To date, only the Ls[a] proteins have been characterized as GPC and GPD variants of apparent M_r increased by about 6,000 that carry blood group GE determinants (Macdonald et al. 1986, 1990).

Webb Variant. The low-frequency antigen Webb (Wb) is a trypsin-sensitive determinant carried by an abnormal form of GPC having an apparent M_r reduced of about 2,700, presumably caused by the absence of the N-glycan chain attached to Asn[8] (Reid et al. 1985; Macdonald and Gerns 1986). Genomic analysis as well as DNA sequencing after reticulocyte RNA amplification have recently revealed that an A→G mutation at nucleotide 23 changed Asn to Ser at position 8, thus removing the single N-glycosylation site of the GPC protein, which in turn may account for the lower molecular weight of the Wb polypeptide seen by immunochemical analysis (Telen et al. 1991b). No other amino acid changes were detected when the entire coding region was sequenced (Chang et al. 1991). Interestingly, abolition of the N-glycan attached to [26]Asn of GPA is responsible for the Mi.I and Mi.II variants, but this is caused by amino acid substitutions at position 28 (Met/Ser, respectively) that destroy the consensus N-glycosylation sequence Asn-X-Thr (see Table 6.2).

TISSUE SPECIFICITY AND PROMOTER STRUCTURE OF THE GE GENE

Expression and Tissue Specificity of GPC. Northern blot analysis with a GPC cDNA probe and cell-surface labeling experiments with murine monoclonal antibodies that are glycosylation-dependent (MR4-130) and -independent (APO-3) have shown that GPC is expressed at the surface of the majority of peripheral blood cells and cell lines with the exception of granulocytes, platelets, and the Raji (B lymphoid) cell line (Le Van Kim et al. 1989). The level of transcription of the GPC gene as well as the glycosylation of the mature GPC were dependent upon the erythroid or nonerythroid origin of the cells investigated. Cells of erythroid origin (K562, HEL, KU812) expressed higher amounts of GPC on the RNA as well as the protein level as compared with the nonerythroid cells such as Jurkat (T lymphoid), U937 (promonocytic), or MEG01 (megakaryocytic). In addition, GPC was glycosylated differently in erythroid cells than in other cells. Peripheral B lymphocytes and HL60 cells, however, exhibited a significant amount of GPC mRNA but barely detectable amounts of surface protein. Whether the biosynthesis or transport of GPC is altered in these cells, as found for the precursors of certain glycophorins of mouse erythroleukemia cells (Ulmer and Palade 1989), is not known.

In contrast to other glycophorins, GPC was already expressed on erythroid progenitors (BFU-E and CFU-E) during normal and leukemic erythroid differentiation (Villeval et al. 1989) and has been detected in all human tissues examined so far (thymus, stomach, breast, adult liver, and kidney).

Primer extension analysis indicates that the GPC mRNA is initiated at three distinct sites that are differently used in erythroid and nonerythroid cells (Le Van Kim et al. 1989). The use of these multiple initiation sites might be involved in the differential level of expression of the GPC gene in various tissues as reported for several other genes such as *c-myc* (Battey et al. 1983), the IL2 receptor (Leonard et al. 1985), IL-6 (Yasukawa et al. 1987), and band 3 (Kopito et al. 1987), but the mechanisms regulating this phenomenon remain poorly understood.

The presence of GPC in a variety of nonerythroid cells and tissues raises the question of the function of this glycoprotein in these cells. This is presently not known, but there is no reported abnormality of nonerythroid cell functions in rare individuals with the erythrocyte deficiency of GPC and GPD, although such potential defects might not have been explored to date. Tissue analogues of erythrocyte membrane proteins (spectrin, actin, ankyrin, protein 4.1) have been recognized for some time (for reviews see Bennett 1985, 1990), which has led to the speculation that these proteins may play a similar cell function by mediating, for instance, association of integral membrane proteins with the cytoskeletal proteins. Whether GPC might also contribute to a similar function requires further investigation.

Promoter Structure of the GPC Gene. Investigation of the 5′ flanking region of the GPC gene has proved an important step to understanding the mechanisms regulating the multiple usage of transcription initiation sites. Indeed, the general *cis*-acting sequences such as TATA and Sp1 binding sites were found upstream from the three initiation sites, and it has been speculated that they regulate the basal transcription activity of the GPC gene in all cells. In addition, sequences homologous to erythroid specific *cis*-acting elements such as GATA-1 binding sites (for reviews see Orkin 1990; Yamamoto et al. 1990) were identified 5′ of the erythroid cap site, suggesting that the promoter region of GPC contains sequences that could bind to specific transcription factors present in erythroid cells but absent in nonerythroid cells (Le Van Kim et al. 1989).

To determine the elements involved in the enhanced expression of the GPC gene in erythroid cells, the nuclear protein factors that interact with the human GPC promoter in erythroid and nonerythroid cells have been explored by DNase I footprinting, gel retardation, and methylation interference assays (Colin et al. 1990). These analyses led to the identification of a novel erythroid/megakaryocyte–specific protein called NFE-6 that binds to a CTCCAGGGGG motif of the GPC promoter. This factor is present in embryonic, fetal, and adult-like human or mouse erythroleukemic cell lines, in a megakaryoblastic cell line (MEG01), but not in lymphoid or nonhematopoietic cell lines. These data, together with the presence of a GATA-1 and NFE-2 binding activity in nuclear extracts of the megakaryocytic cell line (Roméo et al. 1990; Martin et al. 1990) and of potential binding sites for NFE-6 in the promoters of the human GPIIb and GPIbα genes, strongly suggest that erythroid- and megakaryocyte-specific genes might be regulated in part by the same *trans*-acting factors. Presumably NFE-6, like the GATA-1 factor, is tissue- but not stage-specific and is conserved across species. It is proposed that NFE-6 might be involved in the quantitative change in expression of the housekeeping GPC gene related to red cell specialization. The respective role of NFE-6 and GATA-1 in this process, however, requires further investigation.

ACKNOWLEDGMENTS

We wish to thank Alain Vignal, Yves Colin, Caroline Le Van Kim, and Cécile Rahuel (INSERM U76) for critical reading and helpful discussions.

An abridged version of this chapter appeared as an invited review in *Transfusion Medicine Reviews* in 1991.

REFERENCES

Adams, J., M. Broviac, W. Brooks, N. R. Johnson, and P. D. Issitt. 1971. An antibody in the serum of a Wr(a+) individual reacting with an antigen of very high frequency. *Transfusion* 11:290–91.

Alloisio, N., L. Morlé, D. Bachir, D. Guetarni, P. Colonna, and J. Delaunay. 1985. Red cell membrane sialoglycoprotein in homozygous and heterozygous 4.1(−) heredity elliptocytosis. *Biochim. Biophys. Acta* 816:57–62.

Anderson, R. A. 1989. Regulation of protein 4.1-membrane association by a phosphoinositide. In *Red blood cell membranes: Structure, function, clinical implications.* P. Agre and J. C. Parker, eds. 187–236. New York, Marcell Dekker.

Anstee, D. J. 1980. Blood group MNSs-active sialoglycoproteins of the human erythrocyte membrane. In *Immunology of the erythrocyte.* Vol. 43. S. G. Sandler, M. D. Nusbacher, and M. S. Schanfield, eds. 67–98. New York, Alan R Liss.

——— 1981. The blood group MNSs active-sialoglycoproteins. *Sem. Hematol.* 18:13–31.

——— 1990. The nature and abundance of human red cell surface glycoproteins. *J. Immunogenet.* 17:219–25.

Anstee, D. J., and E. Lisowska. 1990. Monoclonal antibodies against glycoproteins and other glycoproteins. *J. Immunogenet.* 17:301–308.

Anstee, D. J., W. J. Mawby, S. F. Parsons, M. J. A. Tanner, and C. Giles. 1982. A novel hybrid sialoglycoprotein in St^a positive human erythrocytes. *J Immunogenet.* 9:51–55.

Anstee, D. J., S. F. Parsons, K. Ridgwell, M. J. A. Tanner, A. H. Merry, E. E. Thomson, P. A. Judson, P. Johnson, S. Bates, and I. D. Fraser. 1984a. Two individuals with elliptocytic red cells lack three minor erythrocyte membrane sialoglycoproteins. *Biochem. J.* 218:615–19.

Anstee, D. J., K. Ridgwell, M. J. A. Tanner, G. L. Daniels, and S. F. Parsons. 1984b. Individuals lacking the Gerbich blood-group antigen have alterations in the human erythrocyte membrane sialoglycoproteins β and γ. *Biochem. J.* 221:97–104.

Battey, J., C. Moulding, R. Taub, W. Murphy, T. Stewart, H. Potter, G. Lenoir, and P. Leder. 1983. The human c-myc oncogene: Structural consequences of translocation into the IgH locus in Burkitt lymphoma. *Cell* 34:779–87.

Beattie, K. M., and K. E. Sigmund. 1987. A Ge-like autoantibody in the serum of a patient receiving gold therapy for rheumatoid arthritis. *Transfusion* 27: 54–57.

Bennett, V. 1985. The membrane skeleton of human erythrocytes and its implications for more complex cells. *Annu. Rev. Biochem.* 54:273–304.

——— 1990. Spectrin-based membrane skeleton: A multipotential adaptator between plasma membrane and cytoplasm. *Physiol. Rev.* 70:1029–65.

Bernstein, P., and J. Ross. 1988. Poly(A), poly(A) binding protein and the regulation of mRNA stability. *Trends in Biological Sciences* 14:373–77.

Bigbee, W. L., R. G. Langlois, M. Vanderlaan, et al. 1984. Binding specificities of eight monoclonal antibodies to human glycophorin A. Studies with M^cM and M^kEn (UK) variant erythrocytes and M– and MN^v–type chimpanzee erythrocytes. *J. Immunol* 133:3149–55.

Blanchard, D. 1990. Human red blood cell glycophorins: Biochemical and antigenic properties. *Transf. Med. Rev.* 4:170–86.

Blanchard, D., J. P. Cartron, P. Rouger, and C. Salmon. 1982. Pj variant, a new hybrid MNSs glycoprotein of the human red cell membrane. *Biochem. J.* 203:419–26.

Blanchard, D., W. Dahr, K. Beyreuther, J. Moulds, and J. P. Cartron. 1987a. Hybrid glycophorins from human erythrocyte membranes: Isolation and complete structural analysis of the novel sialoglycoprotein from St(a+) red cells. *Eur. J. Biochem.* 167:361–66.

Blanchard, D., W. Dahr, M. Hummel, F. Latron, K. Beyreuther, and J. P. Cartron. 1987b. Glycophorins B and C from human erythrocyte membranes: Purification and sequence analysis. *J. Biol. Chem.* 262:5808–11.

Blumenfeld, O. O., A. M. Adamany, K. V. Puglia, and W. W. Socha. 1983. The chimpanzee M blood-group is a variant of the human M-N glycoproteins. *Biochem. Genet.* 21:333–48.

Booth, P. B., and K. McLoughlin. 1972. The Gerbich blood group system especially in Melanesians. *Vox Sang.* 22:73–84.

Breathnach, R., and P. Chambon. 1981. Organization and expression of eukaryotic split genes coding for proteins. *Annu. Rev. Biochem.* 50:349–83.

Bretscher, M. S. 1973. Membrane structure: Some general principle. *Science* 181:622–29.

Brown, W. R. A., A. N. Barclay, C. A. Sunderland, and A. F. Williams. 1981. Identification of a glycophorin-like molecule at the cell surface of rat thymocytes. *Nature* 289:456–60.

Bunn, H. F. and B. G. Forget. 1986. In *Hemoglobin: Molecular, genetic and clinical aspectcs.* J. Dyson, ed. 381–451. Philadelphia, W.B. Saunders.

Burness, A. T. H. 1981. Glycophorin and sialylated components as receptor for viruses. In *Virus receptors. Part 2: Receptors and recognition.* K. Lonberg-Holm and L. Philipson, eds. 63–84. London, Chapman & Hall.

Cartron, J. P., Y. Colin, S. Kudo, M. Fukuda. 1990. Molecular genetics of human erythrocyte sialoglycoproteins, glycophorins A, B, C and D. In *Blood cell biochemistry.* Vol. 1. J. R. Harris, ed. 299–335. New York, Plenum Press.

Cartron, J. P., O. Prou, M. Luilier, and J. P. Soulier. 1983. Susceptibility to invasion by *Plasmodium falciparum* of some human erythrocytes carrying rare blood group antigens. *Br. J. Haematol.* 55:639–47.

Cartron, J. P., A. Tounkara, O. Prou, M. Luilier, and J. P. Soulier. 1984. Wrb antigen not required for invasion of human erythrocytes by *Plasmodium falciparum. Lancet* 2:466–67.

Chang, S., M. E. Reid, J. Conboy, Y. Wai Kan, and N. Mohandas. 1991. Molecular characterization of erythrocyte glycophorin C variants. *Blood* 77: 644–48.

Chasis, J. A., and N. Mohandas. 1986. Erythrocyte membrane deformability and stability: Two distinct membrane properties that are independently regulated by skeletal protein associations. *J. Cell. Biol.* 103:343–50.

Chasis, J. A., N. Mohandas, and S. B. Shohet. 1985. Erythrocyte membrane rigidity induced by glycophorin A–ligand interaction: Evidence for a ligand induced association between glycophorin A and skeletal proteins. *J. Clin. Invest.* 75:1919–26.

Chasis, J. A., M. E. Reid, R. H. Jensen, and N. Mohandas. 1988. Signal transduction by glycophorin A: Role of extracellular and cytoplasmic domains in a modulatable process. *J. Cell Biol.* 107:1351–57.

Colin, Y., V. Joulin, C. Le Van Kim, P. H. Roméo, and J. P. Cartron. 1990. Characterization of a new erythroid megakaryocyte-specific nuclear factor that binds the promoter of house keeping human glycophorin C gene. *J. Biol. Chem.* 265:16729–32.

Colin, Y., C. Le Van Kim, A. Tsapis, M. Clerget, L. d'Auriol, J. London, F. Galibert, and J. P. Cartron. 1989. Human erythrocyte glycophorin C gene structure and rearrangement in genetic variants. *J. Biol. Chem.* 264:3773–80.

Colin, Y., C. Rahuel, J. London, P. H. Roméo, L. d'Auriol, F. Galibert, and J. P. Cartron. 1986. Isolation of cDNA clones for human erythrocyte glycophorin C. *J. Biol. Chem.* 261:229–33.

Contreras, M., C. Green, J. Humphreys, P. Tippett, G. Daniels, P. Teedale, S. Armitage, and A. Lubenko. 1984. Serology and genetics of MNSs-associated antigen Dantu. *Vox Sang.* 46:377–86.

Cook, P. J. L., R. H. Lindenbaum, R. Salonen, A. De La Chapelle, M. G. Daker, K. E. Buckton, J. E. Noades, and P. Tippett. 1981. The MNSs blood group of families with chromosome 4 rearrangements. *Ann. Hum. Genet.* 45:39–47.

Créau-Goldberg, N., J. London, C. Cochet, C. Rahuel, J. P. Cartron, C. Turleau, and J. De Grouchy. 1989. Evidence of genic homology between human and primate glycophorins and localization on homologous chromosomes in the chimpanzee, the gibbon, the baboon and the capuchin monkey. *Cytogenet. Cell. Genet.* 51:981.

Dahr, W. 1986. Immunochemistry of sialoglycoproteins in human red blood cell membranes. In *Recent advances in blood group biochemistry.* V. Vengelen-Tyler and W. J. Judd, eds. 23–65. Arlington, VA, American Association of Blood Banks.

Dahr, W., and J. J. Moulds. 1987. High-frequency antigens of human erythrocyte membrane sialoglycoproteins. IV. Molecular properties of the U antigen. *Biol. Chem. Hoppe Seyler* 368:659–67.

Dahr, W., K. Beyreuther, M. Kordowicz, and J. Kruger. 1982. N-terminal amino acid sequence of sialoglycoprotein D (glycophorin C) from human erythrocyte membranes. *Eur. J. Biochem.* 125:57–62.

Dahr, W., K. Beyreuther, H. Steinbach, W. Gielen, and J. Krüger. 1980. Structure of the Ss blood group antigens. II. A methionine/threonine polymorphism within the N-terminal sequence of Ss glycoprotein. *Hoppe Seyler Z. Physiol. Chem.* 361:895–906.

Dahr, W., D. Blanchard, C. Chevalier, J. P. Cartron, K. Beyreuther, and B. Fournet. 1990. The Mz variety of the St(a+) phenotype: A variant of glycophorin A exhibiting a deletion. *Biol. Chem. Hoppe Seyler* 371:403–10.

Dahr, W., D. Blanchard, S. Kiedrowski, A. Poschmann, J. P. Cartron, and J. Moulds. 1989a. High-frequency antigens of human erythrocyte membrane sialoglycoproteins. VI. Monoclonal antibodies reacting with the N-terminal domain of glycophorin C. *Biol. Chem. Hoppe Seyler* 370:849–54.

Dahr, W., S. Kiedrowski, D. Blanchard, P. Hermand, J. J. Moulds, and J. P.

Cartron. 1987. High-frequency antigens of human erythrocyte membrane sialoglycoproteins. V. Characterization of the Gerbich blood group antigens: Ge2 and Ge3. *Biol. Chem. Hoppe Seyler* 368:1375–83.

Dahr W., J. Moulds, G. Baumeister, et al. 1985. Altered membrane sialoglycoproteins in human erythrocytes lacking the Gerbich blood group antigens. *Biol. Chem. Hoppe Seyler* 366:201–11.

Dahr, W., P. M. Pilkington, H. Reinke, D. Blanchard, and K. Beyreuther. 1989b. A novel variety of Dantu gene complex ($Dantu^{MD}$) detected in a Caucasian. *Blut* 58:247–53.

Dahr, W., G. Uhlenbruck, P. Issitt, and F. H. Allen. 1975b. SDS-polyacrylamide gel electrophoretic analysis of the membrane glycoproteins from S−s−U− erythrocytes. *J. Immunogenet.* 2:249–51.

Dahr, W., G. Uhlenbruck, E. Janssen, and R. Schmalisch. 1977. Different N-terminal amino acids in the M,N glycoprotein from MM and NN erythrocytes. *Hum. Genet.* 35:335–43.

Dahr, W., G. Uhlenbruck, and H. Knott. 1975a. Immunochemical aspects of the MNSs blood group system. *J. Immunogenet.* 2:87–100.

Dahr, W., G. Uhlenbruck, J. Leikola, and W. Wagstaff. 1978. Studies on the membrane glycoprotein defect of En(a−) erythrocytes. III. N-terminal amino acids of sialoglycoproteins from normal and En(a−) red cells. *J. Immunogenet.* 5:117–27.

Daniels G. L., M. E. Reid, D. J. Anstee, et al. 1988. Transient reduction in erythrocyte membrane sialoglycoprotein β associated with the presence of elliptocytes. *Br. J. Haematol.* 70:477–88.

Daniels, G. L., M. A. Shaw, P. A. Judson, M. E. Reid, D. J. Anstee, P. Colpitis, J. Cornwall, B. P. L. Moore, and S. Lee. 1986. A family demonstrating inheritance of the Leach phenotype: A Gerbich-negative phenotype associated with elliptocytosis. *Vox Sang.* 50:117–21.

Daniels, G. R., and P. L. Deininger. 1985. Integration sites preferences of the Alu family and similar repetitive DNA sequences. *Nucleic Acids Res.* 24: 8939–54.

Darnborough, J., I. Dunsford, and J. A. Wallace. 1969. The En^a antigen and antibody: A genetical modification of human red cells affecting their blood grouping reactions. *Vox Sang.* 17:241–55.

Dolan, S. A., L. H. Miller, and T. E. Wellems. 1990. Evidence for a switching mechanism in the invasion of erythrocytes by *Plasmodium falciparum. J. Clin. Invest.* 86:618–24.

El-Maliki, B., D. Blanchard, W. Dahr, K. Beyreuther, and J. P. Cartron. 1989. Structural homology between glycophorins C and D of human erythrocytes. *Eur. J. Biochem.* 183:639–43.

Evans, T., G. Felsenfeld, and M. Reitman. 1990. Control of globin gene transcription. *Annu. Rev. Cell. Biol.* 6:95–124.

Facer, C. A. 1984. Antibodies to red cell glycophorin inhibit invasion by *Plasmodium falciparum. IRSC Med. Sci.* 12:314–15.

Fairbanks, G., T. L. Steck, and D. F. H. Wallach. 1971. Electrophoretic analysis of the major polypeptides of the human erythrocyte membrane. *Biochemistry* 10:2606–17.

Fukuda, M. 1985. Cell surface glycoconjugates as onco-differentiation markers in hematopoietic cells. *Biochim. Biophys. Acta* 780:119–50.

Fukuda, M., and M. N. Fukuda. 1984. Cell surface glycoproteins and carbohydrate antigens in development and differentiation of human erythroid cells. In *The biology of glycoproteins.* R. J. Ivatt, ed. 183–234. New York, Plenum Publishing.

Furthmayr, H. 1978a. Structural comparison of glycophorins and immunochemical analysis of genetic variants. *Nature* 271:519–24.

——— 1978b. Glycophorins A, B, C: A family of sialoglycoproteins. Isolation and preliminary characterisation of trypsin-derived peptides. *J. Supramol. Struct.* 9:79–95.

Furuhjelm, U., G. Myllyla, H. R. Nevanlinna, S. Nordling, A. Pirkola, J. Gavin, A. Gooch, R. Sanger, and P. Tippett. 1969. The red cell phenotype En(a−) and anti-En[a]: Serological and physicochemical aspects. *Vox Sang.* 17:256–78.

Gahmberg, C. G., M. Autero, and J. Hermonen. 1988. Major O-glycosylated sialoglycoproteins of human hematopoietic cells: Differentiation antigens with poorly understood functions. *J. Chem. Biochem.* 37:91–105.

Gahmberg, J. G., M. Jokinen, and L. C. Anderson. 1978. Expression of the major sialoglycoprotein (glycophorin) on erythroid cells in human bone marrow. *Blood* 52:379–87.

Gardner, B., S. F. Parsons, A. H. Merry, and D. J. Anstee. 1989. Epitopes on sialoglycoprotein α: Evidence for heterogeneity in the molecule. *Immunol.* 68:283–89.

Gedde-Dahl, T., A. L. Grimstad, S. Gundersen, and E. Vogt. 1967. A probable crossing-over or mutation in the MNSs blood group system. *Acta Genet.* 17: 193–210.

Giles, C. M. 1982. Serological activity of low frequency antigens of the MNSs system and reappraisal of the Miltenberger complex. *Vox Sang.* 42:256–61.

Greaves, M. F., C. Sieff, and P. A. W. Edwards. 1983. Monoclonal antiglycophorin as a probe for erythroleukemias. *Blood* 61:645–51.

Greenwalt, T. J., T. Sasaki, R. Sanger, J. Sneath, and R. R. Race. 1954. An allele of the S(s) blood group genes. *Proc. Natl. Acad. Sci. U.S.A.* 40: 1126–29.

Hadley, T. J., F. W. Klotz, and L. H. Miller. 1986. Invasion of erythrocytes by malaria parasites: A cellular and molecular overview. *Ann. Rev. Microbiol.* 40:451–77.

Hadley, T. J., F. W. Klotz, G. Pasvol, J. D. Haynes, M. H. McGinnis, Y. Okubo, and L. H. Miller. 1987. Falciparum malaria parasites invade erythrocytes that lack glycophorin A and B (Mk). *J. Clin. Invest.* 80:1190–93.

Hamaguchi H., and H. Cleve. 1972. Solubilization of human erythrocyte membrane glycoproteins and separation of the MN glycoprotein from a glycoprotein with I, S and A activity. *Biochim. Biophys. Acta* 278:271–80.

Hamid, J., and A. T. H. Burness. 1990. The mechanism of production of multiple mRNAs for human glycophorin A. *Nucleic Acids Res.* 18:5829–36.

Harvey, J., S. F. Parsons, D. J. Anstee, B. A. Bradley. 1988. Evidence for the occurrence of human erythrocyte membrane sialoglycoproteins in human kidney endothelial cells. *Vox Sang.* 55:104–108.

Hermentin, P., B. Enders, G. Neunziger, W. Dahr, S. Wilkinson, L. H. Miller, and G. Pasvol. 1984. Wr(a+b−) red blood cells are fully susceptible to invasion by *Plasmodium falciparum.* Lancet 2:466.

High, S., and M. J. A. Tanner. 1987. Human erythrocyte membrane sialoglycoprotein β: The cDNA sequence suggests the absence of a cleaved N-terminal signal sequence. *Biochem. J.* 243:277–80.

High, S., M. J. A. Tanner, E. B. Macdonald, and D. J. Anstee. 1989. Rearrangements of the red cell membrane glycophorin C (sialoglycoprotein β) gene. *Biochem. J.* 262:47–54.

Holman, C. A. 1953. A new rare human blood group antigen (Wr[a]). *Lancet* 2:119.

Huang, C. H., and O. O. Blumenfeld. 1988. Characterization of a genomic hybrid specifying the human erythrocyte antigen Dantu: Dantu gene is duplicated and linked to a δ glycophorin gene deletion. *Proc. Natl. Acad. Sci. U.S.A.* 85:9640–44.

Huang, C. H., and O. O. Blumenfeld. 1991. Molecular genetics of human erythrocyte Mi.III and Mi.VI glycophorins. *J. Biol. Chem.* 266:7248–56.

Huang, C. H., M. L. Guizzo, M. Kikuchi, and O. O. Blumenfeld. 1989a. Molecular genetic analysis of a hybrid gene encoding St[a] glycophorin of the human erythrocyte membrane. *Blood* 74:836–43.

Huang, C. H., K. Johe, J. J. Moulds, P. P. Siebert, M. Fukuda, and O. O. Blumenfeld. 1987. δ Glycoprotein (glycophorin B) gene deletion in two individuals homozygous for the S–s–U– blood group phenotype. *Blood* 70: 1830–35.

Huang, C. H., W. M. Lu, M. E. Boots, M. L. Guizzo, and O. O. Blumenfeld. 1989b. Two types of δ glycophorin gene alterations in S–s–U– individuals. *Transfusion* 29:35S.

Irimura, T., T. Tsuji, K. Togami, K. Yamamoto, and T. Osawa. 1981. Structure of a complex-type sugar chain of human glycophorin A. *Biochemistry* 20: 560–66.

Issitt, P. D. 1981. *The MN blood group system.* Cincinnati, Ohio, Montgomery Scientific Publications.

——— 1985. *Applied blood group serology.* 3rd ed. Miami, Florida, Montgomery Scientific Publications.

Jarolim, P., J. Palek, D. Amato, K. Hassan, P. Sapak, G. T. Nurse, H. L. Rubin, S. Zhai, K. E. Sahr, and S. C. Liu. 1991. Deletion of erythrocyte band 3 gene in malaria-resistant Southeast Asian ovalocytosis. *Proc. Natl. Acad. Sci. U.S.A.* 88:11022–26.

Johe, K. K., A. J. Smith, V. Vengelen-Tyler, and O. O. Blumenfeld. 1989. Amino acid sequence of an α-δ glycophorin hybrid: A structure reciprocal to St[a] δ-α glycophorin hybrid. *J. Biol. Chem.* 264:17486–93.

Jones, G. L., H. M. Edmunson, D. Wesche, and A. Saul. 1991. Human erythrocyte band-3 has an altered N-terminus in malaria-resistant Melanesian ovalocytes. *Biochim. Biophys. Acta* 1096:33–40.

Judd, W. J., P. D. Issitt, B. G. Pavone, J. Anderson, and D. Aminoff. 1979. Antibodies that define NANA-independent MN-system antigens. *Transfusion* 19:12–18.

Kidson C., G. Lamont, A. Saul, and G. T. Nurse. 1981. Ovalocytic erythrocytes from Melanesians are resistant to invasion by malarial parasites in culture. *Proc. Natl. Acad. Sci. U.S.A.* 78:5829–32.

King, M. J., J. Poole, and D. J. Anstee. 1989. An application of immunoblotting in the classification of the Miltenberger series of blood group antigens. *Transfusion* 29:106–12.

Kopito, R. R., M. A. Andersson, and H. F. Lodish. 1987. Multiple tissue-specific sites of transcriptional initiation of the mouse anion antiport gene in erythroid and renal cells. *Proc. Natl. Acad. Sci. U.S.A.* 84:7149–53.

Kozak, M. 1984. Compilation and analysis of sequences upstream from the translational start site in eukaryotic mRNAs. *Nucleic Acids Res.* 12:857–72.

Kozak, M. 1986. Bifunctional messenger RNAs in eukaryotes. *Cell* 47:481–83.

Kozak, M. 1989. The scanning model for translation: An update. *J. Cell. Biol.* 108:229–41.

Krotkiewski, H. 1988. The structure of glycophorins of animal erythrocytes. *Glycoconjugate J.* 5:35–48.

Kudo, S., and M. Fukuda. 1989. Structural organisation of glycophorin A and B genes: Glycophorin B gene evolved by homologous recombination at Alu repeat sequences. *Proc. Natl. Acad. Sci. U.S.A.* 86:4619–23.

Kudo, S., and M. Fukuda. 1990. Identification of a novel human glycophorin, glycophorin E, by isolation of genomic clones and complementary DNA clones utilizing polymerase chain reaction. *J. Biol. Chem.* 265:1102–10.

Kudo, S., D. Chagnovich, A. Rearden, M. G. Mattei, and M. Fukuda. 1990. Molecular analysis of a hybrid gene encoding human glycophorin variant Miltenberger V like molecule. *J. Biol. Chem.* 265:13825–29.

Kyoizumi, S., N. Nakamura, M. Hakoda, A. A. Awa, M. A. Bean, R. H. Jensen, and M. Akiyama. 1989a. Detection of somatic mutations at the glycophorin A locus in erythrocytes of atomic bomb survivors using a single beam flow sorter. *Cancer Res.* 49:581–88.

Kyoizumi, S., N. Nakamura, H. Takebe, K. Tatsumi, J. German, and H. Akiyama. 1989b. Frequency of variant erythrocytes at the glycophorin A locus in two Bloom's syndrome patients. *Mutat. Res.* 214:215–22.

Laemmli, U. K. 1970. Cleavage of structural proteins during the assembly of the head of bacteriophage T4. *Nature* 227:680–81.

Laird-Fryer, B., J. J. Moulds, W. Dahr, Y. O. Min, and D. Chandanayingyong. 1986. Anti-En^{a}FS in the serum of a Mi.VII heterozygote. *Transfusion* 26: 51–56.

Landsteiner, K., and P. Levine. 1927. A new agglutinable factor differentiating individual human bloods. *Proc. Soc. Exp. Biol.* 24:600–602.

Langlois, R. G., W. L. Bigbee, S. Kyoizumi, N. Nakamura, M. A. Bean, M. Akiyama, and R. H. Jensen. 1987. Evidence for increased somatic cell mutations at the glycophorin A locus in atomic bomb survivors. *Science* 236: 445–48.

Lehrman, M. A., J. L. Goldstein, D. W. Russel, and M. S. Brown. 1987. Duplication of seven exons in LDL receptor gene caused by Alu-Alu recombination in a subject with familial hypercholesterolemia. *Cell* 48:827–35.

Levine, P., A. B. Kuhmichel, M. Wigod, and E. Koch. 1951. A new blood factor, s allelic to S. *Proc. Soc. Exp. Biol.* 78:218–20.

Le Van Kim, C., Y. Colin, D. Blanchard, W. Dahr, J. London, and J. P. Cartron. 1987. Gerbich group deficiency of the Ge:1, −2, −3 and Ge: −1, −2,3 types. *Eur. J. Biochem.* 165:571–79.

Le Van Kim, C., Y. Colin, M. T. Mitjavila, M. Clerget, A. Dubart, M. Nakazawa, W. Vainchenker, and J. P. Cartron. 1989. Structure of the promoter region and tissue specificity of the human glycophorin C. *J. Biol. Chem.* 264: 20407–414.

Le Van Kim, C., M.-T. Mitjavila, M. Clerget, J. P. Cartron, and Y. Colin. 1990. An ubiquitous isoform of glycophorin C is produced by alternative splicing. *Nucleic Acids Res.* 18:3076.

Leonard, W. J., J. M. Depper, M. Kanehisa, M. Krönke, N. J. Peffer, P. B. Svettik, M. Sullivan, and W. C. Greene. 1985. Structure of the human interleukin-2 receptor gene. *Science* 230:633–39.

Lisowska, E. 1989. Antigenic properties of human erythrocyte glycophorins. In *Molecular immunology of complex carbohydrates.* A. M. Wu, ed. New York, Plenum Publishing.

Liu, S.-C., S. Zhai, J. Palek, D. E. Golan, D. Amato, K. Hassan, G. T. Nurse, D. Babona, T. Coetzer, P. Jarolim, M. Zaik, and S. Borwein. 1990. Molecular defect of the band 3 protein in Southeast Asian ovalocytosis. *N. Engl. J. Med.* 323:1530–38.

Loken, M. R., C. I. Civin, W. L. Bigbee, R. G. Langlois, and R. H. Jensen. 1987. Coordinate glycosylation and cell surface expression of glycophorin A during normal human erythropoiesis. *Blood* 70:1959–61.

Lowe, R. F. and P. P. Moores. 1972. Red cell factor in Africans of Rhodesia, Malawai, Mozambique and Natal. *Hum. Hered.* 22:344–48.

Lu, W.-M., C.-H. Huang, W. W. Socha, and O. O. Blumenfeld. 1990. Polymorphism and gross structure of glycophorin genes in common chimpanzees. *Biochem. Genet.* 28:399–413.

Lu, Y.-Q., J.-F. Liu, W. W. Socha, R. L. Nagel, and O. O. Blumenfeld. 1987a. Polymorphism of glycophorins in nonhuman primate erythrocytes. *Biochem. Genet.* 25:477–91.

Lu, Y.-Q., M. E. Nichols, N. L. Bigbee, R. L. Nagel, and O. O. Blumenfeld. 1987b. Structural polymorphism of glycophorins demonstrated by immunoblotting techniques. *Blood* 69:618–24.

Macdonald, E. B., and L. M. Gerns. 1986. An unusual sialoglycoprotein associated with the Webb-positive phenotype. *Vox Sang.* 50:112–16.

Macdonald, E. B., J. Condon, D. Ford, B. Fisher, and L. M. Gerns. 1990. Abnormal beta and gamma sialoglycoprotein associated with the low-frequency antigen Ls^a. *Vox Sang.* 58:300–304.

Maeda, N., and O. Smithies. 1986. The evolution of multigene families: Human haptoglobin genes. *Annu. Rev. Genet.* 20:81–108.

Marchesi, V. T., H. Furthmay, and M. Tomita. 1976. The red cell membrane. *Annu. Rev. Biochem.* 45:667–98.

Marchesi, V. T., T. W. Tillack, R. L. Jackson, J. P. Segrest, and R. E. Scott. 1972. Chemical characterization and surface orientation of the major glycoprotein of the human erythrocyte membrane. *Proc. Natl. Acad. Sci. U.S.A.* 69:1445–49.

Markert, M. L., J. J. Hutton, D. A. Wiginton, J. C. States, and R. E. Kaufman. 1988. Adenosine deaminase (ADA) deficiency due to deletion of the ADA gene promoter and first exon by homologous recombination between two Alu elements. *J. Clin. Invest.* 81:1323–27.

Martin, D., L. I. Zon, G. Mutter, and S. H. Orkin. 1990. Expansion of an erythroid transcription factor in megakaryocytic and mast cell lineages. *Nature* 344:444–47.

Matsui, Y., S. Natori, and M. Obinata. 1989. Isolation of the cDNA for mouse glycophorin, erythroid-specific protein. *Gene* 77:325–32.

Mattei, M. G., Y. Colin, C. Le Van Kim, J. F. Mattei, and J. P. Cartron. 1986. Localization of the gene for human erythrocyte glycophorin C to chromosome 2q14-q21. *Hum. Genet.* 74:420–22.

McShane, K., and A. Chung. 1989. A novel human alloantibody in the Gerbich system. *Vox Sang.* 57:205–209.

Metaxas, N. N., and M. Metaxas-Bühler. 1964. MK: An apparently silent allele at the MN locus. *Nature* 202:1123.

Mitchell, G. H., and L. H. Bannister. 1988. Malaria parasite invasion: Interaction with the red cell membrane. *CRC Crit. Rev. Oncol. Hematol.* 8:255–310.

Mitchell, G. H., T. J. Hadley, M. H. McGinnis, F. W. Klotz, and L. H. Miller. 1986. Invasion of erythrocytes by *Plasmodium falciparum* malaria parasites: Evidence for receptor heterogeneity and two receptors. *Blood* 67:1519–21.

Mollison, P. L., C. P. Engelfriet, and M. Contreras. 1987. *Blood transfusion in clinical medicine.* 8th ed. Oxford, Blackwell Scientific.

Müeller, T. J., and M. Morrison. 1981. Glycoconnectin (PAS 2), a membrane attachment site for the human erythrocyte cytoskeleton. In *Erythrocyte membrane 2: Recent clinical and experimental advances.* W. C. Kruckenberg, J. W. Eaton, and G. J. Brewer, eds. 95–112. New York, Alan R Liss.

Murayama, J.-I., H. Utsumi, and A. Hamada. 1989. Amino acid sequence of monkey erythrocyte glycophorin MK: Its amino acid sequence has a striking homology with that of human glycophorin. A. *Biochim. Biophys. Acta* 999: 273–80.

Murray, J. C., K. H. Buetow, R. E. Ferrel, P. D. Siebert, and M. Fukuda. 1988. An RFLP for glyclophorin A (MN) is in linkage disequilibrium with MN and S.s. *Cytogenet. Cell Genet.* 47:149–51.

Nagel, R. L. 1990. Red cell cytoskeletal abnormalities: Implications for malaria. *N. Engl. J. Med.* 323:1558–59.

Nash, G. B., J. Parmar, and M. E. Reid. 1990. Effects of deficiencies of glycophorins C and D on the physical properties of the red cell. *Br. J. Haematol.* 76:282–87.

Orkin, S. H. 1990. Globin gene regulation and switching: Circa 1990. *Cell* 63: 665–72.

Pasvol G., D. J. Anstee, and M. J. A. Tanner. 1984. Glycophorin C and the invasion of red cells by *Plasmodium falciparum.* Lancet 1:907.

Pasvol, G., J. A. Chasis, N. Mohandas, D. J. Anstee, M. J. A. Tanner, and A. H. Merry. 1989. Inhibition of malarial parasite invasion by monoclonal antibodies against glycophorin A correlates with reduction in red cell membrane deformability. *Blood* 74:1836–43.

Pasvol, G., M. Jungery, and D. J. Weatherall, et al. 1982. Glycophorin as a possible receptor for *Plasmodium falciparum. Lancet* 2:947–50.

Petz, L. D., and G. Garratty. 1980. *Acquired immune hemolytic anemias.* New York, Churchill Livingstone.

Pevny, L., M. C. Simon, E. Robertson, W. H. Klein, S. F. Tsai, V. D'Agati, S. H. Orkin, and F. Constantini. 1991. Erythroid differentiation in chimaeric mice blocked by a targeted mutation in the gene for transcription factor GATA-1. *Nature* 349:257–60.

Race, R. R., and R. Sanger. 1975. *Blood groups in man.* 6th ed. Oxford, Blackwell Scientific.

Rahuel, C., J. London, L. d'Auriol, M. G. Mattei, C. Tournamille, C. Skrzynia, Y. Lebouc, F. Galibert, and J. P. Cartron. 1988a. Characterization of cDNA clones for human glycophorin A: Use for gene localization and for analysis of normal and glycophorin A–deficient (Finnish type) genomic DNA. *Eur. J. Biochem.* 172:147–53.

Rahuel, C., J. London, A. Vignal, B. Cherif-Zahar, Y. Colin, P. Siebert, M. Fukuda, and J. P. Cartron. 1988b. Alteration of the genes for glycophorin A and B in glycophorin A deficient individuals. *Eur. J. Biochem.* 177:605–14.

Rahuel, C., J. London, A. Vignal, S. K. Ballas, and J. P. Cartron. 1991. Erythrocyte glycophorin B deficiency may occur by two distinct gene alterations. *Am. J. Haematol.* 37:57–58.

Rahuel, C., A. Vignal, J. London, S. Hamel, P. H. Roméo, Y. Colin, and J. P. Cartron. 1989. Structure of the 5′ flanking region of the glycophorin A gene and analysis of its multiple transcripts. *Gene* 85:471–77.

Rearden, A., H. Phan, T. Dubnicoff, S. Kudo, and M. Fukuda. 1990a. Identification of the crossing-over point of a hybrid gene encoding human glycophorin variant St^a. *J. Biol. Chem.* 265, 16:92259–9263.

Rearden, A., H. Phan, S. Kudo, and M. Fukuda. 1990b. Evolution of the glycophorin gene family in the hominoid primates. *Biochem. Genet.* 28: 209–22.

Reid, E. M., D. J. Anstee, M. J. A. Tanner, K. Rigdwell, and C. T. Nurse. 1987a. Structural relationships between human erythrocyte sialoglycoproteins β and γ and abnormal sialoglycoproteins found in certain rare human erythrocyte variants lacking the Gerbich blood-group antigen(s). *Biochem. J.* 244: 123–28.

Reid, E. M., J. A. Chasis, and N. Mohandas. 1987b. Identification of a functional role for human erythrocyte sialoglycoproteins β and γ. *Blood* 69:1068–72.

Reid, M. E., Y. Takakuwa, J. Conboy, G. Tchernia, and N. Mohandas. 1990. Glycophorin C content of human erythrocytes membrane is regulated by protein 4.1. *Blood* 75:2229–34.

Reid, M. E., M. A. Shaw, G. Rowe, D. J. Anstee, and M. J. A. Tanner. 1985.

Abnormal minor human erythrocyte membrane sialoglycoprotein β in association with the rare blood-group antigen Webb (Wb). *Biochem. J.* 232:289–91.
Robinson, J., C. Sieff, D. Delia, P. A. W. Edwards, and M. Greaves. 1981. Expression of cell-surface HLA-DR, HLA-ABC and glycophorin during erythroid differentiation. *Nature* 289:68–71.
Roméo, P. H., M.-H. Prandini, V. Joulin, V. Mignotte, M. Prenant, W. Vainchenker, G. Marguerie, and G. Uzan. 1990. Megakaryocytic and erythrocytic lineages share specific transcription factors. *Nature* 344:447–49.
Rosenfield R. E., G. V. Haber, J. A. Kissmeyer-Nielson, et al. 1960. Ge, a very common red cell antigen. *Br. J. Haematol.* 6:344–49.
Rountree, J., J. Chen, M. K. Moulds, J. J. Moulds, A. M. Green, and M. J. Telen. 1989. A second family demonstrating inheritance of the Leach phenotype. *Transfusion* 29(Suppl):15S.
Sanger, R., and R. R. Race. 1947. Subdivisions of the MN blood groups in man. *Nature* 160:505.
Sanger, R., R. R. Race, R. J. Walsh, and C. Montgomery. 1948. An antibody which subdivides the human MN blood groups. *Heredity* 2:131–39.
Schnitzer, J. E., J. B. Ulmer, and G. E. Palade. 1990. A major endothelial plasmalemmal sialoglycoprotein, gp60, is immunologically related to glycophorin. *Proc. Natl. Acad. Sci. U.S.A.* 87:6843–47.
Siebert, P. D. and M. Fukuda. 1986a. Isolation and characterization of human glycophorin A cDNA clones by a synthetic oligonucleotide approach: Nucleotide sequence and mRNA structure. *Proc. Natl. Acad. Sci. U.S.A.* 83: 1665–69.
——— 1986b. Human glycophorin A and B are encoded by separate, single copy genes coordinately regulated by a tumor-promoting phorbol ester. *J. Biol. Chem.* 261:12433–36.
——— 1987. Molecular cloning of human glycophorin B cDNA: Nucleotide sequence and genomic relationship to glycoprotein A. *Proc. Natl. Acad. Sci. U.S.A.* 84:6735–39.
Sondag, D., N. Alloisio, D. Blanchard, M. T. Ducluzeau, P. Colonna, D. Bachir, C. Bloy, J. P. Cartron, and J. Delaunay. 1987. Gerbich reactivity in 4.1(−) hereditary elliptocytosis and protein 4.1 level in blood group Gerbich deficiency. *Br. J. Haematol.* 65:43–50.
Springer, G. F., and S. V. Huprikar. 1972. On the biochemical and genetic basis of the human blood-group MN specificities. *Haematologia* 6:81–92.
Steck, T. L. 1974. The organization of proteins in the human red blood cell membrane. *J. Cell Biol.* 62:1–19.
Stoppa-Lyonnet, D., P. Carter, T. Meo, and M. Tosi. 1990. Clusters of intragenic Alu repeats predispose the human C1 inhibitor locus to deleterious rearrangements. *Proc. Natl. Acad. Sci. U.S.A.* 87:1551–55.
Strubin, M., E. O. Long, and B. Mach. 1986. Two forms of the Ia antigen–associated invariant chain result from alternative initiations at two in-phase AUGs. *Cell* 47:619–25.
Taliano, V., R.-M. Guévin, D. Hébert, G. L. Daniels, P. Tippett, D. J. Anstee, W. J. Mawby, and M. J. A. Tanner. 1980. The rare phenotype En(a−) in a French-Canadian family. *Vox Sang.* 38:87–93.
Tanner, M. J. A., D. Anstee, and P. A. Judon. 1977. A carbohydrate-deficient membrane glycoprotein in human erythrocytes of phenotype S−s−. *Biochem. J.* 165:157–61.
Tanner, M. J. A., D. J. Anstee, and W. J. Mawby. 1980. A new human erythrocyte variant (Ph) containing abnormal sialoglycoprotein. *Biochem. J.* 187:493–500.
Tanner, M. J. A., S. High, P. G. Martin, D. J. Anstee, P. A. Judson, and T. J.

Jones. 1988. Genetic variants of human red cell membrane sialoglycoprotein β: Study of the alterations occurring in the sialoglycoprotein β gene. *Biochem. J.* 250:407–14.

Tate, C. G. and M. J. A. Tanner. 1988. Isolation of cDNA clones for human erythrocyte membrane sialoglycoproteins α and δ. *Biochem. J.* 254:743–50.

Tate, C. G., M. J. A. Tanner, P. A. Judson, and D. J. Anstee. 1989. Studies on human red-cell membrane glycophorin A and glycophorin B genes in glycophorin-deficient individuals. *Biochem. J.* 263:993–96.

Telen, M. J., and J. A. Chasis. 1990. Relationship of the human erythrocyte Wr^b antigen to an interaction between glycophorin A and band 3. *Blood* 76: 842–48.

Telen, M. J., C. Le Van Kim, A. Chung, J. P. Cartron, and Y. Colin. 1991a. Molecular basis for elliptocytosis associated with glycophorin C deficiency in the Leach phenotype. *Blood* 78:1603–06.

Telen, M. J., C. Le Van Kim, M. L. Guizzo, J. P. Cartron, and Y. Colin. 1991b. Erythrocyte Webb-type glycophorin C variant lacks N-glycosylation due to an asparagine to serine substitution. *Am. J. Hematol.* 37:51–52.

Thomas, D. B., and R. J. Winzler. 1969. Structural studies on human erythrocyte sialoglycoproteins: Alkali-labile oligosaccharides. *J. Biol. Chem.* 244:5943–46.

Tokunaga, E., S. Sasakama, K. Tamaka, et al. 1979. Two apparently healthy Japanese individuals of type Mk/Mk have erythrocytes which lack both the blood group MN and Ss active sialoglycoproteins. *J. Immunogenet.* 6:383–90.

Tomita, M., and V. T. Marchesi. 1975. Amino-acid sequence and oligosaccharide attachment sites of human erythrocyte glycophorin. *Proc. Natl. Acad. Sci. U.S.A.* 72:2964–68.

Tomita, M., H. Furthmayr, and V. T. Marchesi. 1978. Primary structure of human erythrocyte glycophorin A: Isolation and characterization of peptides and complete amino acid sequence. *Biochemistry* 17:4756–70.

Ullu, E., S. Murphy, and M. Melli. 1982. Human 7SL RNA consists of 140 nucleotide middle repetitive sequence. *Cell* 29:195–202.

Ulmer, J. B. and G. E. Palade. 1989. Anomalies in the translocation and processing of glycophorin precursors in murine erythroleukemia cells. *J. Biol. Chem.* 264:1084–91.

Unger, P., J. L. Procter, J. J. Moulds, M. K. Moulds, D. Blanchard, M. L. Guizzo, L. A. McCall, J. P. Cartron, and W. Dahr. 1987. The Dantu erythrocyte phenotype of the NE variety. II. Serology, immunochemistry, genetics and frequency. *Blut* 54:33–43.

Van Arsdell, S. W., R. A. Denison, L. B. Bernstein, A. M. Weiner, T. Manser, and R. F. Gesteland. 1981. Direct repeats flank three small nuclear RNA pseudogenes in the human genome. *Cell* 26:11–17.

Vengelen-Tyler, V., D. J. Anstee, P. D. Issitt, B. G. Pavone, S. J. Ferguson, W. J. Mawby, M. J. A. Tanner, M. A. Blajchman, and P. Lorque. 1981. Studies on the blood of an Mi.V homozygote. *Transfusion* 21:1–14.

Vignal, A., J. London, C. Rahuel, and J. P. Cartron. 1990a. Promoter sequence and chromosomal organisation of the genes encoding glycophorins A, B and E. *Gene* 95:289–93.

Vignal, A., C. Rahuel, B. El Maliki, C. Le Van Kim, J. London, D. Blanchard, L. d'Auriol, F. Galibert, M. A. Blajchman, and J. P. Cartron. 1989. Molecular analysis of glycophorin A and B gene structure and expression in homozygotes Miltenberger class V (MiV) human erythrocytes. *Eur. J. Biochem.* 84:337–44.

Vignal, A., C. Rahuel, J. London, B. Cherif-Zahar, S. Schaff, C. Hattab, Y. Okubo, and J. P. Cartron. 1990b. A novel gene member of the human glycophorin A and B gene family: Molecular cloning and expression. *Eur. J. Biochem.* 191:619–25.

Villeval, J. L., P. Cramer, F. Lemoine, A. Henri, A. Bettaieb, F. Bernaudin, Y. Beuzard, R. Berger, G. Flandrin, J. Breton-Gorius, and W. Vainchenker. 1986. Phenotype of early erythroblastic leukemia. *Blood* 68:1167–74.

Villeval, J. L., C. Le Van Kim, A. Bettaieb, N. Debili, Y. Colin, B. El Maliki, D. Blanchard, W. Vainchenker, and J. P. Cartron. 1989. Early expression of glycophorin C during normal and leukemic human erythroid differentiation. *Cancer Res* 49:2626–29.

Vnencak-Jones, C. L., J. A. Phillips III, E. Y. Chen, and P. H. Seeburg. 1988. Molecular basis of growth hormone gene deletions. *Proc. Natl. Acad. Sci. U.S.A.* 85:5615–19.

Voss, J. W., T. P. Yao, and M. G. Rosenfeld. 1991. Alternative translation initiation site usage results in two structurally distinct forms of *Pit*-1. *J. Biol. Chem.* 266:12832–35.

Wasniowska, K., Z. Drzeniek, and E. Lisowska. 1977. The amino acids of M and N blood group glycopeptides are different. *Biochem. Biophys. Res. Commun.* 76:385–90.

Wiener, A. S., E. B. Gordon, J. Moor-Jankowski, and W. W. Socha. 1972. Homologues of the human M-N blood types in gorillas and other nonhuman primates. *Haematologia* 6:419–32.

Wiener, A. S., L. J. Unger, and E. B. Gordon. 1953. Fatal hemolytic transfusion reaction caused by sensitization to a new blood factor. *U. J.A.M.A.* 153: 1444–46.

Wise, G. E. 1984. Identification and function of transmembrane glycoproteins: The red cell model. *Tissue Cell* 16:665–76.

Yamamoto, M., L. J. Ko, M. W. Leonard, H. Beug, S. H. Orkin, and J. D. Engel. 1990. Activity and tissue-specific expression of the transcription factor NF-E1 multigene family. *Genes Dev.* 4:1650–62.

Yasukawa, K., T. Hirano, Y. Watanabe, K. Muratini, T. Matsuda, S. Nakai, and T. Kishimoto. 1987. Structure and expression of human B cell stimulatory factor-2 (BSF-2/IL-6) gene. *EMBO J.* 6:2939–45.

Yoshima, H., H. Furthmayr, and A. Kobata. 1980. Structures of the asparagin-linked sugar chains of glycophorin A. *J. Biol. Chem.* 255:9713–18.

7

THE ROLE OF RED CELL GLYCOPHORINS IN REGULATING MEMBRANE FUNCTION

Joel Anne Chasis M.D.
and Narla Mohandas Ph.D.

The human red cell membrane contains at least four distinct sialoglycoproteins, commonly referred to as glycophorins A, B, C, and D (Anstee 1981; Furthmayr 1978a; Dahr 1986). The gene for a fifth glycophorin (E) has been isolated, but it is not known to be expressed (Kudo and Fukuda 1990; Vignal et al. 1990). The primary focus of studies on these molecules has long centered on their role as blood group antigens. A detailed discussion of the molecular biology and antigenic determinants of these molecules is outlined in Chapter 6. Recent studies, however, have begun to define an additional, potentially important, role for these proteins, as regulators of cell shape and membrane mechanical function. In this chapter, we concentrate entirely on this aspect of glycophorin biology.

Although these distinct sialoglycoproteins have all been designated as *glycophorins,* suggesting a common genetic origin, this is partially a misnomer, since recent molecular biologic studies have firmly established that the various glycophorins constitute different gene products (Mattei et al. 1986; Siebert and Fukuda 1987; Tate and Tanner 1988). For example, glycophorins A, B, and C are encoded by three different genes on two different chromosomes. Glycophorins C and D are closely related, arising from the same gene through the use of alternative translational initiation sites (Le Van Kim et al. 1987; Tanner et al. 1988). Early protein sequencing studies and the more recent cloning studies have provided us with a complete understanding of the primary structure of the four glycophorin molecules.

Glycophorin A (GPA), constituting the major membrane sialoglycoprotein of the human red cell, is present at 500,000 to 900,000 copies per cell and is composed of 131 amino-acid residues (Fairbanks et al. 1971; Furthmayr 1978b; Merry et al. 1984, 1986; Dahr 1986; Tomita and Marchesi 1975; Tomita et al. 1978). As a class I transmembrane protein, it contains a single membrane-spanning domain of 22 amino acids with 70 extracellular residues and 39 cytoplasmic residues. The MN blood group antigenic epitopes are localized on the five N-terminal amino acids with the M-phenotype characterized by serine at residue 1 and glycine at residue 5, while the N-phenotype contains leucine at residue 1 and glutamic acid at residue 5 (Furthmayr 1978a; Dahr et al. 1977; Wasniowska et al. 1977). This carbohydrate-rich structure containing 15 O-linked and 1 N-linked sugar chains is the major sialoglycoprotein of the red cell membrane (Marchesi et al. 1972; Tomita et al. 1978). As such, GPA is predominantly responsible for the negative surface charge of the red cell membrane. Glycophorin A is expressed early during terminal erythroid differentiation and has not been detected in nonerythroid tissues (Gahmberg et al. 1978; Cartron et al. 1990).

Glycophorin B (GPB), which is present at 80,000 to 300,000 copies per cell, is composed of 72 residues, only six of which are in the cytoplasmic domain (Furthmayr 1978b; Merry et al. 1986; Dahr 1986). The first 26 N-terminal residues are almost identical to those of the N-phenotype of GPA (Furthmayr 1978b; Dahr et al. 1980). Additional blood group antigenic determinants on GPB include S, s and U (Dahr et al. 1980). There are 11 O-linked sugars on GPB. In contrast to GPA, little is known about the tissue-specific expression of GPB.

Glycophorins C (GPC) and D (GPD) are much less abundant in the red cell membrane than are GPA and GPB. There are approximately 50,000 to 100,000 copies of GPC and 20,000 copies of GPD per cell (Anstee et al. 1984). The polypeptide chain of GPC comprises 128 amino-acid residues, of which approximately 57 are exoplasmic, 24 are membrane spanning, and 47 are cytoplasmic (Blanchard et al. 1987a). As GPD is encoded by the same gene as GPC except for differential utilization of translation initiation sites (methionine-1 for GPC and methionine-22 for GPD), the two polypeptides are identical in the transmembrane and cytoplasmic domains, while the exoplasmic domain of GPD is truncated by 21 amino acids (Blanchard et al. 1987b; Dahr et al. 1989; El-Maliki et al. 1989; Le Van Kim et al. 1987). It is interesting to note that the cytoplasmic domains of these two sialoglycoproteins are the longest of the four glycophorins. The carbohydrate composition of GPC consists of 12 O-linked and one N-linked sugars, while that of GPD consists of just six O-linked sugars. The blood group antigens of the Gerbich class are present on these two glycophorins (Dahr et al. 1987; Reid et al. 1987a). Glycophorin C appears on the cell surface much earlier during erythroid development than GPA (Villeval et al. 1989). Moreover, in contrast to GPA, GPC is expressed on the surface of many nonerythroid cells (Cartron et al. 1990).

Recent cloning of the genes for various glycophorins has not only provided detailed information on the primary structure of these molecules but also has enabled the characterization of naturally occurring mutant forms of these molecules (Fig. 7.1). This information, in association with detailed biophysical characterization of normal and mutant red cells, has

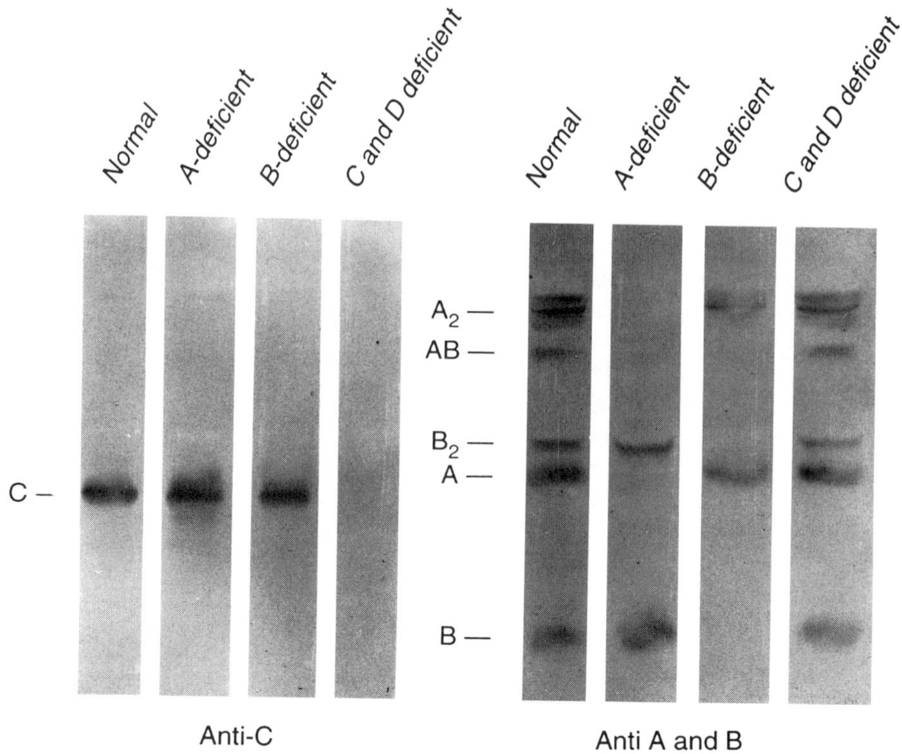

Figure 7.1. A Western blot analysis of red cell membranes lacking various glycophorins. Specific deficiencies of the different sialoglycoproteins were shown in the various phenotypes using anti-GPC and anti-GPA and anti-GPB antibodies. (*Source:* From Reid et al. 1987c.)

enabled us to begin to understand the contributions of GPA and GPC to the regulation of membrane material behavior. In the sections that follow we will review these studies and the new insights they have stimulated.

THE FUNCTION OF GLYCOPHORIN A

Initial serologic screening assays, as well as more recent biochemical and molecular biologic studies, have delineated a group of mutations in the GPA gene. Characterization of the cellular consequences of these mutations has provided crucial leads for understanding the function of GPA. The two mutant phenotypes with complete deficiency of GPA, M^kM^k and En(a−), are particularly relevant in this regard (Tanner and Anstee 1976; Tokunaga et al. 1979). Individuals with these two phenotypes do not have clinically significant anemia; in addition, their red cells display normal discocytic morphology. When membrane material properties of En(a−) red cells were characterized by ektacytometry (Reid et al. 1987c), both membrane deformability and membrane mechanical stability were found to be normal (Fig. 7.2). These findings unequivocally show that GPA has no role in regulating cell shape, membrane deformability, and membrane mechanical stability.

An underappreciated role for GPA is that of bestowing a net negative charge to the red cell membrane through its high sialic acid content. This net negative surface charge is critical for minimizing red cell–red cell interactions and preventing red cell aggregation in circulation. An intriguing associated surface change in red cells lacking GPA [M^kM^k and En(a−) phenotypes] is the increased glycosylation of band 3 resulting from the addition of sialic acid moieties (Gahmberg et al. 1976; Tanner and Anstee 1976; Tokunaga et al. 1979). This posttranslational modification of band 3 partially compensates for the loss of GPA-associated sialic acid moieties. As a consequence, these red cells maintain a net

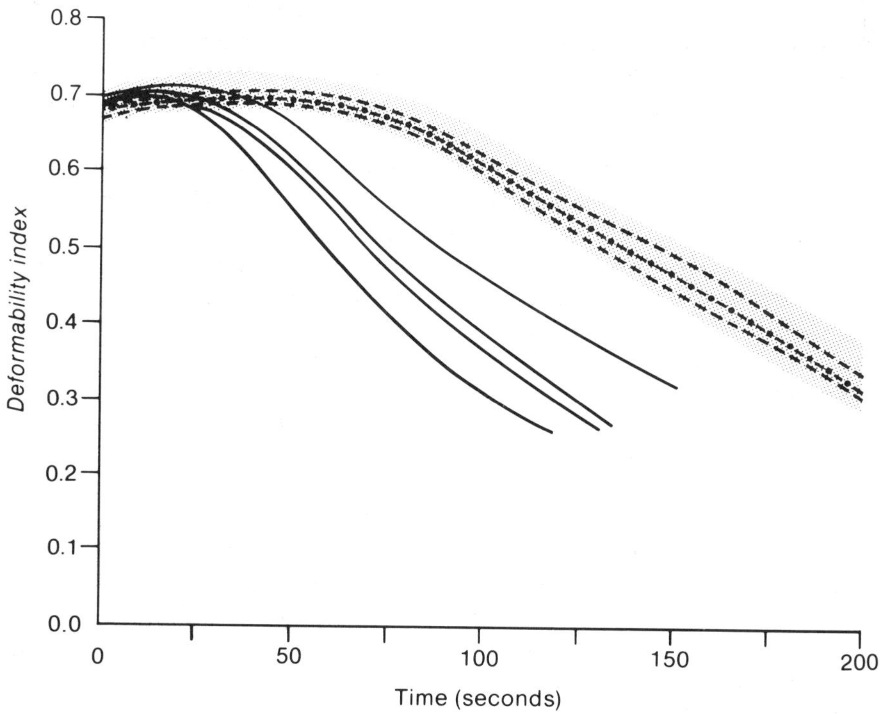

Figure 7.2. The membrane mechanical stability of red cells deficient in various glycophorins. The deformability index of red cell membranes deficient in glycophorins C and D (solid line) decreased more rapidly with time when exposed to constant shear stress than did that of normal red cell membranes (shaded area), implying a decreased mechanical stability. In contrast, the rate of decline of the deformability index of red cell membranes deficient in GPA (-··-) and GPB (---) was normal, implying that these membranes had normal mechanical stability. (*Source:* From Reid et al. 1987c.)

negative surface charge that is only 20 percent less than normal, rather than the 60 percent decrease that would be expected owing to deficiency of GPA. It has been suggested that increased glycosylation of band 3 functionally substitutes for loss of surface charge due to GPA deficiency and accounts for the normal red cell behavior observed in these individuals. Mutations that result in GPA deficiency without a concomitant increase in glycosylation of other membrane proteins may be incompatible with survival. An important function of GPA in the red cell membrane is to prevent cell-cell interactions in the circulation.

While the findings outlined above suggest that GPA in its native state does not have a significant role in regulating either cell shape or membrane material properties, a number of recent studies have shown that after binding of a ligand specific for this protein, profound changes occur in membrane material behavior. The initial observation that led to this series of studies was that binding of the lectin wheat germ agglutinin to the red cell surface inhibited chemically induced echinocytic transformation (Lovrien and Anderson 1980) and markedly reduced red cell membrane deformability (Chasis et al. 1985). Since wheat germ agglutinin binds to a number of red cell surface components in addition to GPA, it was necessary to use ligands specific for GPA to implicate a role for this molecule in the observed membrane changes. After binding of a monoclonal IgG specific for the exoplasmic domain of GPA, a dose-dependent decrease in membrane deformability was induced (Chasis et al. 1985). This alteration in membrane deformability was documented using both ektacytometry and micropipet aspiration technique. To exclude the possibility that the observed membrane changes were induced by formation of an extracellular lattice of cross-linked GPA molecules following binding of divalent IgG, the effect of monovalent Fab fragments on membrane properties was determined. Binding of these monovalent fragments also induced decreased membrane deformability, implying that the observed changes were not the result of formation of an external network lattice (Chasis et al. 1985).

An extensive series of theoretic and experimental studies have shown that membrane deformability is primarily regulated by the organization of the spectrin-based membrane skeletal network (Chasis and Mohandas et al. 1986). We therefore hypothesized that ligand binding induces increased association of the cytoplasmic domain of GPA with the skeletal network, resulting in decreased membrane deformability. A series of experimental approaches were used to validate this hypothesis. As lateral mobility of transmembrane proteins is regulated by the interaction of the cytoplasmic domains of these proteins with the underlying skeletal or cytoskeletal structures, one prediction of the hypothesis is that following ligand-binding the lateral mobility of GPA should be significantly retarded. Using the technique of fluorescence recovery after photobleaching, lateral mobility of GPA molecules in the liganded and nonliganded state was measured. Binding of both intact IgG and its monovalent Fab fragment indeed resulted in a marked decrease in lateral mobility of GPA (Knowles et al. 1990), validating the hypothesis that ligand binding induces increased association of the cytoplasmic domain with the underlying skeletal network. A second prediction of our hypothesis is that ligand binding will not decrease either membrane deformability or lateral mobility of GPA in red cells with a variant GPA lacking a cytoplasmic domain. Such a variant molecule exists in Miltenberger V red cells, which contain no normal GPA molecules, but rather a variant sialoglycoprotein that is a hybrid molecule composed of the exoplasmic domain of GPA and transmembrane and cytoplasmic domains of GPB (Mawby et al. 1981). As a result, this mutant GPA has a significantly truncated cytoplasmic domain of only six amino acids compared with 39 cytoplasmic residues in normal GPA. Since the exoplasmic domain of mutant GPA contains the antigenic epitopes for the anti-GPA antibodies, we were able to measure the effects of ligand binding on membrane properties (Chasis et al. 1988). No significant changes in either membrane deformability or lateral mobility of GPA were noted after ligand binding to Miltenberg V red cells (Fig. 7.3). This series of studies unequivocally established that cytoplasmic domain of GPA is necessary for ligand-induced changes in membrane properties. Based on these findings we proposed the following model for GPA in the red cell membrane (Fig. 7.4). In the native state, the cytoplasmic domain of GPA has little or no interaction with the skeletal network; however, ligand binding induces a conformational change in the cytoplasmic domain that results in its increased association with the skeletal network.

An interesting feature of ligand-induced changes in membrane properties is that the phenomenon is specific for GPA. For example, binding of ligands specific for other red cell surface components, including band 3 and blood group antigens A, B, Rh, and Kell, do not alter membrane properties (Pasvol et al. 1989). An additional interesting feature of the GPA-ligand–induced deformability change is that the extent of deformability decrease can be modulated by varying the ligand binding site on the exoplasmic domain (Fig. 7.5) (Chasis et al. 1988). Binding of a monoclonal antibody to an epitope close to the N-terminus of GPA increased membrane rigidity 5.8-fold; binding to an epitope in the mid-region of the exoplasmic domain resulted in a 10.8-fold increase in membrane rigidity; while binding to an epitope between residues 56 and 67 close to the membrane increased rigidity 18-fold (Fig. 7.6). While the mechanism for this modulatable process has not yet been delineated, we speculate that the extent of conformational change in the cytoplasmic domain depends on the site of ligand binding. We suggest that the closer the binding site is to the bilayer, the larger the extent of conformational change induced and the greater the interaction between the cytoplasmic domain of GPA and the skeletal network.

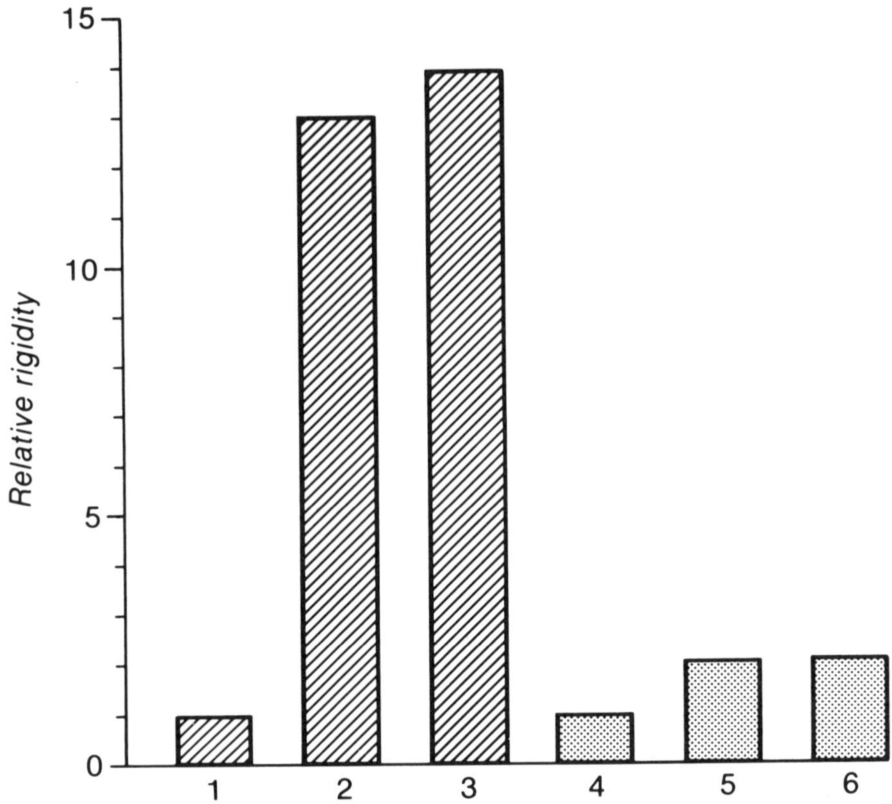

Figure 7.3. The effect of antibodies R10 and 10F7 on the relative rigidity of normal red cell and Miltenberg V red cells. The deformability of nonliganded normal cells (lane 1) and Miltenberg V cells (lane 4) was normal, with a relative rigidity of 1. The relative rigidity of normal cells after R10 (lane 2) and 10F7 (lane 3) binding was 13.1 and 13.9, respectively. The rigidity of Miltenberg red cells after R10 (lane 5) and 10F7 (lane 6) binding increased only minimally. These results imply that marked increases in antibody-induced rigidity require the presence of the cytoplasmic domain of GPA. (*Source:* Reproduced from the *Journal of Cell Biology* (1988) 107:1351–57, by copyright permission of the Rockefeller University Press.)

While these data clearly established that ligand binding induces increased association of the cytoplasmic domain of GPA with the skeletal network, the specific nature of this association is unclear. One association that has received considerable attention is a phosphoinositide modulatable interaction between GPA and protein 4.1, reported by Anderson and Marchesi (1985). However, our finding that ligand binding to GPA induces rigidity in red cells totally deficient in protein 4.1 (Chasis et al. 1985) implies that the proposed interaction between protein 4.1 and GPA plays no part in the observed membrane changes. What remains to be elucidated is whether the observed membrane changes are the result of a specific protein-protein interaction or whether changes in the confor-

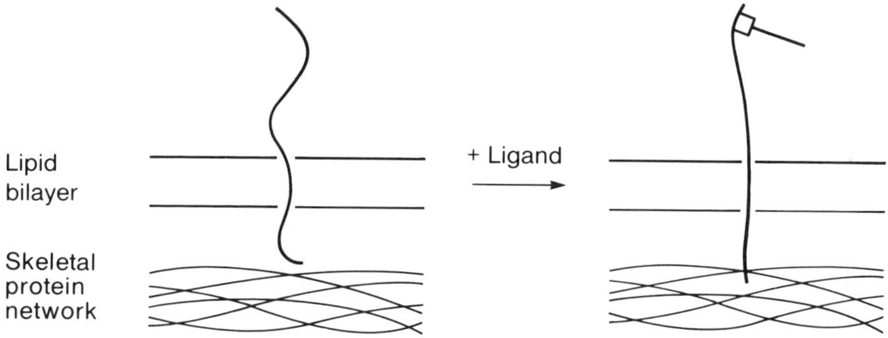

Figure 7.4. A model of the effect of ligand binding on GPA. In the nonliganded state, the cytoplasmic domain of GPA is free-floating and not associated with the skeletal protein network. Ligand binding induces a conformational change that causes the cytoplasmic domain of glycophorin to come into close contact with the skeletal protein lattice, resulting either in entanglement in the lattice or in a specific protein-protein interaction with a component of the lattice. Both these occurrences would cause increased membrane rigidity. Individual protein components of the skeletal protein network have not been delineated, since the exact nature of the interaction of liganded GPA with any one specific component is unclear at present. (*Source:* Reproduced from the *Journal of Cell Biology* (1988) 107:1351–57, by copyright permission of the Rockefeller University Press.)

mation of the cytoplasmic domain of GPA allows this domain to become physically entangled with the dense underlying skeletal lattice. The nature of this interaction, as well as the physiologic relevance of this inducible alteration in membrane properties, are two of the critical unanswered questions in GPA biology.

There is also considerable interest and debate concerning an interaction between GPA and the other major red cell transmembrane protein, band 3. Both these proteins have been shown to be constituents of the intramembranous particles seen in freeze-fracture electron microscopy of red cell membrane (Tillack et al. 1972; Pinto da Silva and Nicolson 1974). Moreover, it has been noted that rotational mobility of band 3 molecules are affected by antibody-induced cross-linking of GPA (Nigg et al. 1980). Recent studies on Wr^b antigen expression showed that monoclonal antibodies specific for this antigen immunoprecipitated both GPA and band 3 and reacted by radioimmunoassay only with cells that expressed both of these proteins (Telen and Chasis 1990). These data strongly suggest that both transmembrane proteins are involved in the expression of Wr^b and, considered with earlier studies, suggest that at least some portion of band 3 and GPA molecules are closely associated in the red cell membrane.

While much remains to be learned regarding ligand-induced membrane changes and GPA–band 3 associations in the membrane, it can be categorically stated that a major physiologic function of GPA is to bestow negative surface charge to the membrane, thus minimizing cell-cell interactions.

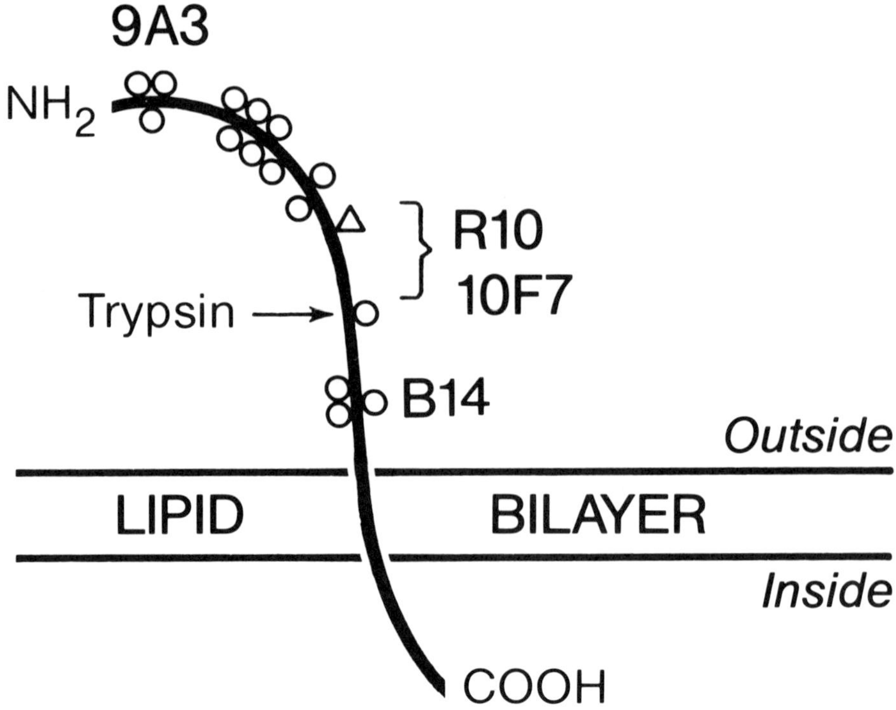

Figure 7.5. A schematic drawing of GPA with the antibody binding sites. The peptide backbone with its 15 O-linked (○) and one N-linked (△) tetrasaccharides is shown traversing the lipid bilayer. The blood group antigens M and N are determined by variations within the first five amino acids in the amino terminal end of the molecule. The monoclonal antibody 9A3 has anti-M specificity and binds to the amino terminus. Antibodies R10 and 10F7 bind in the mid-region of the extracellular portion of GPA distal to the site of trypsin cleavage. Antibody B14 detects an epitope closely adjacent to the lipid bilayer, between residues 56 and 57. (*Source:* Reproduced from the *Journal of Cell Biology* (1988) 107:1351–57, by copyright permission of the Rockefeller University Press.)

THE FUNCTION OF GLYCOPHORIN C

As with GPA, a number of mutations involving the GPC gene result in red cells that either are completely deficient in GPC or contain a variant form of the sialoglycoprotein (Anstee et al. 1984; Colin et al. 1989; High et al. 1989; Chang et al. 1991). The characterization of the cellular consequences of these mutations has provided crucial leads for understanding the function of GPC (Reid et al. 1987b, 1987c). The Leach phenotype, characterized by a complete deficiency of GPC, does not cause clinically significant anemia. However, the red cells do exhibit both altered cell shape, predominantly elliptocytic (Anstee et al. 1984), and marked abnormalities in membrane properties (Reid et al. 1987c). Ektacytometric measurements of membrane properties revealed a decreased

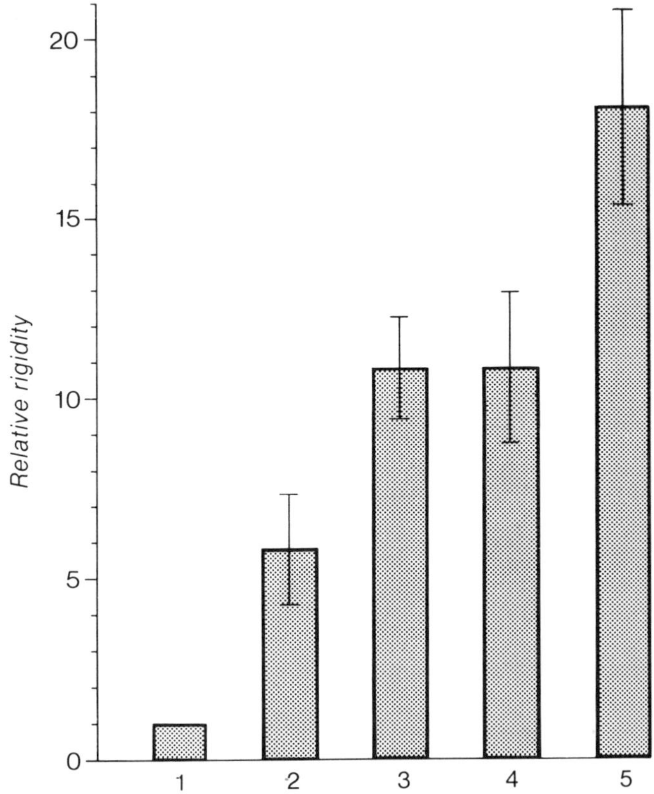

Figure 7.6. The maximal relative rigidity of MM red cells induced by antibodies 9A3, 10F7, R10, and B14. Antibody binding to different regions of GPA induces different degrees of increase in the membrane rigidity. Control red cells with no bound antibody (lane 1) have normal deformability and a relative rigidity of 1. The binding of 9A3 (lane 2) produces cells with a relative rigidity of 5.8 + 1.5; 10F7 (lane 3), cells with a relative rigidity of 10.8 + 1.4; R10 (lane 4), cells with a relative rigidity of 10.8 + 2.1; and B14 (lane 5), cells with a relative rigidity of 18.2 + 2.7. (*Source:* Reproduced from the *Journal of Cell Biology* (1988) 107:1351–57, by copyright permission of the Rockefeller University Press.)

membrane deformability and a marked reduction in membrane mechanical stability (see Fig. 7.2). When the same blood samples were analyzed by micropipet analysis of individual cells, the abnormality in deformability was not detected, revealing the limitations of that technique (Nash et al. 1990). These abnormalities in cell shape and membrane properties are in dramatic contrast to the normal discocytic morphology and normal membrane properties of GPA-deficient red cells. The findings with Leach phenotype red cells imply that GPC has a critical role in regulating the shape of the red cell and the properties of membrane material.

A series of GPC mutant phenotypes characterized not by quantitative deficiency of the sialoglycoprotein but by qualitative defects in the exoplasmic domain of the polypeptide have also been identified (Colin et al.

1989; High et al. 1989; Chang et al. 1991). Cellular characterization of these mutant phenotypes with an abnormal exoplasmic domain but a normal cytoplasmic domain has enabled us to define the role of various domains in regulating membrane function. The Yus phenotype is characterized by a deletion of 19 amino acids (N-terminal amino acids 17 to 35), the Gerbich phenotype by a deletion of 28 amino acids (N-terminal amino acids 36 to 63), and the Webb phenotype by a substitution of serine for asparagine at position 8. Thus the Yus, Gerbich, and Webb phenotypes all have mutations limited to the region of the gene encoding the exoplasmic domain, while the primary structure of the cytoplasmic domains in these variant cells is normal (Chang et al. 1991). Red cells with these variant forms of GPC, in contrast to red cells of the Leach phenotype, have normal discocytic morphology and exhibit normal membrane deformability and mechanical stability (Fig. 7.7) (Reid et al. 1987b). The normal membrane properties of these phenotypes, in the context of a structurally normal cytoplasmic domain, implies that the cytoplasmic

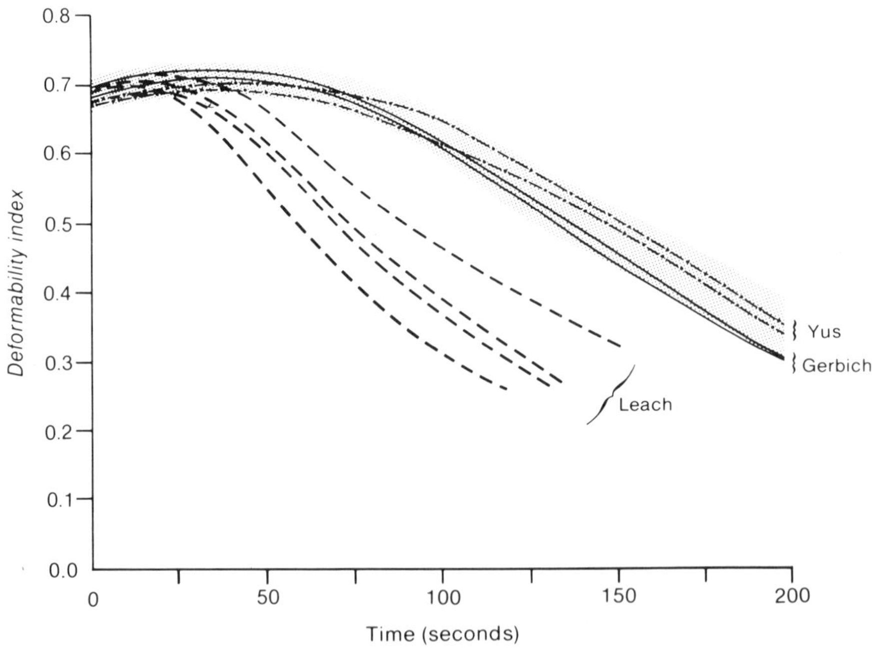

Figure 7.7. The membrane mechanical stability of red cells with various mutant GPC polypeptides. The deformability index of resealed membranes prepared from red cells of the Leach phenotype (dashed line) decreased more rapidly with time than did normal membranes (shaded area), implying a decreased mechanical stability. In contrast, the rate of decline of the deformability index of membranes of the Gerbich and Yus phenotypes was normal, implying that these membranes had normal mechanical stability. (*Source:* From Reid et al. 1987b.)

domain of GPC is critical for maintaining normal shape and regulating membrane properties.

As discussed previously, the interaction of the cytoplasmic domains of integral proteins with the spectrin-based skeletal network has a regulatory role in modulating membrane material properties. Having identified a role for the cytoplasmic domain of GPC in this regard, the next issue to be addressed is the nature of interaction between the cytoplasmic domain and the components of the skeletal network. Mueller and Morrison originally suggested a specific interaction between the cytoplasmic domain of GPC and protein 4.1 based on the finding that nonionic detergents do not extract GPC from normal membranes but do extract this sialoglycoprotein from membranes deficient in the skeletal component protein 4.1 (Müeller and Morrison 1981). Subsequent studies by several investigators have validated this hypothesis, including experiments by Elliot and Ralston that glycophorin C and protein 4.1 co-purify after extraction from the red cell membrane (Elliot and Ralston 1984). Furthermore, a number of studies have shown that the GPC content of the red cell membrane is related to the protein 4.1 content (Alloisio et al. 1985; Reid et al. 1990; Sondag et al. 1987). Specifically, flow cytometry showed that the GPC content of membranes with 50 percent deficiency of protein 4.1 was 44 percent of normal, while it was only 9 percent of normal in membranes totally deficient in protein 4.1. Molecular analysis of both GPC and protein 4.1 genes in these individuals showed only an abnormality in the protein 4.1 gene, implying that GPC deficiency in these membranes is not the result of a primary defect in the sialoglycoprotein itself but is secondary to protein 4.1 deficiency (Reid et al. 1990). It was inferred from these data that GPC may be anchored within the lipid bilayer through its association with protein 4.1. Direct support for an anchoring role for protein 4.1 has recently been provided by a series of experiments in which detergent extractability of GPC was examined in protein 4.1–deficient red cells (1) in their native state and (2) after reconstitution with exogenously purified protein 4.1 (Reid et al. 1990). Whereas GPC was readily extractable from native protein 4.1–deficient membranes, this sialoglycoprotein was retained with the spectrin-based network following reconstitution of these deficient membranes with purified protein 4.1 (Fig. 7.8). These protein 4.1 reconstitution experiments provide the most convincing evidence to date that this skeletal protein serves as an anchor for GPC in the red cell membrane. Although no direct binding studies have yet evaluated the interaction between the cytoplasmic domain of GPC and protein 4.1, the accumulated evidence to date with the mutant red cells strongly suggests such an interaction does indeed take place and that it is physiologically relevant.

As outlined in our discussion of GPA, Anderson and Marchesi (1985) have suggested an interaction between protein 4.1 and GPA modulated by phosphoinositides. While these provocative studies have generated

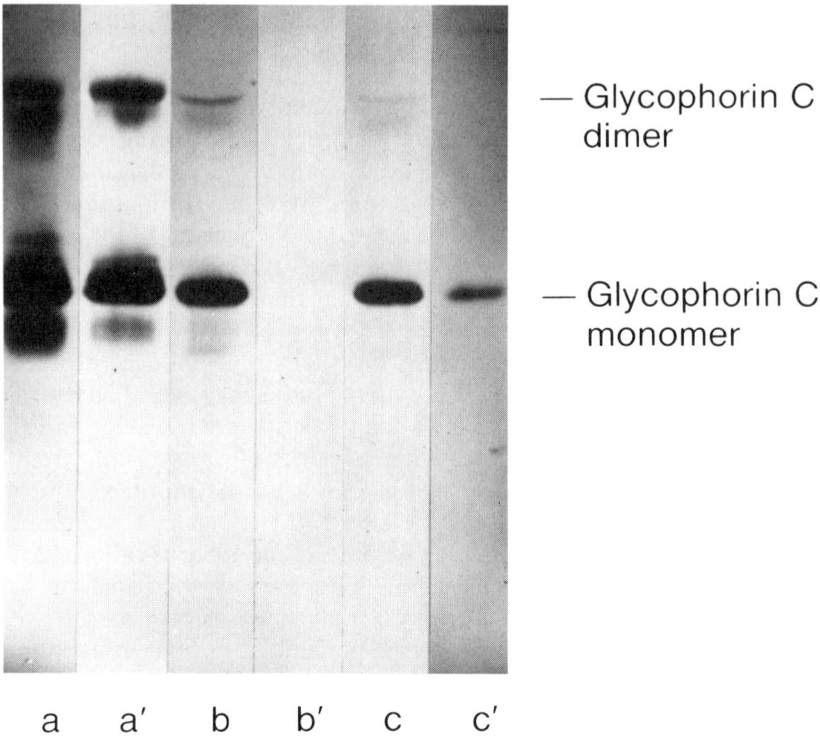

Figure 7.8. A Western blot analysis using anti-GPC antibody on membranes and detergent-extracted membrane skeletons from protein 4.1–deficient red cells before and after reconstitution with purified protein 4.1. The first two lanes show the presence of GPC in membranes (lane a) and detergent-extracted membrane skeletons (lane a′) from normal red cells. Lane b shows that GPC is present in totally protein 4.1–deficient membranes but absent from detergent-extracted membrane skeletons prepared from these membranes (lane b′). The last two lanes show the results of tests on protein 4.1–deficient membranes that have been reconstituted with exogenous protein 4.1. Glycophorin C is present in both the membrane (lane c) and the detergent-extracted membrane skeletons (lane c′). (*Source:* From Reid et al. 1990.)

considerable interest and debate, we believe that the conclusions from these studies must be considered with a certain degree of caution. In particular, there is a significant concern that the glycophorin preparations used in these binding studies may have contained GPC as well as GPA. As evidence continues to accumulate regarding the interaction between GPC and protein 4.1, it is critical that these binding studies be performed with well-characterized preparations of GPA to ascribe unequivocally an interaction between this major sialoglycoprotein and protein 4.1. Finally, it is difficult to assign a physiologically important role for the proposed interaction between GPA and protein 4.1 in light of the observed normal membrane behavior of cells completely deficient in GPA.

While much remains to be learned regarding the molecular nature of the interaction between GPC and protein 4.1, it can be categorically stated that GPC plays a functionally important part in regulating red cell shape and membrane properties, and that protein 4.1 serves as a membrane anchor for this sialoglycoprotein.

CONCLUSIONS AND SPECULATIONS

The evidence accumulated to date has identified some important and previously unsuspected functions for various red cell sialoglycoproteins. Glycophorin A is the key membrane constituent involved in bestowing negative surface charge, which is critical for minimizing cell-cell interactions in the circulation. While this sialoglycoprotein in its native state does not appear to have a role in regulating either cell shape or membrane material properties, ligand binding to this surface component induces profound increases in membrane rigidity. This ligand-binding–induced change in membrane properties is the result of increased association of the cytoplasmic domain of GPA with the skeletal network. This inducible change in membrane behavior can be considered to be a form of signal transduction akin to ligand-induced changes in cellular functions noted in granulocytes and platelets. Detailed molecular characterization of the mechanism involved in GPA signal transduction may provide insights into novel cell communication pathways.

In contrast to GPA, GPC in the native state appears to have a critical role in regulating cell shape, membrane deformability, and membrane mechanical stability. The regulation of these membrane functions appears to be through the interaction of the cytoplasmic domain of GPC with protein 4.1. The finding of GPC and protein 4.1 in a wide variety of nonerythroid cells raises the possibility that the interaction between these two proteins may have important but as yet undefined functions in these types of cells.

The observation that GPA and GPC, in addition to carrying specific blood group antigenic determinants, also regulate membrane function leads us to speculate that other membrane proteins that are currently viewed solely as antigenic determinants may also have other important functional roles. Defining the functions of these various red cell membrane integral proteins is a challenge that lies ahead of us.

REFERENCES

Alloisio, N., L. Morle, D. Bachir, D. Guetarni, D. Colonna, and J. Delaunay. 1985. Red cell membrane sialoglycoprotein in homozygous and heterozygous 4.1(−) hereditary elliptocytosis. *Biochem. Biophys. Acta* 816:57.

Anderson, R. A. and V. T. Marchesi. 1985. Regulation of the association of membrane skeletal protein 4.1 with glycophorin A by polyphosphoinositide. *Nature* 318:295.

Anstee, D. J. 1981. The blood group MNSs-active sialoglycoproteins. *Semin. Hematol.* 18:13.

Anstee, D. J., S. F. Parsons, K. Ridgwell, M. J. A. Tanner, A. H. Merry, E. E. Thomson, P. A. Judson, P. Johnson, S. Bates, and I. D. Fraser. 1984. Two individuals with elliptocytic red cells lack three minor erythrocyte membrane sialoglycoproteins. *Biochem. J.* 218:615–19.

Blanchard, D., W. Dahr, M. Hummel, F. Latron, K. Beyreuther, and J. P. Cartron. 1987a. Glycophorin B and C from human erythrocyte membranes: Purification and sequence analysis. *J. Biol. Chem.* 262:5808–11.

Blanchard, D., B. El-Maliki, P. Hermand, W. Dahr, and J. P. Cartron. 1987b. Structural homology between glycophorins C and D, two minor glycoproteins of the human erythrocyte membrane carrying blood group Gerbich antigen. In *Proceedings of the Ninth International Symposium on Glycoconjugates.* F54. Lille, France.

Cartron, J. P., Y. Colin, S. Kudo, and M. Fukuda. 1990. Molecular genetics of human erythrocyte sialoglycoproteins glycophorins A, B, C and D. In *Blood cell biochemistry*. Vol. 1. J. R. Harris, ed. 322. New York, Plenum Publishing.

Chang, S., M. E. Reid, J. Conboy, Y. W. Kan, and N. Mohandas. 1991. Molecular characterization of erythrocyte glycophorin C variants. *Blood* 77: 644–48.

Chasis, J. A., N. Mohandas, and S. B. Shohet. 1985. Erythrocyte membrane rigidity induced by glycophorin A-ligand interaction: Evidence for a ligand-induced association between glycophorin A and skeletal proteins. *J. Clin. Invest.* 75:1919–26.

Chasis, J. A., and N. Mohandas. 1986. Erythrocyte membrane deformability and stability: Two distinct membrane properties that are independently regulated by skeletal protein associations. *J. Cell Biol.* 103:343–50.

Chasis, J. A., M. E. Reid, R. H. Jensen, and N. Mohandas. 1988. Signal transduction by glycophorin A: Role of extracellular and cytoplasmic domains in a modulatable process. *J. Cell Biol* 107:1351–57.

Colin, Y., C. Le Van Kim, A. Tsapis, M. Clerget, L. d'Auriol, J. London, and J. P. Cartron. 1989. Human erythrocyte glycophorin C: Gene structure and rearrangement in genetic variants. *J. Biol. Chem.* 264:3773.

Dahr, W., G. Uhlenbruck, E. Janssen, and R. Schmalisch. 1977. Different N-terminal amino acids in the M,N glycoprotein from MM and NN erythrocytes. *Hum. Genet.* 35:335–43.

Dahr, W., K. Beyreuther, H. Steinbach, W. Gielen, and J. Kruger. 1980. Structure of the Ss blood group antigens. II. A methionine/threonine polymorphism within the N-terminal sequence of the Ss glycoprotein. *Hoppe Seyler Z. Physiol. Chem.* 361:895–906.

Dahr, W. 1986. Immunochemistry of sialoglycoproteins in human red blood cell membranes. In *Recent advances in blood group biochemistry*. V. Vengelen-Tyler and W. J. Judd, eds. 23–65. Arlington, Va: American Association of Blood Banks.

Dahr, W., S. Kiedrowski, D. Blanchard, P. Hermand, J. J. Moulds, and J. P. Carton. 1987. High-frequency antigens of human erythrocyte membrane sialoglycoproteins. V. Characterization of the Gerbich blood group antigens. Ge2 and Ge3. *Biol. Chem. Hoppe Seyler* 368:1375–83.

Dahr, W., D. Blanchard, S. Kiedrowski, A. Poschmann, J. P. Cartron, and J. Moulds. 1989. High-frequency antigens of human erythrocytes membrane sialoglycoproteins. VI. Monoclonal antibodies reacting with the N-terminal domain of glycophorin C. *Biol. Chem. Hoppe Seyler* 370:849–54.

Elliot, C., and G. B. Ralston. 1984. Solubilization of human erythrocyte band 4.1 protein in non-ionic detergent Tween-20. *Biochem. Biophys. Acta* 775:313.

El-Maliki, B., D. Blanchard, W. Dahr, K. Beyreuther, and J. P. Cartron. 1989.

Structural homology between glycophorins C and D of human erythrocytes. *Eur. J. Biochem.* 183:639–43.

Fairbanks, G., T. L. Steck, and D. F. H. Wallach. 1971. Electrophoretic analysis of the major polypeptides of the human erythrocyte membrane. *Biochemistry* 10:2602–17.

Furthmayr, H. 1978a. Glycophorins A, B, C: A family of sialoglycoproteins. Isolation and preliminary characterization of trypsin-derived peptides. *J. Supramol. Struct.* 9:79–95.

——— 1978b. Structural comparison of glycophorins and immunochemical analysis of genetic variants. *Nature* 271:519–24.

Gahmberg, C. G., G. Myllyla, J. Leikola, A. Pirkola, and S. Nordling. 1976. Absence of the major sialoglycoprotein in the membrane of human En(a−) erythrocytes and increased glycosylation of band 3. *J. Biol. Chem.* 251: 6108–16.

Gahmberg, C. G., M. Jokinen, and L. C. Andersson. 1978. Expression of major sialoglycoprotein (glycophorin) on erythroid cells in human bone marrow. *Blood* 52:379–87.

High, S., M. J. A. Tanner, E. B. Macdonald, and D. J. Anstee. 1989. Rearrangements of the red-cell membrane glycophorin C (sialoglycoprotein β) gene: A further study of the alterations in the glycophorin C gene. *Biochem. J.* 262:47.

Knowles, D., J. A. Chasis, E. Evans, and N. Mohandas. 1990. Decreased lateral mobility of glycophorin A following ligand binding: Implications for a signal transduction process involving the cytoplasmic domain. *Blood* 76(Suppl. 1):10a.

Kudo, S., and M. Fukuda. 1990. Identification of a novel glycophorin, glycophorin E, by isolation of genomic clones and complementary DNA clones using polymerase chain reaction. *J. Biol. Chem.* 265:1102–10.

Le Van Kim, C., Y. Colin, D. Blanchard, W. Dahr, J. London, and J. P. Cartron. 1987. Gerbich group deficiency of the Ge:1,−2,−3 and Ge:1,−2,−3 types. *Eur. J. Biochem.* 165:571–79.

Lovrien, R. E., and R. A. Anderson. 1980. Stoichiometry of wheat germ agglutinin as a morphology controlling agent and as a morphology protective agent for the human erythrocyte. *J. Cell Biol.* 85:534–48.

Marchesi, V. T., T. W. Tillack, R. L. Jackson, J. P. Segrest, and R. E. Scott. 1972. Chemical characterization and surface orientation of the major glycoprotein of the human erythrocyte membrane. *Proc. Natl. Acad. Sci. U.S.A.* 69:1445–49.

Mattei, M. G., Y. Colin, C. Le Van Kim, J. F. Mattei, and J. P. Cartron. 1986. Localization of the gene for human erythrocyte glycophorin C to chromosome 2, q14-q21. *Hum. Genet.* 74:420.

Mawby, W. J., D. J. Anstee and M. J. A. Tanner. 1981. Immunochemical evidence for hybrid sialoglycoproteins of human erythrocytes. *Nature* 291: 161–62.

Merry, A. H., E. E. Thompson, D. J. Anstee, and F. Stratton. 1984. The quantification of erythrocyte antigen sites with monoclonal antibodies. *Immunology* 51:793–800.

Merry, A. H. J., C. Hodson, E. Thomson, G. Maallinson, and D. J. Anstee. 1986. The use of monoclonal antibodies to quantify the levels of sialoglycoproteins a and d variant sialoglycoproteins in human erythrocyte membranes. *Biochem. J.* 233:93–98.

Mueller, T. J. and M. Morrison. 1981. Glycoconnectin (PAS 2); a membrane attachment site for the human erythrocyte cytoskeleton. In *Erythrocyte membranes II: Recent clinical and experimental advances.* G. Brewer and J. Eaton, eds. 85. New York: Alan R Liss.

Nash, G. B., Parmar, J., and Reid, M. E. 1990. Effects of deficiency of glycophorins C and D on the physical properties of the red cell. *Brit. J. Haem.* 76:282–87.

Nigg, E. A., C. Bron, M. Girardet, and R. J. Cherry. 1980. Band 3–glycophorin A association in erythrocyte membrane demonstrated by combining protein diffusion measurements with antibody-induced cross-linking. *Biochemistry* 19:1887.

Pasvol, G., J. A. Chasis, N. Mohandas, D. J. Anstee, M. J. A. Tanner, and A. H. Merry. 1989. Inhibition of malaria parasite invasion by monoclonal antibodies against glycophorin A correlates with reduction in red cell membrane deformability. *Blood* 74:1836–43.

Pinto da Silva, P., and G. L. Nicolson. 1974. Freeze-etch localization of concanavalin A receptor to the membrane intercalated particles of human erythrocyte ghost membranes. *Biochim. Biophys. Acta* 363:311–19.

Reid, E. M., D. J. Anstee, M. J. A. Tanner, K. Ridgwell, and C. T. Nurse. 1987a. Structural relationships between human erythrocyte sialoglycoproteins β and γ and abnormal sialoglycoproteins found in certain rare human erythrocyte variants lacking the Gerbich blood group antigen(s). *Biochem. J.* 244: 123–28.

Reid, M. E., D. J. Anstee, R. H. Jensen, and N. Mohandas. 1987b. Normal membrane function of abnormal β-related erythrocyte sialoglycoproteins. *Br. J. Haematol.* 67:467.

Reid, M. E., J. A. Chasis, and N. Mohandas. 1987c. Identification of a functional role for human erythrocyte sialoglycoproteins β and γ. *Blood* 69:1068–72.

Reid, M. E., Y. Takakuwa, J. Conboy, G. Tchernia, and N. Mohandas. 1990. Glycophorin C content of human erythrocyte membrane is regulated by protein 4.1. *Blood* 75:2229–34.

Siebert, P. D., and M. Fukuda. 1987. Molecular cloning of human glycophorin B cDNA: Nucleotide sequence and relationship to glycophorin A. *Proc. Natl. Acad. Sci. U.S.A.* 84:6735. (Erratum *Proc. Natl. Acad. Sci. U.S.A.* 1988;85:421.

Sondag, D., N. N. Alloisio, D. Blanchard, M. T. Ducluzeau, P. Colonna, D. Bachir, C. Bloy, J. P. Cartron, and J. Delaunay. 1987. Gerbich reactivity in 4.1(−) hereditary elliptocytosis and protein 4.1 level in blood group Gerbich deficiency. *Br. J. Haematol.* 65:43–50.

Tanner, M. J. A., and D. J Anstee. 1976. The membrane change in En(a−) human erythrocytes: Absence of the major erythrocyte sialoglycoprotein. *Biochem. J.* 153:271.

Tanner, M. J. A., S. High, P. G. Martin, D. J. Anstee, P. A. Judson, and T. J. Jones. 1988. Genetic variants of human red-cell membrane sialoglycoprotein β: Study of the alterations occurring in the sialoglycoprotein-b gene. *Biochem. J.* 250:407–14.

Tate, C. G., and M. J. A. Tanner. 1988. Isolation of cDNA clones for human erythrocyte membrane sialoglycoproteins α and δ. *Biochem. J.* 254:743.

Telen, M., and J. A. Chasis. 1990. Relationship of the human erythrocyte Wr^b antigen to an interaction between glycoprotein A and band 3. *Blood* 76: 842–48.

Tillack, T. W., R. E. Scott, and V. T. Marchesi. 1972. The structure of erythrocyte membrane studied by freeze-etching. II. Localization of receptors for phytohemagglutinin and influenza virus to the intramembranous particles. *J. Exp. Med.* 135:1209–27.

Tokunaga, E., S. Sasakawa, K. Tamaka H. Kawamata, C. M. Giles, E. W. Ikin, J. Poole, D. J. Anstee, W. Mawby, and M. J. A. Tanner. 1979. Two apparently healthy Japanese individuals to type MkMk have erythrocytes which lack both the blood group MN and Ss-active sialoglycoproteins. *J. Immunogenet.* 6:383.

Tomita, M. and V. T. Marchesi. 1975. Amino-acid sequence and oligosaccharide attachment sites of human erythrocyte glycophorin. *Proc. Natl. Acad. Sci. U.S.A.* 72:2964–68.

Tomita, M., H. Furthmayr, and V. T. Marchesi. 1978. Primary structure of human erythrocyte glycophorin A. Isolation and characterization of peptides and complete amino acid sequence. *Biochemistry* 17:4756–70.

Vignal, A., C. Rahuel, J. London, B. Cherif-Zahar, S. Schaff, C. Hattub C, Y. Okubo, and J. P. Cartron. 1990. A novel gene member of the glycophorin A and B gene family: Molecular cloning and expression. *Eur. J. Biochem.* 191: 619–25.

Villeval, J. L., C. Le Van Kim, A. Bettaieb, N. Debili, Y. Colin, B. El-Maliki, D. Blanchard, W. Vainchenker, and J. P. Cartron. 1989. Early expression of glycophorin C during normal and leukemic human erythroid differentiation. *Cancer Res.* 49:2626:29.

Wasniowska, K., Z. Drzeniek, and E. Lisowoska. 1977. The amino acids of M and N blood group glycopeptides are different. *Biochem. Biophys. Res. Commun.* 76:385–90.

8

THE USE OF MONOCLONAL ANTIBODIES TO DETERMINE THE DISTRIBUTION OF RED CELL SURFACE PROTEINS ON CELLS AND TISSUES

David J. Anstee, Ph.D.,
Christopher H. Holmes, Ph.D.,
Philip A. Judson, Ph.D.,
and Michael J. A. Tanner, Ph.D.

Since the original studies of Kohler and Milstein (1975), numerous monoclonal antibodies have been raised to surface proteins of the human red blood cell. This chapter summarizes our studies using some of these monoclonal antibodies to investigate the occurrence of red cell surface proteins on other human cells and tissues.

THE REACTIVITY OF MONOCLONAL ANTIBODIES WITH HEMOPOIETIC CELLS

The pattern of reactions obtained with monoclonal antibodies to several different red cell surface proteins is summarized in Table 8.1. Antibodies to blood group–active glycoproteins that express MNSs, Gerbich, Rh, Kell, and LW antigens are relatively red cell–specific in peripheral blood, and their reactivity with hemopoietic cell lines is, for the most part, restricted to those lines with erythroid/myeloid characteristics (K562, HEL, HL60, U937). In contrast, CD55 [decay-accelerating factor (DAF)], which carries Cromer blood group antigens, and CD44, which carries In^a/In^b blood group antigens, have a wide pattern of reactivity. A similar pattern is observed for antibodies to CD47, CD58 (LFA-3), and CD59 (HRF20). Blood group antigens have not, as yet, been assigned to these glycoproteins. The wide distribution of CD55 and CD59 is consistent with their general role in the inhibition of autologous complement activation (Hadam 1989b, 1989c), while the broad reactivity found for CD44 and CD58 reflects their involvement in cell adhesion interactions (Stoll et al. 1989; Shaw and Johnson 1989). CD47 is a widely distributed glycoprotein of unknown function that shows reduced expression in red cells of the rare Rh_{null} phenotype (Avent et al. 1988; Hadam 1989a; Spring et al. 1989).

During the maturation of erythroid cells in bone marrow, the major red cell proteins appear in the order glycophorin C (GPC), Rh, glycophorin A (GPA), band 3 (reviewed in Telen 1990). Glycophorin C and Rh are found in progenitor cells [burst forming units–erythroid (BFU-E) and colony forming units–erythroid (CFU-E), respectively], while GPA and band 3 first appear in the erythroid precursor cells (pronormoblast and basophilic normoblast, respectively).

THE REACTIVITY OF MONOCLONAL ANTIBODIES WITH FETAL LIVER

The mammalian liver is a major site of hemopoiesis during development; in humans, erythropoiesis is established in the liver by about 40 days after ovulation (Emura et al. 1983). Immunostaining studies using anti–red cell antibodies on sections of human fetal liver reveal marked differences in the developmental expression of blood group polypeptides during the hepatic phase of erythropoiesis. For example, the red cell surface proteins band 3 (Wainwright et al. 1989), Rh (Avent et al. 1988), GPA, and GPC (Fig. 8.1a) are widely expressed on erythropoietic cells in first- and second-trimester human fetal liver (Table 8.2). By contrast, other red cell components appear to be absent (CD58) or show very restricted expression (Kell, LW, CD55) at this stage of development. Glycoprotein CD55, for example, is largely confined to cells of the megakaryocyte rather than the red cell lineage (Holmes et al. 1990) in the early fetal liver. On the other hand, Kell antigen cannot be detected in first-trimester fetal liver (Fig. 8.1b), although by the second trimester the product is detectable in isolated hemopoietic cells.

With the exception of CD59 and CD47, which show a very wide tissue distribution in adult life (see Table 8.3), most of the red cell proteins are restricted to hemopoietic cells in the fetal liver and show no expression on developing hepatic epithelial cells (see Table 8.2).

THE REACTIVITY OF MONOCLONAL ANTIBODIES WITH NONHEMOPOIETIC CELLS AND TISSUES

The two most abundant proteins on the surface of the red cell (band 3 and GPA) have very restricted tissue distribution (see Table 8.3). However, in addition to red cells, erythroid band 3 has been localized to a subset of epithelial cells in the collecting tubules of human kidney (Wagner et al. 1987; Wainwright et al. 1989). These cells, the type A intercalated cells, are involved in acid secretion from the kidney. A form of erythroid band 3 that has a truncated N-terminus is found on the basolateral

Table 8.1. The Reactivity of Monoclonal Antibodies to Red Cell Surface Proteins with Other Hemopoietic Cells and Hemopoietic Cell Lines

Red Cell Surface Protein	Blood Group Antigen	Reactivity with Peripheral Blood Cells			
		Lymphocytes	*Granulocytes*	*Monocytes*	*Platelets*
GPA/GPB (n = 1)	MNSs			2	1
GPA (n = 1)		0	0	0	nd
GPC (n = 2)	Gerbich	1	0	0	0
Rh polypeptides 30K/50K (n = 2)	Rh	0	0	0	0
Kell (n = 3)	Kell	0	0	0	0
LW (n = 2)	LW	0	0	1	nd
CD44 (n = 11)	In^a/In^b	3	3	3	0
CD58 (LFA-3) (n = 2)	nk	2	3	3	1
CD55 (DAF) (n = 5)	Cromer	1	2	2	1
CD59 (HRF20) (n = 2)	nk	2	3	2	1
CD47 (n = 6)	nk	3	3	3	2

Note: Performed by immunohistochemical staining (see Fig. 8.1).
Key: 0 = <10% cells positive; 1 = 10–50% cells positive; 2 = 50–90% cells positive; 3 = >90% cells positive; n = number of different monoclonal antibodies used; nd = not done; and nk = not known.

membrane of these cells (Drenckhahn et al. 1989; Fig. 8.1d). Antibodies to GPA also react with some cells in the kidney (Fig. 8.1e), although the identity of these cells is unclear. An antibody to GPC shows a broader tissue reactivity profile, staining not only kidney but also brain and ileum cells (Reid et al. 1990). Glycophorin C interacts with the red cell skeleton through protein 4.1, and the absence of either GPC (Anstee et al. 1984) or protein 4.1 (Feo et al. 1981) is associated with defects in the shape and deformability of the red cell. Analogues of protein 4.1 are known to occur in other tissues (Bennett 1985), so the broad expression of GPC may reflect its general involvement in the maintenance of cytoskeletal association. The wide distribution of GPC has also been noted by Northern blot analysis in kidney (High and Tanner 1987) and in many other tissues (Le Van Kim et al. 1989). A restricted distribution is observed for the minor red cell proteins Kell and LW.

The expression of Cromer-related blood group antigens on a number of adult surface epithelia, including skin and tongue, and on the placental trophoblast epithelium (Table 8.3) has functional implications, since these antigens are known to be carried on the complement regulatory protein decay-accelerating factor (DAF, CD55) (Parsons et al. 1988; Telen et al. 1988). Decay-accelerating factor has an important role in protecting red cells from damage by autologous complement by inhibiting the assembly of and accelerating the decay of C3 and C5 convertases of both classic and alternative pathways. Decay-accelerating factor may function in a similar fashion on epithelial surfaces, where its expression has been noted

Reactivity with Hemopoietic Cell Lines								
K562	*HEL*	*HL60*	*U937*	*IM9*	*EBV-LCL*	*RAJI*	*DAUDI*	*MOLT 4*
0	0				0/1	0		0
2	2	0	0		0	0		0
3	3	0	3	0	1	0	0	0
0	1/2	0	0	0	0	0	0	0
0/1	0	0/1	0		0/1	0/1		0
0	0	0	2	nd	0	0	0	0
1	3	3	3	3	3	3	1	3
3	3	1	2	nd	1	3	1	2
2	1	1	2	2	2	2	1	0
3	1	2	1	2	3	2	1	3
3	3	3	3	nd	3	3	3	3

previously (Medof et al. 1987), although some other, noncomplement-related activity is also possible. The expression of DAF on placental trophoblasts correlates precisely with the anatomically complex course of the fetomaternal interface, suggesting that the molecule may protect the semiallogeneic human conceptus from maternal complement-mediated attack (Holmes et al. 1990). A further complement-regulatory protein, CD59 (HRF20), which acts after CD55 in the complement cascade, protecting human red cells from serum complement by directly restricting the membrane assembly and lytic activity of human C5b-9 proteins, is virtually ubiquitously expressed in human tissues (see Table 8.3 and Fig. 8.1c). This widespread distribution across a spectrum of tissues is also evident for CD47, a 47- 52- kDa glycoprotein in red cells of unknown function (see Table 8.3, Fig. 8.1f).

Glycoproteins CD44 and CD58 are both expressed on a broad range of hemopoietic cells (see Table 8.1). Glycoprotein CD44 is also broadly expressed in nonhemopoietic tissues, whereas CD58 expression appears sparse (see Table 8.3). Available evidence concerning the function of these molecules is consistent with such a tissue distribution. Glycoprotein CD58 is a ligand for CD2, and CD58-CD2 interaction has a well-described role in cell-cell interactions relevant to immune recognition (Makgoba et al. 1989). In contrast, CD44 is a receptor for hyaluronate, which functions not only in lymphocyte activation and homing but also in matrix adhesion. Recent studies have identified two isoforms of CD44: one hemopoietic and the other epithelial (Stamenkovic et al. 1991).

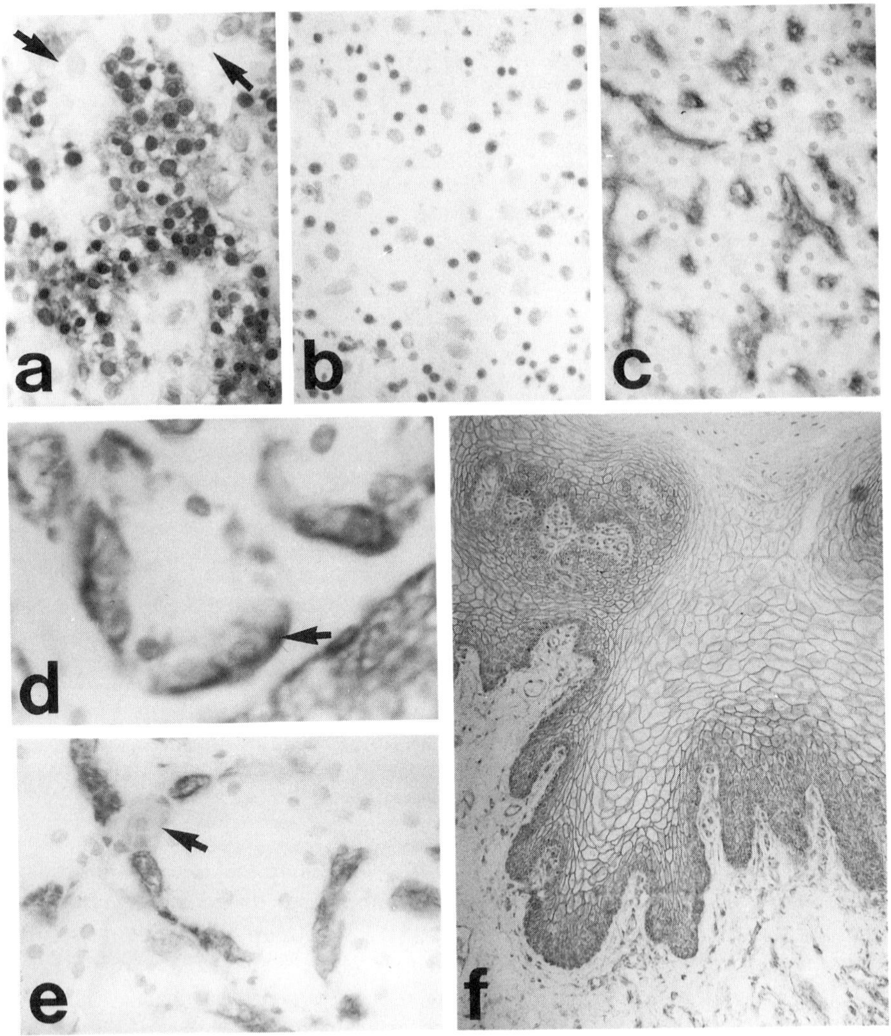

Figure 8.1. The reactivity of monoclonal antibodies to red cells with fetal and adult liver and with nonhemopoietic tissues. **a.** Antibody BGRL100 against GPC stains clusters of hemopoietic cells, most of which are erythroid, in fetal liver at about 6 weeks' gestation. Fetal hepatocytes (arrows) are negative. (×160.) **b.** There is no reactivity in an adjacent section from the same specimen stained with an antibody to Kell (BRIC203), suggesting that early hepatic erythropoietic cells do not express this product. (×160.) **c.** Adult liver sinusoidal cells show intense reactivity with an antibody to CD59 (BRIC229). (×100.) **d.** An antibody to band 3 (BRIC155) stains tubular epithelial cells in the adult kidney. Reactivity appears particularly associated with the basolateral membrane (arrow). (×400.)
e. Antibody BRIC163 to GPA stains isolated cells (arrow) in the adult kidney, although their identity is unknown. (×400.) **f.** Antibody BRIC125 against CD47 stains the epithelium of the tongue. (×40.)

Table 8.2. The Reactivity of Monoclonal Antibodies to Red Cell Surface Proteins with Fetal Liver

		Reactivity with Hemopoietic Cells in		Reactivity with Nonhemopoietic Cells in	
Red Cell Surface Protein	Blood Group Antigen	*1st Trimester*	*2nd Trimester*	*1st Trimester*	*2nd Trimester*
GPA (*n* = 3)	MN	+	+	−	−
GPC (*n* = 3)	Gerbich	+	+	−	−
Band 3 (*n* = 1)	ABH, Ii	+	+	−	−
Rh polypeptides 30K 50K (*n* = 2)	Rh	+	+	−	−
Kell (*n* = 1)	Kell	−	+/−	−	−
LW (*n* = 1)	LW	−	+/−	−	−
CD44 (*n* = 6)	In[a]/In[b]	+*	+*	−	−
CD58 (*n* = 1)	nk	−	−	−	−
CD55 (*n* = 3)	Cromer	+†	+†	−	−
CD59 (*n* = 2)	nk	+	+	+	+
CD47 (*n* = 3)	nk	+	+	+/−	+

*Some cells positive.
†Very few cells positive.
Key: n = number of different monoclonal antibodies used; nk = not known; + = positive reaction; − = negative reaction.

Table 8.3. The Reactivity of Monoclonal Antibodies to Red Cell Surface Proteins with Nonhemopoietic Tissue

Red Cell Surface Protein	Blood Group Antigen	Brain		Gastrointestinal Tract						Blood Vessels	Skin	Spleen	Liver	Kidney		Placenta (term trophoblast)
		Cortex	*Cerebellum*	*Tongue*	*Trachea*	*Stomach*	*Gall-bladder*	*Pancreas*	*Ileum*					*Cortex*	*Medulla*	
GPA (*n* = 1)*	MNSs	–	–	–	–	–	–	–	–	–	–	–	–	+	–	–
GPC (*n* = 1)*	Gerbich	–	+	–	nd	–	nd	–	+	+	nd	nd	–	+	+	nd
Band 3 (*n* = 1)*	ABH/Ii	–	–	–	–	–	–	–	–	–	–	–	–	–	+	–
Kell (*n* = 1)	Kell	–	–	–	–	–	–	–	–	+	–	–	–	–	–	–
LW (*n* = 1)	LW	–	–	–	–	–	–	–	–	–	nd	–	nd	–	–	+/–
CD44 (*n* = 5)	In^a/In^b	+	+	+	+	+	–	+/–	+	+	+	$+^{W}$	+	$-/+^{W}$	$-/+^{W}$	+/–
CD58 (*n* = 1)	nk	–	–	+/–	–	–	–	–	+/–	nd	+	–	W/–	–	W	–
CD55 (*n* = 2)	Cromer	–	–	+	–	–	–	–	–	nd	+	+	–	–	W	+
CD59 (*n* = 1)	nk	+	+/W	+	+	+	+	+	+	nd	+	+/–	+/–	+	+	+
CD47 (*n* = 1)	nk	+	+	+	+/–	+	+	+/–	+	nd	+	+	+/–	+	+/–	+

*Results obtained with monoclonal antibodies specific for the cytoplasmic domains of the proteins.
Key: *n* = number of different monoclonal antibodies used; nk = not known; nd = not done; + = positive reaction; – = negative reaction; W = weak.

DISCUSSION

When monoclonal antibodies with well-defined specificities on one cell (in this case, the red cell) are used to investigate other cells and tissues, the interpretation of a positive or a negative reaction requires extreme caution. A positive reaction does not necessarily mean that the red cell protein is present. Monoclonal antibodies recognize a single epitope and may cross-react with similar epitopes on proteins that are otherwise totally unrelated to the red cell protein against which the antibody was made.

The importance of using more than one monoclonal antibody when interpreting data obtained from experiments that rely on antibody screening is illustrated in the case of antibody BRIC127, which is specific for GPA in red cells (Gardner et al. 1989). During attempts to isolate GPA cDNA clones from human fetal liver expression libraries, BRIC127 reacted strongly with cDNA clones, which, by sequencing and homology alignment, proved to encode peroxisomal 3-oxoacyl-CoA thiolase (Fairbairn and Tanner 1989). A comparison of the sequence of this protein with that of GPA revealed that the region comprised of residues 208 to 218 (REKQDTFALAS) of a peroxisomal 3-oxoacyl-CoA thiolase was homologous to residues 28 to 38 (THKRDTYAATP) of GPA. The residues underlined in the two sequences would be located close together in the same relative positions in either an alpha helix or type I beta bend (Fairbairn 1987). Epitope mapping of BRIC127 on GPA suggests that tyrosine 34 is involved in the epitope (Gardner et al. 1989). The results suggest therefore that the underlined residues form an important part of the BRIC127 epitope.

Thorpe (1989) described the reactivity of three of six human monoclonal anti-Ds with nonerythroid tissues from both D-positive and D-negative individuals. The antibody that showed the broadest tissue reactivity (MAD-2) was subsequently shown to recognize the intermediate filament protein vimentin (Thorpe 1990).

One way of minimizing this problem is to use several monoclonal antibodies that react with different epitopes on the target red cell protein. If antibodies to all the different epitopes give positive reactions on a given cell or tissue, then the probability that the red cell protein or a closely related protein is present is clearly higher than if a single antibody is used. The numbers of different monoclonal antibodies used for each protein described in this chapter are given in the tables. In some cases (e.g., CD44), several antibodies known to detect at least three different epitopes were used. In other cases (Kell and LW; Tables 8.2 and 8.3), a single antibody was used and the interpretation must, ipso facto, be less secure. Unequivocal confirmation of the presence of a red cell or related protein will need further study. Immunoblotting and/or immunoprecipitation experiments can demonstrate that the reactivity results from interaction with a protein of the same or similar molecular weight. [It should be noted that the same polypeptide in different tissues may have different molecular weights because of different glycosylation patterns (Parekh et al. 1987) and that glycosylation may differ between fetal and adult forms of the same protein (Cunningham et al. 1987; Fukuda and Fukuda 1984).] If nucleic acid probes are available for the red cell protein under study, then an examination of the reactive tissue for the expression of corresponding RNA and sequencing of the cDNA provides an unambiguous answer.

A negative reaction cannot necessarily be interpreted as unequivocal evidence for the lack of expression of a red cell protein in a given cell or tissue. Many monoclonal antibodies are raised to epitopes on the extracellular domains of red cell proteins. Since these extracellular domains are almost invariably glycosylated [the 30-kDa Rh polypeptide is an exception (Gahmberg 1983)], it is frequently the case that these covalently bound carbohydrate moieties influence the binding of monoclonal antibodies either directly by forming part of the epitope or indirectly by stabilizing the tertiary structure of the protein (Mallinson et al. 1986; Parsons et al. 1987). Since (as described above) glycosylation patterns may vary for the same polypeptide in different tissues or during development, it is possible that false-negative reactions may be obtained with such monoclonal antibodies. Antibodies to GPA and GPC have been used to aid the diagnosis of erythroleukemia (reviewed in Telen 1990). The choice of antibody for this purpose is critical, as the epitopes recognized by many antibodies to GPA and GPC are dependent on the glycosylation state of the glycoproteins and altered glycosylation of GPA and GPC may occur in malignant cells. Where red cell proteins have a cytoplasmic domain, this problem can sometimes be overcome by using monoclonal antibodies to these domains, which almost invariably lack carbohydrate. The results in Table 8.3, which summarizes the tissue distribution of band 3, GPA, and GPC, were obtained with antibodies to cytoplasmic domains. It should be noted, however, that some intracellular proteins, including band 4.1, have been found to be glycosylated by O-N-acetyl glucosamine (Holt et al. 1987; Inaba and Maedl 1989).

This chapter has been confined to a discussion of monoclonal antibodies specific for red cell proteins rather than for blood group antigens expressed upon red cell proteins. Monoclonal antibodies with blood group specificity have been extensively studied in two international workshops (Rouger et al. 1987; Messeter and Johnson 1990). The majority of the antibodies examined in these workshops had specificities for antigens of the AB(H), Rh, or MN blood group systems. Antigens of the AB(H) system, in contrast to those of the Rh and MN systems, are exclusively carbohydrate in nature and as such their expression is not confined to a particular polypeptide. Antigens of the Rh and MN systems are expressed on the Rh polypeptides and glycophorins A and B, respectively.

Our decision to focus on red cell proteins rather than red cell antigens is deliberate. Blood group antigens are useful markers for protein polymorphism, but monoclonal antibodies that define monomorphic determinants are more useful for investigating the tissue distribution and development of red cell proteins. The red cell proteins that we have discussed fall into two broad groups: those with restricted distribution (band 3, GPA, Rh, Kell, LW) and those with a broad distribution (GPC, CD44, CD47, CD55, CD58, CD59).

Red cell proteins with a restricted distribution are not necessarily confined to erythroid cells. Band 3 and GPA are found in kidney cells, and there is tentative evidence (see Table 8.3) that LW may occur in placenta. It is interesting to note that band 3, GPA, and the Rh polypeptides are the most abundant polypeptides at the red cell surface (reviewed in Anstee 1990), a feature that would be consistent with important functions relevant to a highly specialized cell. In contrast, proteins with a broader tissue distribution would be expected to carry out functions common to a number of cell types. The available evidence suggests that this is the case: CD55 and CD59 regulate autologous complement activation, CD44 and CD58 are involved in cell-cell interactions, and GPC may have a general role in the maintenance of cytoskeletal associations. These results show that monoclonal antibodies can provide information relevant to an understanding of the functional importance of red cell proteins both in mature and immature red cells and in cells and tissues generally.

ACKNOWLEDGMENT

We thank Mrs. Sherrie Ayles for typing the manuscript.

REFERENCES

Anstee, D. J. 1990. Blood group-active surface molecules of the human red blood cell. *Vox Sang.* 58:1–20.

Anstee, D. J., S. F. Parsons, K. Ridgwell, et al. 1984. Two individuals with elliptocytic red cells apparently lack three minor erythrocyte membrane sialoglycoproteins. *Biochem. J.* 218:615–19.

Avent, N. D., P. A. Judson, S. F. Parsons, G. Mallinson, D. J. Anstee, M. J. A. Tanner, P. R. Evans, E. Hodges, A. G. Maciver, and C. H. Holmes. 1988. Monoclonal antibodies that recognise different membrane proteins that are deficient in Rh_{null} human erythrocytes. *Biochem. J.* 251:499–505.

Bennett, V. 1985. The membrane skeleton of human erythrocytes and its implications for more complex cells. *Ann. Rev. Biochem.* 54:273–304.

Cunningham, B. A., J. S. Hemperly, B. A. Murray, et al. 1987. Neural cell adhesion molecule—structure, Ig-like domains, cell surface modulation and alternate RNA splicing. *Science* 236:799–806.

Drenckhahn, D., S. Wagner, T. Jons, M. Oelmann, and R. Koob. 1989. In *Anion transport protein of the red blood cell membrane.* N. Hamasaki and M. L. Jennings, eds. 165–75. Amsterdam, Elsevier Science Publishers.

Emura, I., M. Sikiya, and Y. Ohnishi. 1983. Two types of immature erythrocyte series in the human fetal liver. *Arch. Histol. Jap.* 46:631–43.

Fairbairn, L. J. 1987. Ph.D. thesis, University of Bristol.

Fairbairn, L. J., and M. J. A. Tanner. 1989. Complete cDNA sequence of human foetal liver peroxisomal-3-oxoacyl-CoA thiolase. *Nucleic Acids Res.* 17:3588.

Feo, C. J., S. Fisher, J. P. Piau, M. J. Gronge, and G. Tchernia. 1981. Premiere observations de l'absence d'une proteine de la membrane erythrocytaire (band 4.1) dans un cas anemie elliptocytaire familiale. *Nouv. Rev. Fr. Hematol.* 22:315.

Fukuda, M., and M. N. Fukuda. 1984. Cell surface glycoproteins and carbohydrate antigens in development and differentiation of human erythroid cells. In *The biology of glycoproteins.* R. J. Ivatt, ed. 183–234. New York, Plenum Publishing.

Gahmberg, C. 1983. Molecular characterization of the human red cell Rho(D) antigen. *EMBO J.* 2:223–27.

Gardner, B., S. F. Parsons, A. H. Merry, and D. J. Anstee. 1989. Epitopes on sialoglycoproteins α: Evidence for heterogeneity in the molecule. *Immunology* 68:283–89.

Hadam, M. R. 1989a. Cluster report: CD47. In *Leucocyte typing IV.* W. Knapp, B. Dorken, W. R. Gilks, et al., eds. 658–60. Oxford, Oxford University Press.

———. 1989a. Cluster report: CD59. ibid. 720–22.

———. 1989c. Cluster report: CD55. ibid. 694–97.

High, S., and M. J. A. Tanner. 1987. Human erythrocyte sialoglycoprotein β: cDNA sequence suggest the absence of a cleared N-terminal signal. *Biochem. J.* 243:277–80.

Holmes, C. H., K. L. Simpson, S. D. Wainwright, C. G. Tate, et al. 1990. Preferential expression of the complement regulatory protein decay accelerating factor at the fetomaternal interface during pregnancy. *J. Immunol.* 144:3099–3105.

Holt, G. D., R. S. Haltiwanger, C. R. Torres, and G. W. Hart. 1987. Erythrocytes contain cytoplasmic glycoproteins. *J. Biol. Chem.* 262:14847–50.

Inaba, M., and Y. Maedl. 1989. O-N-Acetyl-D-glucosamine moiety on discrete peptide of multiple 4.1 isoforms regulated by alternative pathways. *J. Biol. Chem.* 264:18149–55.

Kohler, G., and C. Milstein. 1975. Continuous cultures of fused cells secreting antibody of predefined specificity. *Nature* 256:495–97.

Le Van Kim, C., Y. Colin, M.-T. Mitjavila, et al. 1989. Structure of the promoter region and tissue specificity of the human glycophorin C gene. *J. Biol. Chem.* 264:20407–14.

Makgoba, M.-W., M. E. Sanders, and S. Shaw. 1989. The CD2-LFA-3 and LFA-ICAM pathways: Relevance to T cell recognition. *Immunol. Today* 10:1417–22.

Mallinson, G., P. G. Martin, D. J. Anstee, et al. 1986. Identification and partial characterisation of the human erythrocyte membrane component(s) that express the antigens of the LW blood group system. *Biochem. J.* 234:649–52.

Medof, M. E., E. I. Walter, J. L. Rutgers, D. M. Knowles, and V. Nussenzweig. 1987. Identification of the complement decay-accelerating factor (DAF) on epithelium and glandular cells and in body fluids. *J. Exp. Med.* 165:848–64.

Messeter, L., and U. Johnson. 1990. Proceedings of the second international workshop on monoclonal antibodies against human red blood cells and related antigens. *J. Immunogenet.* 17:213–357.

Parekh, R. B., A. G. D. Tse, R. A. Dwek, A. F. Williams, and T. W. Rademacher. 1987. Tissue-specific N-glycosylation, site-specific oligosaccharide patterns, and lentil lectin recognition of rat Thy-1. *EMBO J.* 6:1233–44.

Parsons, S. F., G. Mallinson, P. A. Judson, et al. 1987. Evidence that the Lu^b antigen is located on red cell membrane glycoproteins of 85 and 78 Kd. *Transfusion* 27:61–63.

Parsons, S. F., F. A. Spring, A. H. Merry, et al. 1988. In *Proceedings of the Twentieth Congress of the International Society of Blood Transfusion*. 116. British Blood Transfusion Society, Plymouth Grove, Manchester, United Kingdom.

Reid, M. E., W. J. Mawby, M. L. Scott, R. E. Mushens, M.-J King, and C. H. Holmes. 1990. Use of a monoclonal antibody to the C-terminus of glycophorin C to study the distribution of the glycoprotein in human tissues. *Transfusion Med.* 1(Supp. 1):66.

Rouger, P., D. J. Anstee, and C. Salmon. 1987. First international workshop on monoclonal antibodies against human red blood cells and related antigens. *Revue Francaise de Transf. Immuno-hematologie.* Volumes 30 and 31.

Shaw, S., and J. P. Johnson. 1989. Cluster report: CD58. In *Leucocyte typing IV*. W. Knapp, B. Dorken, W. R. Gilks, et al., eds. 714–16. Oxford, Oxford University Press.

Spring, F. A., P. A. Judson, and D. J. Anstee. 1989. Reactivity of CD47 antibodies with human red cells. ibid. 660–61.

Stamenkovic, I., A. Aruffo, M. Amiot, and B. Seed. 1991. The hemopoietic and epithelial forms of CD44 are distinct polypeptides with different adhesion potentials for hyaluronate-bearing cells. *EMBO-J.* 10:343–48.

Stoll, M., R. Dalchau, and R. E. Schmidt. 1989. Cluster report: CD44. In *Leucocyte typing IV*. W. Knapp, B. Dorken, W. R. Gilks, et al., eds. 619–22. Oxford, Oxford University Press.

Telen, M. J. 1990. Expression of human erythrocyte membrane protein antigens during erythroid differentiation. In *Blood cell biochemistry,* Vol. 1. J. R. Harris, ed., 27–40. New York, Plenum Publishing.

Telen, M. J., S. E. Hall, A. M. Green, J. J. Moulds, and W. F. Rosse. 1988. Identification of human erythrocyte blood group antigens on decay-accelerating factor (DAF) and erythrocyte phenotype negative for DAF. *J. Exp. Med.* 167:1993–98.

Thorpe, S. J. 1989. Detection of Rh-D–associated epitopes in human and animal tissues using human monoclonal anti-D antibodies. *Br. J. Haematol.* 73:527–36.

———. 1990. Reactivity of a human monoclonal antibody against Rh(D) with the intermediate filament protein vimentin. *Br. J. Haematol.* 76:116–20.

Wagner, S., R. Vogel, R. Lietzke, R. Koob, and D. Drenckhahn. 1987. Immunochemical characterisation of a band 3–like anion exchanger in the collecting duct of human kidney. *Am J. Physiol.* 253:F213–21.

Wainwright, S. D., M. J. A. Tanner, G. E. M. Martin, J. E. Yendle, and C. H. Holmes. 1989. Monoclonal antibodies to the membrane domain of the human erythrocyte anion transport protein: Localisation of the C-terminus to the cytoplasmic side of the membrane and distribution of the protein in some human tissues. *Biochem. J.* 258:211–20.

II

DISEASES AND PROTEIN BLOOD GROUP ANTIGENS

9

HEMOLYTIC DISEASE OF THE NEWBORN

Nevin C. Hughes-Jones, M.D., Ph.D.

Hemolytic disease of the newborn (HDN) is a condition in which the lifespan of the infant's red cells is shortened by the action of specific antibodies derived from the mother by placental transfer. The effect on the infant is extremely variable: some infants appear to be normal, while others die in utero. The most common cause of severe hemolytic disease is the anti-D antibody of the Rh system, and the next commonest is anti-c, also of the Rh system. Other antibodies that may be found are anti-Kell and anti-Duffy. Antibodies of other specificities are extremely rare, although almost all specificities of IgG antibodies have been implicated.

Ruth Darrow in 1938 first postulated that in this disease the child's red cells might be destroyed by an immune reaction, although she thought that the incompatible antigen was fetal hemoglobin. The breakthrough came in 1939 when Levine and Stetson described a woman who, following a stillbirth, had a severe transfusion reaction when transfused with her husband's blood. An antibody was found in the woman's serum that agglutinated the red cells of her husband, and it was correctly surmised that this antibody would also react with the fetal red cells. In the following year, Landsteiner and Wiener (1940) showed that rabbits injected with the blood of Rhesus monkeys formed antibodies that agglutinated not only the monkey's red cells but also about 85 percent of red cells from Caucasians as well. Those people whose red cells were agglutinated by the anti-Rhesus serum were designated as Rh-positive. Levine and colleagues (1941) finally demonstrated that the Rh antigen described by Landsteiner and Wiener was also implicated in HDN. It is interesting to note that it was later realized (Levine et al. 1961) that the antibody found in rabbits by Landsteiner and Wiener was in fact specific for a completely different antigen, now termed LW. For reasons that are not at all clear, the rabbit anti-LW reacts more strongly with Rh-positive than with Rh-negative red cells; undoubtedly some phenotypic relationship exists between the Rh and LW antigens, even though the genes for the Rh system are on chromosome 1 and those for LW are on chromosome 19.

Over the following few years, other antibodies were found in humans that were clearly related to the Rh system, and it was Fisher (1943) who finally postulated the existence of three pairs of allelomorphic genes *Dd, Cc,* and *Ee,* situated close together on the chromosome. People designated as Rh-positive carried the D antigen, and Rh-positive is synonymous with D-positive.

The Rh D antigen is found only on human cells and therefore the mothers can only be immunized either by the transfer of cells from the fetus or by a mismatched transfusion; of these two, transfer of cells from the fetus is by far the most important. It is possible to demonstrate the presence of fetal red cells in the mother's circulation by the simple process of making a blood smear. If the smear is dipped into a low-ionic-strength solution at acid pH the maternal adult hemoglobin elutes out, but fetal hemoglobin is insoluble and remains within the fetal cell, which can therefore be readily demonstrated by microscopy (Kleihauer and Betke 1960). With this test it has been possible to demonstrate the presence of fetal red cells in the first and second trimester, although at that time the numbers are extremely low. In the third trimester, the presence of fetal red cells is more common and about 3 to 4 percent of all mothers can be shown to have fetal red cells at some time. However, the greatest transfer occurs during labor, and about 50 percent of all mothers can be shown to have fetal red cells in their circulation at that time. About 20 percent of all women have more than 0.1 mL of fetal red cells, about 1 percent of women have more than 3 mL, and 0.3 percent have more than 10 mL.

Approximately 17 percent of all Caucasians are Rh-negative and thus it can be calculated, taking into account that fathers may be homozygous or heterozygous, that about 1 in 10 of all pregnancies will be an Rh-negative woman with an Rh-positive fetus. The chance of having a second Rh-positive pregnancy is less, however, being only 8 percent, reduced by the fact that the chance of a *Dd* heterozygote father handing on the *D* gene a second time is only 1 in 4. Thus the incidence of HDN should be about 8 percent of the population—that is, about half of all the babies born to Rh-negative Caucasian women pregnant for the second time. In fact the incidence is far less than this, being only about 1 percent of all Caucasian women. The reason for this low number is almost certainly twofold: first, the volume of red cells transferred is frequently too low to induce an immune response, and second, it is known that 10 to 20 percent of all Rh-negative people are nonresponders—that is, they are tolerant to the D antigen (Mollison et al. 1987). For these reasons, approximately 6 percent of Rh-negative women undergo primary immunization from the first Rh-positive fetus, but only in about half of these can the anti-D be detected 3 to 6 months postpartum. In the remainder, the antibody appears only as a result of secondary stimulation during the second pregnancy (Mollison et al. 1987).

As the release of fetal red cells into the mother occurs mainly at the time of labor, HDN is uncommon in a first pregnancy. Anti-D is found in only about 1.5 percent of Rh-negative primiparas from about the thirty-fifth week on. The antibody concentration is almost always low, and the disease is usually mild in the first born.

PLACENTAL TRANSFER OF ANTIBODIES

Only IgG antibodies bring about HDN, as it is only this class that is transferred across the placenta by means of an Fc receptor on the plasma membrane of the placenta (van der Meulen et al. 1980). Transfer does not occur in any significant amount until the twenty-fourth week of pregnancy, and is relatively slow. Gitlin and associates (1964) found that even 12 days after the injection of labelled IgG into the mother, its concentration in the serum of the fetus was only about 40 percent of that in the maternal circulation. Both IgG1 and IgG3 antibodies are transferred, although there is evidence that IgG1 levels in the fetus may rise sooner than levels of IgG3 (Schur et al. 1973).

The slow rate of transfer across the placenta may be the rate-limiting step in the attachment of maternal anti-D to the fetal red cells. Thus, biologic variation in the rate of anti-D transfer could account in part for the common observation that the correlation is poor between maternal anti-D levels and the severity of hemolysis.

IgG SUBCLASS OF ANTI-D AND SEVERITY OF DISEASE

Anti-D molecules belong predominantly to subclasses IgG1 and IgG3 (Natvig and Kunkel 1968), although IgG2 and IgG4 are occasionally present, sometimes in relatively high concentrations. There is evidence from autoimmune hemolytic anemias that the IgG3 subclass is the most potent in bringing about red cell destruction, the IgG1 class being considerably less active (Engelfriet et al. 1981).

In most antisera containing anti-D, IgG1 is the predominant subclass. Shaw and colleagues (1988) investigated subclass distribution in blood donors (mainly female); after addition of the plasma to D-positive red cells, they found that the amount of IgG1 anti-D on the cells was on average 84 percent that of the total anti-D that had been bound. A similar result was found by Gorick and Hughes-Jones (1991).

The relationship between subclass and severity of HDN is not at all clear. Two recent reports found that the more severe forms of the disease occurred when both subclasses were present (Zupanska et al. 1989; Pollock and Bowman 1990). However, in both reports the interpretation is complicated by the fact that the total concentration of the antibodies was higher when both classes were present in the sera than when anti-D of only a single class was present; thus the greater severity seen in the presence of both classes could have been due to a dosage effect, although synergistic activity cannot be excluded. Some synergistic action between the two subclasses has been demonstrated for phagocytosis in vitro (Hadley and Kumpel 1989).

An attempt has been made to correlate severity with the total amount of anti-D on cord red cells. Although in general the higher the anti-D density on the red cell surface, the greater the severity, there was a considerable amount of variation in severity for any given anti-D concentration (Hughes-Jones et al. 1967). The subclass distribution was not investigated.

A relatively good correlation has been found between severity and antibody-dependent cell-mediated cytotoxicity tests using monocytes. With only a few exceptions, a strongly positive result indicated serious disease in the infant, whereas all the results that showed low activity were correlated with mild disease (Ouwehand et al. unpublished). Urbaniak and colleagues (1984) made similar observations using lymphocytes.

It is probable that the severity of the disease results from a number of different factors. As there is always biologic variation in the intensity of each of these factors, outcome varies considerably in individual cases. These varying factors are concentration and subclass of IgG anti-D, rate of placental transfer, Rh phenotype of the child (resulting in different antigen densities on the red cells), the ability of the child's hemopoietic system to respond to anemia, and the maturity of the bilirubin excretory mechanism. This multiplicity of factors makes it unlikely that severity will ever be able to be predicted accurately.

CLINICAL FEATURES

As mentioned above, the severity of the disease can vary greatly. At one end of the scale are infants who, although they have anti-D on their red cells, are not anemic at birth and who never become jaundiced owing to excessive red cell destruction. Moderately affected babies may or may not be anemic at birth, but hemoglobin concentration falls rapidly after birth and jaundice develops within a few hours. The rate of rise of bilirubin concentration depends partly on the rate of red cell destruction and partly on the extent of maturity of the bilirubin excretory mechanism. The danger posed by high bilirubin levels is possible damage to the brainstem (kernicterus), which can result in spasticity and death from respiratory failure. Infants that survive are usually mentally retarded.

The most severely affected infants become very anemic in utero, develop cardiac failure, and are stillborn. The stillbirth rate is approximately 15 percent of all infants with HDN; death may occur from the twentieth week on.

TREATMENT

Before the discovery of the Rh blood group system, infants were transfused with the father's D-positive blood (if ABO compatible), and the mortality rate was about 40 percent. Following the discovery of the Rh system, transfusion with Rh-negative blood combined with induction of labor two to three weeks before term resulted in a reduction in mortality to about 20 percent. The major breakthrough came with the introduction by Diamond (1947) of exchange transfusion through the umbilical vein. In the best hands, 99 percent survival has been reported (Shapiro 1964). When stillbirth threatens to occur so early in pregnancy that the child is unlikely to survive outside the womb, intrauterine transfusion is possible, using guidance by fiberoptics.

PROPHYLAXIS

Levine (1943) observed that the incidence of HDN was more frequent in women mated to men who were ABO compatible—that is, ABO incompatibility appeared to confer protection. Race and Sanger (1950) suggested that this protection resulted from the rapid destruction of the fetal red cells by the maternal anti-A or anti-B before they had brought about immunization. Stern and associates (1961) were the first to demonstrate that D-positive red cells coated in vitro with anti-D and injected into Rh-negative subjects were not antigenic. A group in Liverpool under the leadership of Cyril Clarke had the idea that the injection of anti-D into the mother would have an effect similar to that of anti-A and anti-B. They initially used IgM anti-D, but this proved to be ineffective (Finn et al. 1961); they then found that IgG anti-D was effective (Clarke et al. 1963). A New York group independently had similar ideas about the use of anti-D (Freda and Gorman 1962; Freda et al. 1964, 1966), although their reason for trying this method was based on the well-established observation that antigen-antibody complexes were far less antigenic than antigen alone. These latter authors also introduced the idea of injecting small volumes of pure IgG anti-D preparations intramuscularly, which was far more convenient and safer than infusions of whole serum.

The dose of anti-D used in obstetric practice varies between countries. An extensive clinical trial was carried out in the United Kingdom in which four doses—20, 50, 100, and 200 μg—were given on a random basis (Medical Research Council 1974). The incidence of immunization to the D antigen at the end of the second pregnancy following injection into primigravidas was 2.9 percent, 1.5 percent, 1.1 percent, and 1.5 percent, respectively, as set against an expected incidence of about 17 percent. The results suggest that the 20-μg dose may not be adequate, although the result was not significantly different from that found for the other three doses. As a result of this trial, a dose of 100-μg of anti-D is used in the United Kingdom. The suppressive dose of anti-D depends on the amount of Rh-positive cells present in the circulation, and it has been recommended (WHO 1971) that the standard dose should be 25 μg of anti-D per milliliter of red cells; thus, 100 μg is deemed to be immuno-suppressive for up to 4 mL of fetal red cells. It has been estimated that 0.7 percent of all women have more than 4 mL of fetal red cells in their circulation, and these women should receive additional anti-D. The number of fetal cells in the maternal circulation can be estimated by the Kleihauer technique.

The small failure rate of about 1.5 percent in Rh-negative women found in the United Kingdom trial after the second pregnancy is typical of results found elsewhere (see Mollison et al. 1987), suggesting a success rate of about 90 percent. Almost all the failures are due to primary immunization occurring during the first or second pregnancies, the incidence for this being about 0.7 percent for each pregnancy. The incidence of immunization during pregnancy can be reduced further (the extent of protection exceeding 95 percent) by giving anti-D at 28 weeks (Bowman 1984) or at 28 and 34 weeks (Tovey et al. 1983). Despite this, immunization still occurs in a small number of mothers. These failures are probably due to the occurrence of an unrecognized transplacental hemorrhage greater than 4 to 5 mL. Despite the occasional failure, the reduction of immunization by well over 95 percent is a remarkable achievement for prophylactic medicine.

The incidence of total deaths from HDN in the United Kingdom has fallen from 300 to 400 each year during the years 1960 to 1965 to a number that has now stablized at 20 to 40 each year (Clarke et al., 1987). The introduction of passive immunization procedures has played a large part in this reduction of mortality, but there has also been a considerable contribution from improvement in exchange transfusion and from the improvement in survival of children after premature delivery; the reduction in mortality has also been aided by the smaller size of today's families.

REFERENCES

Bowman, J.M. 1984. Controversies in Rh prophylaxis. In *Haemolytic disease of the newborn.* G. Garratty, ed. 67–85. Arlington, Va., American Association of Blood Banks.

Clarke, C. A., W. T. Donohoe, R. B. McConnell, J. C. Woodrow, R. Finn, J. R. Krevans, W. Kulke, D. Lehane, and P. M. Sheppard. 1963. Further experimental studies on the prevention of Rh haemolytic disease. *B.M.J.* 1:979–84.

Clarke, C. A., A. G. Whitfield, and P. L. Mollison. 1987. Deaths from Rh haemolytic disease in England and Wales in 1984 and 1985. *B.M.J.* 294:1001.

Darrow, R. R. 1938. Icterus gravis (erythroblastosis) neonatorum: An examination of etiologic considerations. *Arch. Pathol.* 25:378–417.

Diamond, L. K. 1947. Erythroblastosis foetalis or haemolytic disease of the newborn. *Proc. R. Soc. Med.* 40:546–50.

Engelfriet, C. P., A. E. G. K. von dem Borne, F. W. van der Meulen, A. Fleer, D. Roos, and W. H. Ouwehand. 1981. Immune destruction of red cells. In *A seminar on immune-mediated cell destruction.* Chicago; American Association of Blood Banks.

Finn, R., C. A. Clarke, W. T. A. Donohoe, R. B. McConnell, P. M. Sheppard, D. Lehane, and W. Kulke. 1961. Experimental studies on the prevention of Rh haemolytic disease. *B.M.J.* 1:1486–90.

Fisher, R. A. 1943. Cited by Race, R. R. 1944. An incomplete antibody in human serum. Nature 153:771–72.

Freda, V. J. and J. G. Gorman. 1962. Current Concepts: Antepartum management of Rh haemolytic disease. *Bull. Sloane Hosp. Women N.Y.* 8:147–58.

Freda, V. J., J. G. Gorman, and W. Pollack. 1964. Successful prevention of experimental Rh sensitization in man with an anti-Rh gamma$_2$-globulin antibody preparation: A preliminary report. *Transfusion* 4:26–32.

———. 1966. Rh factor: Prevention of immunization and clinical trial on mothers. *Science* 151:828–30.

Gitlin, D., J. Kumate, J. Urrusti, and C. Morales. 1964. The selectivity of the human placenta in the transfer of plasma proteins from mother to fetus. *J. Clin. Invest.* 43:1938–51.

Gorick, B. D., and N. C. Hughes-Jones. 1991. Relative functional binding activity of IgG1 and IgG3 anti-D in IgG preparations. *Vox Sang.* 61:251–254.

Hadley, A. G., and B. M. Kumpel. 1989. Synergistic effect of blending IgG1 and IgG3 monoclonal anti-D in promoting the metabolic response of monocytes to sensitized red cells. *Immunology* 67:550–52.

Hughes-Jones, N. C., M. J. Hughes, and W. Walker. 1967. The amount of anti-D on red cells in haemolytic disease of the newborn. *Vox Sang.* 12:279–85.

Kleihauer, E., and K. Betke. 1960. Praktische Anwendung des Nachweises von Hb-F-haltigen Zellen in fixierten Blutausstrichen. *Internist* 1:292–95.

Landsteiner, K., and A. S. Wiener. 1940. An agglutinable factor in human blood recognized by immune sera for Rhesus blood. *Proc. Soc. Exp. Biol. Med.* 43:223.

Levine, P. 1943. Serological factors as possible causes in spontaneous abortions. *J. Hered.* 34:71–80.

Levine, P., L. Burnham, E. M. Katzin, and P. Vogel. 1941. Role of iso-immunization in pathogenesis of erythroblastosis fetalis. *Am. J. Obstet. Gynecol.* 42:925–37.

Levine, P., M. Celano, R. Fenichel, W. Pollack, and H. Singher. 1961. A "D-like" antigen in Rhesus monkey, human Rh-positive and human Rh-negative red blood cells. *J. Immunol.* 87:747–52.

Levine, P., and R. Stetson. 1939. An unusual case of intra-group agglutination. *J.A.M.A.* 113:126–27.

Medical Research Council. 1974. Report of a working party on the use of anti-D immunoglobulin for the prevention of isoimmunization of Rh-negative women during pregnancy. *B.M.J.* 2:75–80.

Mollison, P. L., C. P. Engelfriet, and M. Contreras. 1987. *Blood transfusion in clinical medicine.* Oxford; Blackwell Scientific Publications.

Natvig, J. B., and H. G. Kunkel. 1968. Genetic markers of human immunoglobulins: The Gm and Inv systems. *Ser. Haematol.* 1:66–96.

Pollock, J. M., and J. M. Bowman. 1990. Anti-Rh(D) IgG subclasses and severity of Rh haemolytic disease of the newborn. *Vox Sang.* 59:176–79.

Race, R. R., and R. Sanger. 1950. *Blood groups in man.* Oxford; Blackwell Scientific Publications.

Schur, P. H., E. Alpert, and C. Alper. 1973. Gamma G subgroups in human fetal, cord and maternal sera. *Clin. Immunol. Immunopathol.* 2:62–66.

Shapiro, M. 1964. Safer exchange transfusion with citrated blood. Communication to the Tenth Congress of the International Society for Blood Transfusion, Stockholm.

Shaw, D. R., M. E. Conley, F. J. Knox, M. B. Khazaeli, and A. F. Lobuglio. 1988. Direct quantitation of IgG subclasses 1, 2 and 3 bound to red cells by Rh (D) antibodies. *Transfusion* 28:127–31.

Stern, K., H. S. Goodman, and M. Berger. 1961. Experimental isoimmunization to haemo-antigens in man. *J. Immunol.* 87:189–98.

Tovey, L. A. D., A. Townley, B. J. Stevenson, and J. Taverner. 1983. The Yorkshire antenatal anti-D immunoglobulin trial in primigravidae. *Lancet* 2:244–46.

Urbaniak, S. J., M. A. Greiss, R. J. Crawford, and M. J. C. Fergusson. 1984. Prediction of the outcome of Rhesus haemolytic disease of the newborn: Additional information using an ADCC assay. *Vox Sang.* 46:323–29.

van der Meulen, J. A., T. C. McNabb, N. Haeffner-Cavaillon, M. Klein, and K. J. Dorrington. 1980. The Fc receptor on human placental plasma membrane. I. Studies on the binding of homologous and heterologous immunoglobulin G. *J. Immunol.* 124:500–507.

WHO. 1971. Prevention of Rh sensitization. Technical Report Series. *468.*

Woodrow, J. C. 1980. Rh immunization and its prevention. Ser. Haematol. 3: No. 3.

Zupanska, B., E. Brojer, Y. Richards, B. Lenkiewicz, H. Seyfried, and P. Howell. 1989. Serological and immunological characteristics of maternal anti-Rh(D) antibodies in predicting the severity of haemolytic disease of the newborn. *Vox Sang.* 56:247–53.

10

RED CELL ANTIGEN SPECIFICITIES AND AUTOIMMUNE HEMOLYTIC ANEMIAS

Don L. Siegel Ph.D., M.D.
and Leslie E. Silberstein, M.D.

The hallmark of the human immune system is its ability to distinguish self from nonself. When red cells from one individual are transfused into another, subtle differences in antigenic composition can be recognized and may result in the production of antibodies specific for the foreign antigens. Indeed, the use of such alloantibody-containing sera as immunohematologic reagents led to the discovery and initial characterization of most, if not all, of the blood group antigens discussed in this book.

Occasionally, however, the mechanism of immunologic tolerance breaks down and an individual can begin to produce antibodies directed against his or her own erythrocytes. Autoimmune hemolytic anemia (AIHA) is a group of disorders in which these red cell autoantibodies result in accelerated red cell destruction. Because the red cell antigens to which these autoantibodies bind are typically antigens common to all red cells, the ability to provide compatible blood for patients with clinically significant anemias is a challenging problem in transfusion medicine. To address this problem, research in this area has focused on identifying the relevant antigenic structures and characterizing on a molecular level the nature of the corresponding autoimmune response.

CLINICAL AND SEROLOGIC ASPECTS

Autoimmune hemolytic anemia comprises three major clinical disorders characterized by the serologic behavior of the associated autoantibodies: *cold AIHA, warm AIHA,* and *paroxysmal cold hemoglobinuria (PCH)* (Siegel and Silberstein 1991). In warm AIHA, autoantibodies attach to the patient's red cells optimally at 37°C and can result in splenic sequestration and extravascular hemolysis. This is the most common form of AIHA, and the production of these autoantibodies may be idiopathic (i.e., unassociated with any other disease) or secondary to lymphoproliferative disorders, collagen vascular diseases, immune deficiency syndromes, infections, or drug therapy (Pruzanski and Shumak 1977). The autoantibodies are generally of the IgG class and appear to bind to antigens common to all normal red cells.

Autoimmune hemolytic anemia caused by autoantibodies that preferentially bind to a patient's red cells in the cold (typically room temperature and below) are of two types. In cold AIHA (cold agglutinin disease), IgM autoantibodies, usually directed against the red cell I antigen (also i and Pr) occur spontaneously, during the course of a lymphoproliferative disorder, or as a postinfectious complication of a mycoplasma pneumonia or infectious mononucleosis (Janney et al. 1978; Rosenfield et al. 1965). Patients with this disease may have cold agglutinin titers in the thousands or even millions compared with normal individuals who may have low-titer (<32) IgM cold agglutinins. Because of the low thermal binding properties of the IgM autoantibodies, in vivo they appear to bind to red cells and fix complement in the peripheral circulation, where temperatures fall below ~32°C. As the cells return to warmer parts of the circulation, the IgM dissociates, leaving the cells coated with only complement. Complement activation may then lead to intravascular hemolysis.

Paroxysmal cold hemoglobinuria, like cold agglutinin disease, is caused by cold-reactive autoantibodies that react with red cells in cooler parts of the body, cause complement to irreversibly bind to cells, and then elute off the erythrocyte surface when warmed. However, in PCH, the autoantibodies are IgG molecules usually directed at P blood group antigens (Worlledge and Rousso 1965) and are present in relatively low titers (<64). Because the presence in serum of these biphasic IgG antibodies may be difficult to detect by standard serologic methods, specialized tests that use in vitro hemolysis as an indicator of IgG-induced complement sensitization can be used (e.g., the Donath-Landsteiner test) (Donath and Landsteiner 1904). Paroxysmal cold hemoglobinuria may be idiopathic or secondary to syphilis or viral infection.

Although PCH is the rarest form of AIHA, historically it was the first type recognized, probably because of its graphic clinical presentation: the sudden onset of shaking chills, back and leg pain, abdominal cramps, high fever, and the passage of black urine. Reports in the medical literature began to appear in the mid-1800s that described attacks of hemoglobinuria after exposure to cold (Harley 1865; Hassall 1865). In 1879, Rosenbach reported how he had induced hemoglobinuria by immersing his patient's feet in ice water, and 2 years later Paul Ehrlich (1881) reported his observation of hemolysis and erythrophagocytosis in the blood obtained from the chilled finger of a patient with the disease.

For the next 50 years, laboratory investigation into the biology of AIHA was limited to the study of rare, lytic antibodies, or to cold-reactive IgM autoantibodies that would directly agglutinate red cells in vitro owing to their multivalent, red cell–bridging properties. The introduction of the antiglobulin test in 1945 by Coombs and associates and its subsequent application in patients with acquired hemolytic anemia in 1946 (Boorman et al. 1946) enabled the detection of the more common warm-reacting IgG antibodies on patients' cells. These studies firmly established the importance of red cell autoantibodies in the pathogenesis of AIHA.

AUTOANTIBODY SPECIFICITIES

TARGETS FOR COLD-REACTIVE AUTOANTIBODIES

I/i Blood Group Specificity. Cold-reactive anti–red cell autoantibodies typically bind to carbohydrate structures on membrane glycolipids and/or glycoproteins. The majority of cold agglutinins are IgM immunoglobulins directed at I/i blood group antigens (Wiener et al. 1956; Dacie 1967). This antigen system comprises oligosaccharide chains composed of repeating N-acetyllactosamine (Gal[β1→4]GlcNAc[β1→3]) units (Feizi 1980) linked to ceramide or the membrane glycoproteins band 3 and band 4.5 (Childs et al. 1978; Fukuda et al. 1979) (Fig. 10.1). The best available evidence indicates that the difference between I and i antigens relates to branching of the oligosaccharide chain; anti-i antibodies recognize a linear N-acetyllactosamine oligosaccharide while anti-I antibodies recognize a similar chain that is also branched (Niemann et al. 1978; Watanabe et al. 1979; Feizi et al 1979). There appears to be a developmentally regulated transition in expression of the I/i antigens; fetal and newborn red cells express mostly i antigen while adult red cells demonstrate the opposite pattern (Marsh 1961) (see Fig. 10.1). This transition appears to involve the acquisition of a "branching enzyme" [a(β1→6)-N-acetylglucaminyl transferase] (Watanabe and Hakomori 1976). It is of interest to note that the conversion of the unbranched i structure to a branched one coincides

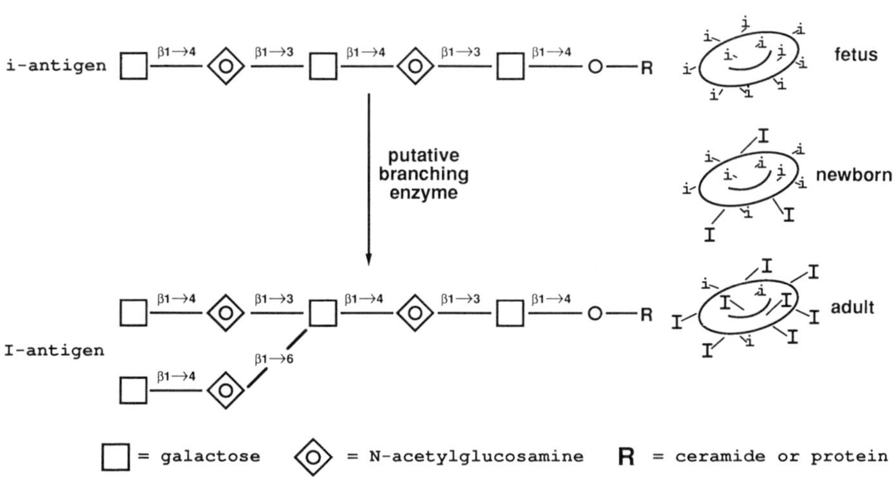

Figure 10.1. The structure and expression of human red cell I/i blood group antigens.

temporally with the switch from fetal to adult hemoglobin synthesis, which has led some researchers to suggest that these processes may be related (Hakomori 1981).

I and i antigens are also present on human granulocytes, macrophages, platelets, and lymphocytes, and antibodies to these antigens can be lymphocytotoxic (Pruzanski and Shumak 1977; Dunstan et al. 1985). In addition, they are variably expressed on nonhuman red cells (Wiener et al. 1965) and cultured cell lines of several animal species (Toh et al. 1979; Childs et al. 1979). On human B-lymphocytes, the I/i antigens appear to be carried on a family of high-molecular weight glycoproteins (~200 kDa) known as the *leukocyte common antigen* (T200 or CD45) (Omary et al. 1980), while on normal T cells, lower-molecular-weight (128 to 140 kDa) sialoglycoproteins express I/i-related structures (Childs and Feizi 1981; Childs et al. 1983). The presence of I/i-related antigens on CD45 is of particular interest since CD45, recently identified as a protein tyrosine phosphatase involved in regulating lymphocyte activation and proliferation (for review see Thomas 1989), can exist as isoforms abnormally distributed on cells in autoimmune disease (Rose et al. 1985; Yamashita et al. 1989). The finding that antibodies to CD45 on T or B cells can either inhibit or augment lymphocyte activity in vitro, depending on what other membrane receptors are nearby (Sanders et al. 1988), raises interesting questions regarding the effect(s) that autoantibodies to I/i-blood group antigens may have on lymphocyte function in vivo.

Pr-Blood Group Specificity. The term "Pr" refers to a group of red cell antigens defined serologically to possess the following characteristics: inactivation by Proteases, equivalent expression on adult and newborn red cells, and inactivation by neuraminidase (Marsh and Jenkins 1968; Roelcke 1969). Anti-Pr antibodies were originally divided into the subclasses Pr_1, Pr_2, Pr_3, and Pr_a based on their reactivity with various animal red cells and by hemagglutination inhibition experiments with chemically modified human red cell sialoglycoprotein preparations (Roelcke et al. 1976). Although the biochemistry of this blood group system is still not completely understood, the best available evidence indicates that the Pr antigens comprise O-linked sialylated oligosaccharide structures that reside within the N-terminal 26 amino acid residues of glycophorins A and B (GPA and GPB) (Ebert et al. 1979; Anstee 1981; Uemura et al. 1984). This is based in part on the findings that anti-Pr antisera fail to agglutinate neuraminidase-treated human red cells and are inhibited by the O-linked sialotetrasaccharides isolated from red cell sialoglycoprotein preparations. That they are located on GPA and GPB (and not GPC) is based on the observation that anti-Pr reactivity is dramatically reduced with En(a−) erythrocytes (which lack GPA) and totally eliminated with homozygous M^kM^k red cells (which lack GPA and GPB but have normal amounts of GPC) (Anstee 1980). Like the I/i-blood group antigens, Pr antigens have

Table 10.1. P Blood Group Antigens

Pk	Gal(α1$\rightarrow$4)Gal(β1$\rightarrow$4)Glc-ceramide
P	GalNAc(β1$\rightarrow$3)Gal(α1$\rightarrow$4)Gal(β1$\rightarrow$4)Glc-ceramide
P_1	Gal(α1$\rightarrow$4)Gal(β1$\rightarrow$4)GlcNAc(β1$\rightarrow$3)Gal(β1$\rightarrow$4)Glc-ceramide

Key: Gal = galactose; Glc = glucose; GalNac = N-acetylgalactosamine.

been found on human lymphocytes, granulocytes, and monocytes (Pruzanski et al. 1980) as well as on kidney, liver, stomach, pancreas, lung, and brain tissue (Romer et al. 1979). The significance of these findings has not been reported to date. Other targets for cold-reacting IgM autoantibodies include the Gd (for glycolipid-dependent) gangliosides (Roelcke et al. 1977) and other neuraminidase- and/or protease-sensitive antigens referred to as Sa, Lud, Fl, Vo, and Li (see Mollison et al. 1988).

P Blood Group Specificity. As noted in the previous section, complement-fixing, cold-reactive IgG autoantibodies characteristic of PCH are directed at the P blood group system. The P antigens comprise three glycosphingolipids—P^k, P, and P_1—which are structurally and biosynthetically related (Naiki and Marcus 1975) (Table 10.1). Gal(β1$\rightarrow$4)Glc-ceramide serves as a common precursor with the P^k and P_1 antigens sharing the common disaccharide Gal(β1$\rightarrow$4Gal(β1$\rightarrow$4)-R at the nonreducing end of the glycosphingolipid. The presence of P blood group antigens on red cell membrane polypeptides has not been demonstrated.

TARGETS FOR WARM-REACTIVE AUTOANTIBODIES

In contrast to our understanding of the antigens recognized by cold-reacting erythrocyte autoantibodies, the precise structures to which warm-reacting IgG autoantibodies bind has remained elusive. A major difficulty in studying this disease on a molecular level has been the inability to obtain sufficient quantities of the relevant autoantibody molecules (see next section). Consequently, our knowledge of the specificity of warm autoantibodies is limited to that provided by serologic observation and the analysis of minute quantities of immunoglobulin molecules eluted off the surface of patient red cells.

Rh-Related Specificities. Many serologic studies have suggested that warm-reacting autoantibodies are directed at Rh blood group antigens in a majority of cases by virtue of their "pan-reactivity" with all red cell phenotypes except Rh_{null} cells, which lack all Rh components (Wiener and Vos 1963; Issitt and Pavone 1978; Petz and Garratty 1980). This pattern of reactivity has led to the notion of a common "Rh-core" structure to which these antibodies are directed. However, what these serologic observations mean in molecular terms is not at all clear. For example, it is possible that these autoantibodies do not bind to Rh antigens per se, but to Rh antigens in combination with some other ubiquitous red cell membrane component(s) (Victoria et al. 1990; Agre and Cartron 1991). Alternatively, the autoantigens may not be Rh-related at all since Rh_{null} cells, which are misshapen and fragile (Sturgeon 1970) and display a variety of membrane transport defects (Lauf and Joiner 1976), have decreased expression of other blood group antigens including S, s, U, and N (Dahr et al. 1987). In a small number of cases, a "relative Rh-specificity" can be observed in which antisera are pan-reactive but display increased reactivity against cells possessing certain Rh antigens such as Rh(e). In still fewer cases, autoantibodies specific for particular Rh antigens have been described (Högman et al. 1960; Sachs 1985). In these situations, red cells lacking the corresponding Rh antigen have been found to survive in vivo better than those that express the antigen.

Other Specificities. Warm-reacting autoantibodies with specificities apparently unrelated to the Rh system include autoanti-Kell (Marsh et al. 1979), autoanti-Jk^a (van Loghem and van der Hart 1954), autoanti-N (Dube et al. 1975), autoanti-S (Allessandrino et al. 1984), and a number of others (see Mollison et al. 1988). Recently, hemolysis in a patient with warm AIHA presumably mediated by an autoantibody directed against the red cell cytoskeletal protein band 4.1 was reported (Wakui et al. 1988); however, the patient's serum also contained other red cell autoantibodies, including anti-S. In addition, the patient's brother, who had no evidence of hemolytic anemia, had the band 4.1 autoantibody as well, so the significance of these findings remains difficult to interpret.

THE IMMUNE RESPONSE TO RED CELL AUTOANTIGENS

Much of what we currently know about the immunobiology of AIHA is from work on cold-agglutinin disease. This form of AIHA has been more amenable to study for several reasons. First, as noted above, the red cell antigens to which the cold-reacting autoantibodies bind have been well characterized. Second, certain properties of these autoantigens more easily permit the investigator to determine the specificity of the cold-reacting autoantibody under study. For example, the differential expression of I/i antigens on adult and newborn cells can be used to distinguish between anti-I or anti-i specificities, and the reaction of antisera with protease-treated, neuraminidase-treated, or untreated red cells can be used to identify Pr specificity. This contrasts sharply with the behavior of warm-reacting autoantibodies, which are nearly always pan-reactive or demonstrate a "relative-specificity" toward Rh blood group–related structures that themselves are not well understood. A third reason cold AIHA has served as a model system for AIHA is because pathologic cold agglutinins often exist as serum IgM paraproteins, large quantities of which can be isolated for study. In addition, it has proved possible to establish autoantibody-secreting B-cell clones in vitro from patients with cold agglutinin disease by Epstein-Barr virus (EBV) transformation, a technique that has been exploited to provide a continuous source of biologic material for analysis (Silberstein et al. 1988; Silberstein et al. 1989a). Attempts to apply this approach for the in vitro production of warm-reactive autoantibodies has not been reliably successful, which may relate to a relative resistance of IgG-producing B cells to EBV transformation as noted in other systems (Brown and Miller 1982; Casali et al. 1987; Andrzejewski et al. 1989).

STRUCTURAL STUDIES OF COLD AGGLUTININS

I/i Blood Group Specific Autoantibodies. Initial studies of the structure of these antibodies focused on the constant regions of the immunoglobulin molecules. The composition of nearly all anti-i and anti-I autoantibodies are IgMκ, although IgM cold agglutinins with associated λ light chains have been described (see Mollison et al. 1988). More recently, attention has focused on the structural diversity of the variable regions of these autoantibodies through the use of antiidiotypic reagents and by direct nucleotide sequencing of the rearranged immunoglobulin variable-region genes. Idiotypic variation results from differences in amino acid sequence in both heavy- and light-chain variable regions, and antiidiotypic antibodies can be used to recognize variable-region determinants within or outside the antigen combining site (see Silberstein and Spitalnik 1991b for a recent review of the genetic basis for antibody diversity). Through the use of such antiidiotypic antisera, cross-reactive idiotypes were found among red cell autoantibodies (Williams et al. 1968). This cross-reactivity appeared to be restricted to red cell autoantibodies with similar specificities. For example, antiidiotypic antibodies raised against anti-Pr cold agglutinins generally did not cross-react with anti-I cold agglutinins, and vice versa. A structural basis for this idiotypic cross-reactivity could not be fully appreciated at the time because of insufficient data on variable-region gene usage that had been derived from amino acid sequences limited to the first framework region (Gergely et al. 1973). Subsequent studies by Stevenson and associates (1989) described a monoclonal antiidiotypic antibody termed "9G4" that recognized an idiotypic determinant present on the heavy chain of both anti-I and anti-i cold agglutinins as well as on neoplastic B cells secreting cold agglutinins. This suggested that the heavy-chain variable regions of anti-I and anti-i may share some of the same structural elements. Through collaborative studies between several laboratories (Pascual et al. 1991; Silberstein et al. 1991a), the

9G4 idiotope has been found on 47 of 48 pathogenic anti-I/i cold agglutinins studied to date. A structural basis for this cross-reactive idiotype was suggested by Silverman et al. (1988), who used primary sequence-dependent polyclonal antibodies to heavy-chain variable-region determinants to show that both the anti-I and anti-i cold agglutinins are derived from a distinct subset of V_H4 family genes (Silberstein et al. 1991a). More recently, the establishment of EBV-transformed B-cell lines secreting either anti-I or anti-i autoantibodies has allowed for nucleotide sequence analyses of the entire expressed variable-region genes to further assess the molecular basis for the autoimmune response (Pascual et al. 1991; Silberstein et al. 1991a). Collectively, the work from two laboratories studying four anti-I and four anti-i cold agglutinins indicates that anti-I as well as anti-i cold agglutinins likely derive from the same $V_H4.21$ (or closely related) gene segments (Silberstein et al. 1991a). Furthermore, protein sequencing of another anti-I cold agglutinin has also indicated $V_H4.21$ usage (Leoni et al. 1991).

In contrast, the variable-region genes used by the anti-I/i *light* chains do not demonstrate such restriction. While the anti-I cold agglutinin light chains appear to derive from the VκIII gene family, the anti-i cold agglutinins use light chains from a number of different Vκ families including VκIII (Silberstein et al. 1991a). To ask whether the anti-I/i light chains that use VκIII might exhibit similar idiotypic cross-reactivity as observed for the heavy chains, a panel of eight VκIII light chain–dependent monoclonal antiidiotypic antibodies was raised against an anti-I autoantibody expressing V_H4 and VκIII genes (Jefferies et al., unpublished data). Significant idiotypic heterogeneity was observed among VκIII-expressing cold agglutinin light chains. In addition, the idiotypic heterogeneity could be ascribed to the use of at least three different VκIII gene segments, as well as to somatic diversification of the germline-encoded genes.

The remarkable restriction in the variable-region genes used for the anti-I/i heavy chains, yet diversification in the associated light-chain variable-region gene usage, suggests a model for the relative contributions of heavy and light chains to antigen binding. The V_H sequence would be required for the global interaction with the I/i antigen complex, while the V_L sequence would confer the fine specificity that distinguishes between these distinct yet related carbohydrate structures. This model for cold agglutinin binding to the I/i antigens is currently being tested through the use of bacterial expression systems that permit the mixing and matching of heavy and light chains from different immunoglobulin molecules (see below). From a practical standpoint, the similarities in idiotypic structure among cold agglutinin heavy-chain variable regions and the ability to generate antiidiotypic antibodies specific for these structures suggest exciting potential therapeutic applications for these reagents in down-regulating the production of autoantibodies or inhibiting or inhibiting the growth of an underlying malignancy (Stevenson et al. 1990).

In the study by Silberstein and colleagues described above (1991a), the expressed variable region genes were also examined for the number and pattern of somatic mutations to evaluate the potential role for antigen-mediated selection. It was determined that both the V_H and V_L genes encoding the anti-i antibody were identical to germline sequences, whereas numerous base pair differences were noted in the anti-I response. Compared with its most likely germline precursor, V_H4.21, the V_H gene encoding anti-I had only three amino acid differences, two located in framework regions and one in a complementarity determining region (CDR, or region of antigen contact). In contrast, the V_L sequence of anti-I had a relatively high number of amino acid substitutions (relative to the total number of silent mutations) when compared with its likely precursor germline sequence. These amino acid changes resulted from a *nonrandom* distribution of replacement mutations in the CDRs. Taken together, these results provide evidence that positive selection by antigen led to the accumulation of amino acid substitutions in the light chain of the anti-I antibody studied. If this proves to be a universal feature of anti-I cold agglutinins, it may represent a consequence of differential regulation of the immune responses to the related I/i antigens. Perhaps the high expression of i antigen on fetal red cells mediates tolerance to i, either by clonal anergy or deletion of B cells with anti-i specificity. The expression of I antigen occurs much later in development, so immunologic tolerance for I may differ from that for i. With respect to B-cell function, it was recently demonstrated that IgM autoantibodies found in patients with Wiskott-Aldrich syndrome, a rare X-linked recessive immunodeficiency disorder, often have anti-i cold agglutinin activity, are encoded by the V_H4.21 gene, and recognize a subpopulation of human B cells present early in B-cell ontogeny (Grillot-Courvalin et al., unpublished data). This same early B-cell population is also recognized by anti-i cold agglutinins isolated from patients with cold agglutinin disease (Silberstein et al. 1991a). These studies suggest the possibility that the gene product encoded by this highly conserved germline V_H4.21 gene may have a physiologic role in B-cell development and/or differentiation.

Pr Blood Group Specific Autoantibodies. With respect to isotype, similar to anti-I/i cold agglutinins, IgMκ predominates, although anti-Pr_1 specificities have been more often associated with IgAκ (see Mollison et al. 1988). In contrast to the structural uniformity of anti-I cold agglutinins discussed above, substantial structural differences occur in the two anti-Pr_2 cold agglutinins that have been sequenced (Wang et al. 1973; Silberstein et al. 1989b). In the latter case, the heavy-chain variable region was 88 percent homologous to a V_H1 germline gene, while the light-chain variable region was 97 percent homologous to a VκIII germline gene. Antiidiotypic antibodies raised against the anti-Pr_2 cold agglutinin from this patient did not show cross-reactivities with red cell autoantibodies from other individuals having anti-Pr or different specificities and were thus unique to this patient's anti-Pr_2 autoantibody (Jefferies et al. 1990).

STRUCTURAL STUDIES OF WARM-REACTIVE AUTOANTIBODIES

With respect to the structure of warm-reactive IgG red cell autoantibodies, the little information we have is limited to the constant regions of the antibodies. For example, warm autoantibodies that cause immune hemolysis are thought to belong to the IgG1 and IgG3 subclasses (Mollison et al. 1988). Because multiple subclasses can exist simultaneously in a given patient (LePetit et al. 1976), the antibodies are considered to be polyclonal, although there is evidence to suggest that they can be restricted with respect to their Gm allotype (Litwin et al. 1973) and/or light-chain type (Leddy and Bakemeir 1965). There is currently no published information on the structure of the variable regions of these autoantibodies.

FUTURE DIRECTIONS

Clearly, more information is needed regarding the structures of the warm-reactive IgG autoantibodies. Because of the difficulty in establishing stable clonal B-cell lines that secrete warm red cell autoantibodies, alternative approaches may be required. Currently, our laboratory is using several recently developed nonmammalian expression systems to create human immunoglobulin libraries from which red cell autoantibodies can be selected. These systems involve the transfection of *Escherichia coli* with human heavy-chain/light-chain constructs that lead to the bacterial secretion of immunoglobulin Fab fragments. Alternatively, heavy-chain/light-chain epitopes that bind antigen can be expressed as part of the viral coat proteins of bacteriophage particles (see Winter and Milstein 1991 for a review of these methods). It is anticipated that the generation of appropriate amounts of clonal red cell autoantibodies using these methods will permit both the analysis of their genetic make-up as well as the identification of the relevant autoantigen molecules. If we find that the warm-reactive IgG autoantibodies are in fact directed at Rh-related structures, it would be of interest to compare their V_H and V_L sequences with the recently published sequences of two human monoclonal Rh(D) *allo*antibodies (Hughes-Jones et al. 1990).

As noted above, we are also using these nonmammalian expression systems to mix and match the heavy and light chains from our anti-I and anti-i cold agglutinins to assess the relative contributions to antigen binding of each chain. The results of these studies will not only identify the immunoglobulin structures that confer the fine specificity required to distinguish between the I/i antigens, two structurally similar carbohydrate structures, but may allow for the future design of antiidiotypic reagents that may have diagnostic or therapeutic value. Applications might include the down-regulation of the production of autoantibodies (Kelose et al. 1980), the development of synthetic peptides with idiotypic specificity for use in active immunization (Campbell et al. 1987), the inhibition in growth of an underlying malignancy (Miller et al. 1982; Meeker et al. 1985; Lowder et al. 1987), or the purging of autologous bone marrow of residual tumor (Anderson et al. 1987).

The issue of what makes an autoantibody "clinically significant," that is, pathologic, is another area worthy of investigation. It is well known that normal individuals without any evidence of immune hemolysis can have high-titer cold agglutinins in their serum or warm-reactive "Rh-specific" autoantibodies coating their circulating red cells. Despite attempts to correlate antibody subclass, complement-fixing ability, or antibody titer with the presence or absence of hemolysis, it remains unclear what structural properties distinguish "benign" autoantibodies from hemolytic ones (Garratty 1987; Rosse and Adams 1980; Schreiber et al. 1977). In this regard, our laboratory has recently isolated an EBV-transformed anti-I-producing B-cell clone from a normal individual who has a one quarter titer nonpathologic cold agglutinin. Interestingly, unlike all the pathologic anti-I/i autoantibodies we have studied thus far that have shown V_H-gene restriction to a $V_H4.21$ variable gene segment, the heavy chain of this benign autoantibody is encoded by a gene from the V_H3 family. In addition, the 9G4 antiidiotypic antibody (see above) does not bind to it. Further studies of this and other nonpathologic cold agglutinins may allow us to determine how the genetic make-up of an autoantibody confers pathogenicity.

Finally, there is the question of the functional significance of these autoantigens. As discussed in the accompanying chapters, ascribing functions to the various red cell antigens has been a difficult task. In the context of autoimmunity, determining the significance of having circulating autoantibodies directed at some of these antigens adds another dimension of complexity. The observation that these autoantigens are not restricted to red cells but are also present on lymphocyte membrane polypeptides may indicate that these autoantigens have a role in immune regulation.

REFERENCES

Agre, P., and J.-P Cartron. 1991. Molecular biology of the Rh antigens. *Blood* 78:551–63.

Allessandrino, E. P., L. Costamagna, A. Pagani, and M. Coronelli. 1984. Late appearance of autoantibody anti-S in autoimmune hemolytic anemia. *Transfusion* 24:369–70.

Anderson, K. C., J. Ritz, F. Takvorian, et al. 1987. Hematologic engraftment and immune reconstitution post-transplantation with anti-B1 purged autologous bone marrow. *Blood* 69:597–604.

Andrzejewski, C., P. J. Young, J. Goldman, S. L. Spitalnik, and L. E. Silberstein. 1989. Production of human IgM warm-reacting red cell monoclonal autoantibodies by EBV transformation. *Transfusion* 29:196–200.

Anstee, D. J. 1980. Blood group MNSs-active sialoglycoproteins of the human erythrocyte membrane. In *Immunobiology of the erythrocyte. Proceedings of the Eleventh American Red Cross Scientific Symposium.* 67–98. New York, Alan R Liss.

———. 1981. The blood group MNSs-active sialoglycoproteins. *Semin. Hematol.* 18:13–27.

Boorman, K. E., B. E. Dodd, and J. F. Loutit. 1946. Hemolytic icterus (acholuric jaundice) congenital and acquired. *Lancet* 1:812–14.

Brown, N. A., and G. Miller. 1982. Immunoglobulin expression by human B lymphocytes clonally transformed by EBV. *J. Immunol.* 128:24–29.

Campbell, M. J., E. Carroll, S. Kon, et al. 1987. Idiotype vaccination against murine B cell lymphoma: Humoral and cellular responses elaborated by tumor-derived immunoglobulin M and its molecular subunits. *J. Immunol.* 139:2825–33.

Casali, P., S. E. Burastero, M. Nakamura, et al. 1987. Human lymphocytes making rheumatoid factor and antibodies to ssDNA belong to Leu-1 positive B-cell subset. *Science* 236:77–81.

Catron, A. J., G. G. Brownlee, L. M. Staudt, and W. Gerhard. 1986. Structural and functional implications of a restricted antibody response to a defined antigen on the influenza virus hemagglutinin. *EMBO J.* 5:1577–87.

Childs, R. A., R. Dalchau, P. Seudder, et al. 1983. Evidence for the occurrence of O-glycosidically linked oligosaccharides of poly-N-acetyllactosamine type on the human leucocyte common antigen. *Biochem. Biophys. Res. Commun.* 110:424–31.

Childs, R. A. and T. Feizi. 1981. Differences in carbohydrate moieties of high molecular weight glycoproteins of human lymphocytes of T and B origins revealed by monoclonal autoantibodies with anti-I and anti-i specificities. *Biochem. Biophys. Res. Commun.* 102:1158–64.

Childs, R. A., T. Feizi, M. Fukuda, et al. 1978. Blood group I activity associated with band 3, the major intrinsic membrane protein of human erythrocytes. *Biochem. J.* 173:333–36.

Childs, R. A., A. Kapadia, and T. Feizi. 1979. In *Glycoconjugates.* ed. R. Schauer, ed. 518–19. Stuttgart, Georg Thieme.

Coombs, R. R. A., A. E. Mourant, and R. R. Race. 1945. A new test for the detection of weak and incomplete Rh agglutinins. *Br. J. Exp. Pathol.* 26:255–66.

Dacie, J. V. 1967. *The haemolytic anaemias congenital and acquired.* 2nd ed. Part III: *Secondary or symptomatic haemolytic anaemias.* 719–809. London, Churchill Livingstone.

Dahr, W., M. Kordowicz, J. Moulds, et al. 1987. Characterization of the Ss sialoglycoprotein and its antigens in Rh_{null} erythrocytes. *Blut* 54:13–24.

Donath J., and K. Landsteiner. 1904. Über paroxysmale Hämoglobinurie. *Munchen Med. Wopprchenshr.* 51:1590–93.

Dube, V. E., R. F. House, J. Moulds, and H. F. Polesky. 1975. Hemolytic anemia caused by auto anti-N. *Am. J. Clin. Pathol.* 63:828–31.

Dunstan, R. A., M. B. Simpson, and M. J. Borowitz. 1985. Heterogenous distribution of antigens on human platelets demonstrated by fluorescence flow cytometry. *Br. J. Haematol.* 61:603–10.

Ebert, W., J. Fey, C. Gärtner, et al. 1979. Isolation and partial characterization of the Pr autoantigen determinants. *Mol. Immunol.* 16:413–19.

Ehrlich, P. 1881. Über paroxysmal Hämoglobinurie. *Z. Klin. Med.* 3:383.
Feizi, T., R. A. Childs, K. Watanabe, and S. Hakomori. 1979. Three types of blood group I specificities among monoclonal anti-I autoantibodies revealed by analogues of a branched erythrocyte glycolipid. *J. Exp. Med.* 149:975–80.
Feizi, T. 1980. Structural and biological aspects of blood group I and i antigens on glycolipids and glycoproteins. *Rev. Franç. Transfus. Immunohématol.* 23:563–77.
Fukuda, M., M. N. Fukuda, and S. Hakomori. 1979. The developmental change and genetic defect in carbohydrate structures of band 3 glycoprotein of human erythrocyte membranes. *J. Biol. Chem.* 254:3700–3703.
Garratty, G. 1987. The significance of IgG on the red cell surface. *Transfus. Med. Rev.* 1:47–57.
Gergely, J., A. C. Wang, and H. H. Fudenberg. 1973. Chemical analyses of variable regions of heavy and light chains of cold agglutinins. *Vox Sang.* 24:432–40.
Hakomori, S. 1981. Blood group ABH and Ii antigens of human erythrocytes: Chemistry, polymorphism, and their developmental change. *Semin. Hematol.* 18:39–62.
Harley, G. 1865. Notes of two cases of intermittent haematuria with remarks upon their pathology and treatment. *Lancet* 1:568.
Hassall, A. H. 1865. On intermittent or winter haematuria. *Lancet* 11:368.
Högman, C., J. Killander, and S. Sjölin. 1960. A case of idiopathic autoimmune haemolytic anaemia due to anti-e. *Acta Paediatr. Scand.* 49:270.
Hughes-Jones, N. C., J. M. Bye, D. Beale, and J. Coadwell. 1990. Nucleotide sequence and three-dimensional modelling of the V_H and V_L domains of two human monoclonal antibodies specific for the D antigen of the human Rh-blood-group system. *Biochem. J.* 268:135–40.
Issitt, P. D., and B. G. Pavone. 1978. Critical reexamination of the specificity of auto-anti Rh antibodies in patients with a positive direct agglutinin test. *Br. J. Haematol.* 38:63–74.
Janney, F. A., L. T. Lee, and C. Howe. 1978. Cold hemagglutinin cross-reactivity with *Mycoplasma pneumoniae*. *Infect. Immunol.* 22:29–33.
Jefferies, L. C., F. K. Stevenson, J. Goldman, I. M. Bennett, S. L. Spitalnik, and L. E. Silberstein. 1990. Anti-idiotypic antibodies specific for a pathologic anti-Pr_2 cold agglutinin. *Transfusion* 30:495–502.
Kelose, G., M. Reth, and K. Rajewsky. 1980. Control of idiotype expression by monoclonal anti-idiotype antibodies. *Immunol. Rev.* 52:74–88.
Lauf, P. K., and C. H. Joiner. 1976. Increased potassium transport and oubain binding in human Rh_{null} red blood cells. *Blood* 48:457–68.
Leddy, J. P., and R. F. Bakemeir. 1965. Structural aspects of human erythrocytes autoantibodies. I. L chain types and electrophoretic dispersion. *J. Exp. Med.* 121:1–17.
Leoni, J., J. Ghiso, F. Goni, and B. Frangione. 1991. The primary structure of the Fab fragment of protein KAU, a monoclonal immunoglobulin M cold agglutinin. *J. Biol. Chem.* 266:2836–42.
LePetit, J. C., L. Rivat, N. Francois, C. Ropart, and C. P. Brizard. 1976. Expression of genetic markers of erythrocyte IgG autoantibodies in autoimmune hemolytic anemia. *Vox Sang.* 31:183–90.
Litwin, S. D., S. Balaban, and M. E. Eyster, 1973. Gm allotype preference in erythrocyte IgG antibodies of patients with autoimmune hemolytic anemia. *Blood* 42:241–46.
Lowder, J. H., T. C. Meeker, M. Campbell, et al. 1987. Studies on B lymphoid

tumors treated with monoclonal anti-idiotypic antibodies: Correlation with clinical responses. *Blood* 69:199–210.

Marsh, W. L. 1961. Anti Ii: A cold antibody defining the I's relationship in human red cells. *Br. J. Haematol.* 7:200–209.

Marsh, W. L., and W. J. Jenkins. 1968. Anti Sp_1: The recognition of a new cold auto-antibody. *Vox Sang.* 15:177–86.

Marsh, W. L., R. Øyen, E. Alicea, et al. 1979. Autoimmune hemolytic anemia and the Kell blood groups. *Am. J. Hematol.* 7:155–62.

Miller, R. A., D. G. Maloney, R. Warnke, and R. Levy. 1982. Treatment of B-cell lymphoma with monoclonal anti-idiotypic antibodies. *N. Engl. J. Med.* 306:517–22.

Meeker, T. C., J. Lowder, D. G. Maloney, et al. 1985. A clinical trial of anti-idiotypic therapy for B cell malignancy. *Blood* 65:1349–63.

Mollison, P. L., C. P. Engelfreit, and M. Contreras. 1988. *Blood transfusion in clinical medicine.* 8th ed. Oxford, Blackwell Scientific Publications.

Naiki, M., and D. M. Marcus. 1975. An immunochemical study of the human blood group P_1, P and P_k glycosphingolipid antigens. *Biochemistry* 14:4837–41.

Niemann, H., K. Watanabe, S. Hakomori, et al. 1978. Blood group i and I activities of "lacto-N-nor-hexaosylceramide" and its analogues: The structural requirements for i-specificities. *Biochem. Biophys. Res. Commun.* 81:1286–93.

Omary, M. B., I. S. Trowbridge, and H. A. Battifora. 1980. Human homologue of mouse T200 glycoprotein. *J. Exp. Med.* 152:842–52.

Pascual, V., K. Victor, D. Leisz, et al. 1991. Nucleotide sequence analysis of the V regions of two IgM cold agglutinins: Evidence that the V_H4-21 gene segment is responsible for the major cross-reactive idiotype. *J. Immunol.* 146:4385–91.

Petz, L. D., and G. Garratty. 1980. *Acquired hemolytic anemia.* New York, Churchill Livingstone.

Pruzanski, W., D. H. Cowan, and D. M. Parr. 1974. Clinical and immunological studies of IgM cold agglutinins with lambda type light chains. *Clin. Immunol. Immunopathol.* 2:234–45.

Pruzanski, W., D. Roelcke, M. Armstrong, and M. S. Manly. 1980. Pr and Gd antigens on human B and T lymphocytes and phagocytes. *Clin. Immunol. Immunopathol.* 15:631–41.

Pruzanski, W., and K. H. Shumak. 1977. Biological activity of cold-reacting antibodies. *N. Eng. J. Med.* 297:538–42, 583–89.

Roelcke, D. 1969. A new serological specificity in cold antibodies of high titre: Anti-HD. *Vox Sang.* 16:76–79.

Roelcke, D., W. Ebert, and H. P. Giesen. 1976. Anti Pr_3: Serological and immunchemical identification of a new anti-Pr subspecificity. *Vox Sang.* 30:122–33.

Roelcke, D., W. Riesen, H. P. Geisen, and W. Ebert. 1977. Serological identification of the new cold agglutinin specificity anti Gd. *Vox Sang.* 33:304–306.

Romer, W., H. P. Seelig, V. Lenhard, and D. Roelcke. 1979. The distribution of I/i, Pr, and Gd antigens in mammalian tissues. *Invest. Cell Pathol.* 2:157–62.

Rose, L. M., A. H. Ginsberg, T. L. Rothstein, et al. 1985. Selective loss of a subset of T helper cells in active multiple sclerosis. *Proc. Natl. Acad. Sci. U.S.A.* 82:7389–93.

Rosenbach, O. 1879. Zur Lehre von der periodischen Hämoglobinurie. *Dtsch. Med. Wochenschr.* 5:613.

Rosenfield, R. E., R. J. Schmidt, R. C. Calvo, and M. H. McGinniss. 1965. Anti-i, a frequent cold agglutinin in infectious mononucleosis. *Vox Sang.* 10:631–34.

Rosse, W. F., and J. P. Adams. 1980. The variability of hemolysis in the cold agglutinin syndrome. *Blood* 56:409–16.

Sachs, V. 1985. Anti-C as a sole autoantibody in autoimmune hemolytic anemia. *Transfusion* 25:587–88.

Sanders, M. E., M. W. Makgoba, and S. Shaw. 1988. *Immunol. Today* 9:195–99.

Schreiber, A. D., B. S. Herskovitz, and M. Goldwein. 1977. Low-titer cold-hemagglutinin disease: Mechanism of hemolysis and response to corticosteroids. *N. Engl. J. Med.* 296:1490–94.

Siegel, D. L., and L. E. Silberstein. 1991. Acquired hemolytic anemia. In *Current diagnosis*. 8th ed. R. B. Conn, ed. 559–63. Philadelphia, W. B. Saunders.

Silberstein, L. E., J. Goldman, J. A. Kant, and S. L. Spitalnik. 1988. Comparative biochemical and genetic characterization of clonally related human B-cell lines secreting pathogenic anti-Pr_2 cold agglutinins. *Arch. Biochem. Biophys.* 264:244–52.

Silberstein, L. E., L. C. Jefferies, J. Goldman, and S. L. Spitalnik. 1989a. Production of carbohydrate-specific human monoclonal antibodies in vitro. *Methods Enzymol.* 179:299–304.

Silberstein, L. E., L. C. Jefferies, J. Goldman, et al. 1991a. Variable region gene analysis of pathologic human autoantibodies to the related i and I red blood cell antigens. *Blood* 78:2372–86.

Silberstein, L. E., S. Litwin, and C. E. Carmack. 1989b. Relationship of variable region genes expressed by a human B-cell lymphoma secreting pathologic anti-Pr_2 erythrocyte autoantibodies. *J. Exp. Med.* 169:1631–43.

Silberstein, L. E., and S. L. Spitalnik. 1991b. Blood group antigens and antibodies. In *Principles of transfusion medicine*. E. C. Rossi, T. L. Simon and G. S. Moss, eds. 63–78. Baltimore, Williams & Wilkins.

Silverman, G. J., F. R. Goni, J. Fernandez, et al. 1988. Distinct patterns of heavy chain variable region subgroup use by human monoclonal autoantibodies of different specificity. *J. Exp. Med.* 168:2361–66.

Stevenson, F. K., A. J. George, and M. J. Glennie. 1990. Antiidiotypic therapy of leukemias and lymphomas. *Chem. Immunol.* 48:126–66.

Stevenson, F. K., G. J. Smith, J. North, T. J. Hamblin, and M. J. Glennie. 1989. Identification of normal B-cell counterparts of neoplastic cells which secrete cold agglutinins of anti-I and anti-i specificity. *Br. J. Haematol.* 72:9–15.

Sturgeon, P. 1970. Hematologic observations on the anemia associated with blood type Rh_{null}. *Blood* 36:310–20.

Thomas, R. 1989. The leukocyte common antigen family. *Annu. Rev. Immunol.* 7:339–69.

Toh, B. H., T. A. Diggle, and S. H. Koh. 1979. I: Blood Group Antigens on Fibroblast Cell Surfaces. *Clin. Immunol. Immunopathol.* 12:177–82.

Uemura, K., D. Roelcke, N. Yoshitaka, and T. Feizi. 1984. The reactivity of human erythrocyte autoantibodies anti-Pr_2, and Gd, Fl, and Sa with gangliosides in a chromatogram binding assay. *Biochem. J.* 219:865–74.

van Loghem, J. J., and M. van der Hart. 1954. Varieties of specific auto-antibodies in acquired hemolytic anemia. *Vox Sang.* 4:2.

Victoria, E. J., S. W. Pierce, M. J. Branks, and S. P. Masouredis. 1990. IgG red blood cell autoantibodies in autoimmune hemolytic anemia bind to epitopes on red blood cell membrane band 3 glycoprotein. *J. Lab. Clin. Med.* 115:74–88.

Wakui, H., H. Imai, and R. Kobayashi. 1988. Autoantibodies against erythrocyte protein band 4.1 in a patient with autoimmune hemolytic anemia. *Blood* 72:408–11.

Wang, A. C., H. H. Fudenberg, J. V. Wells, and D. Roelcke. 1973. A new subgroup of the human kappa chain variable region associated with anti-Pr cold agglutinins. *Nature New Biol.* 243:126–28.

Watanabe, K., and S. Hakamori. 1976. Status of blood group carbohydrate chains in autogenesis and oncogenesis. *J. Exp. Med.* 144:644–53.

Watanabe, K., S. Hakomori, R. A. Childs, et al. 1979. Characterization of a blood group I-active ganglioside: Structural requirements for I and i specificity. *J. Biol. Chem.* 254:3221–28.

Wiener, A. S., J. Moore-Jankowski, E. B. Gordon, and J. Davis. 1965. The blood factors I and i in primates including man and in lower species. *Am. J. Phys. Anthropol.* 23:389–96.

Weiner, A. S., L. T. Unger, L. Cohen, et al. 1956. Type-specific cold autoantibodies as a cause of acquired hemolytic anemia and hemolytic transfusion reactions: Biologic test with bovine red cells. *Ann Intern. Med.* 44:221–40.

Weiner, W., and G. H. Vos. 1963. Serology of acquired hemolytic anemia. *Blood* 22:606–13.

Williams, R. C., H. G. Kunkel, and J. D. Capra. 1968. Antigenic specificities related to the cold agglutinin activity of gamma M globulins. *Science* 161:379–81.

Winter, G., and C. Milstein. 1991. Man-made antibodies. *Nature* 349:293–99.

Worlledge, S. M., and C. Rousso. 1965. Studies on the serology of PCH with special reference to its relationship with the P blood group system. *Vox Sang.* 10:293–98.

Yamashita, Y., I. Yasuyuki, and O. Toshiaki. 1989. Poly [N-acetyllactosamine]-type sugar chain in CD45 antigens of abnormal T cells of Ipr mice are different from those of normal T cells and B cells. *Mol. Immunol.* 26:905–13.

11

PHOSPHATIDYLINOSITOL-GLYCAN LINKED PROTEINS AND THEIR RELATIONSHIP TO PAROXYSMAL NOCTURNAL HEMOGLOBINURIA AND BLOOD GROUP ANTIGENS

Wendell F. Rosse, M.D.
and Marilyn J. Telen, M.D.

Cell surface proteins that are integral to the membrane are anchored to the lipid bilayer by a hydrophobic interaction. For many proteins, the hydrophobic interactions are provided by a sequence of about 23 amino acids that are hydrophobic and that form an (alpha) helix of about 3½ turns, a length sufficient to span the lipid bilayer. This segment is usually near the carboxyl terminus, which is cytoplasmic; in exceptional cases, it may be near the amino terminus, which is cytoplasmic.

Recently, two other means of hydrophobic interaction have been described. One involves the posttranslational addition of fatty acid chains, usually palmitate, at specific cysteine residues. Myristate is added to the N-terminal glycine of a subset of membrane proteins during translation. These lipids are inserted into the lipid bilayer, and the attached protein is thus stabilized on the membrane surface.

Another way in which proteins are held to the membrane involves a specific structure, the so-called phosphatidylinositol-glycan anchor PI–glycan (Low 1989; Rosse 1990a) (Fig. 11.1). This anchor consists of a diacyl or alkylacyl glycerol bridge attached to inositol through a phosphate group (Low 1987). To the inositol is attached a molecule of deacetylated aminoglucose and three other saccharide groups, usually containing at least one mannose. A molecule of ethanolamine is attached to the last sugar group and the protein is covalently bound through its carboxyl terminus to the ethanolamine by an amide linkage. The fatty acids of the molecule are inserted into the membrane and the protein is thus held in place.

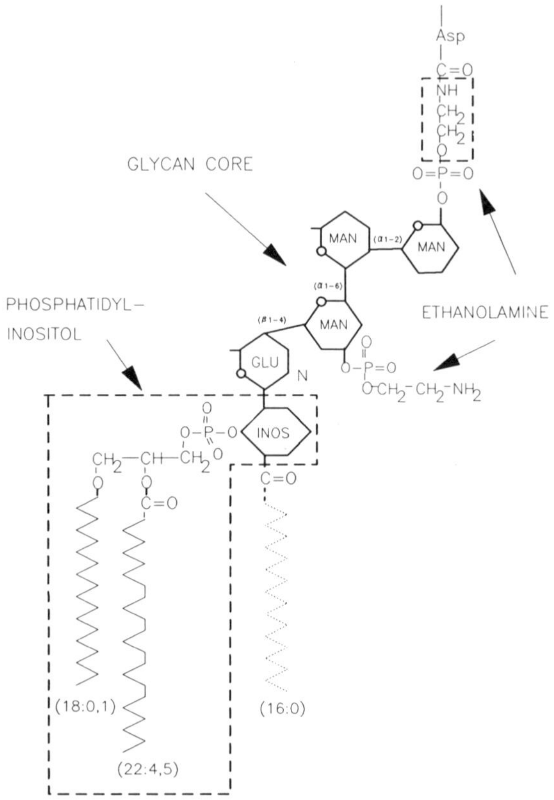

Figure 11.1. The general structure of the phosphatidylinositol-glycan anchor. Phosphotidylinositol is joined to a glycan core consisting of a molecule of N-glucosamine and three molecules of mannose. The structure ends in an ethanolamine that may be affixed by an amide bond to the carboxyl terminal amino acid of the protein. Side chains consisting of a palmitate affixed to the inositol group and ethanolamine affixed to the first mannose may be present.

This type of anchor is widely distributed among animals. Although the details of structure vary somewhat from species to species and even from cell type to cell type within a single species, the general structure is sufficiently preserved that antibodies made to the anchor of the trypanosome cross-react with the mammalian anchor (Davitz et al. 1987a). In trypanosomes, which use this structure for the main surface glycoproteins of the membrane, the anchoring lipids are always two myristyl groups, a fatty acid that is not otherwise employed in the construction of the cell membrane (Ferguson et al. 1985). In addition, a complex of four galactose molecules is added to the structure after the protein has been attached. In mammals, the fatty acids are often attached by an acyl bond to the second carbon of the glycerol molecule and by an alkyl bond to the third carbon (Roberts et al. 1988; Roberts et al. 1987). The first is frequently a molecule of 22 carbons with four or five unsaturated bonds and the latter a molecule of 18 carbons with or without a single unsaturated bond. There is usually a second ethanolamine group attached to one of the sugars and, in the case of the human red cell, a palmitate is attached to the inositol by an acyl linkage.

The biosynthesis of proteins anchored in this way has been studied in the trypanosome (Masterson et al. 1989; Doering et al. 1990). The phosphatidylinositol-glycan anchor is made separately in the endoplasmic reticulum by a series of steps, as shown in Figure 11.2. The protein is synthesized by ribosomes attached to the endoplasmic reticulum and is secreted into the cisterna of the endoplasmic reticulum, where it is immediately attached to the preformed anchor, presumably by a "transamidating enzyme" (Fig. 11.3). The signal for the enzyme is given by a

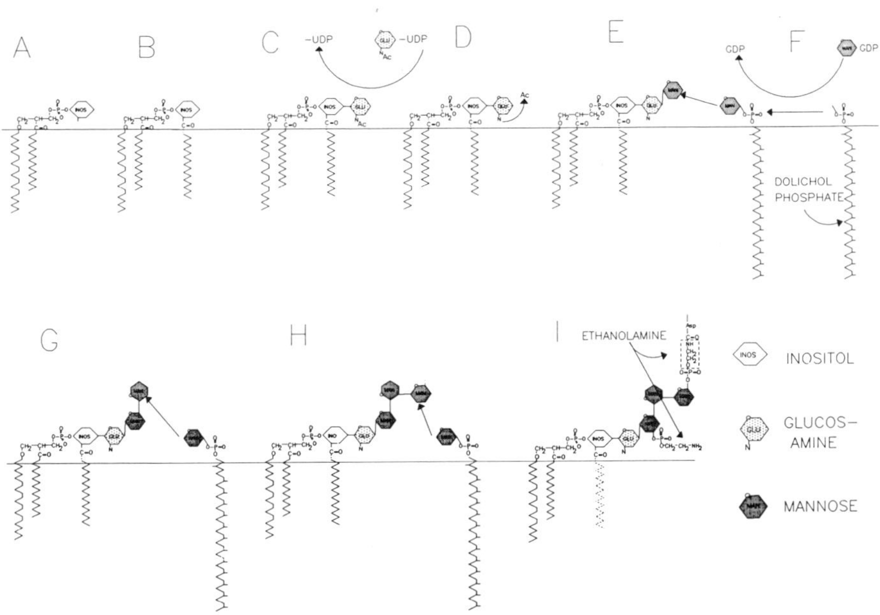

Figure 11.2. The proposed biosynthesis of the phosphatidylinositol-glycan anchor. **A.** Phosphatidylinositol is inserted into the inner leaflet of the membrane of the endoplasmic reticulum. **B.** An acyl group (usually palmitate) is added; it is not known exactly when in the sequence this is done. **C.** A molecule of N-acetylglucosamine (N-Glu) is enzymatically added from UDP-(N-Glu). **D.** The N-Glu molecule is deacetylated. **E.** Mannose is added in a (1,4) linkage; the source of the mannose is dolichol-phosphate-mannose (Dol-P-Man). **F.** Dol-P-Man is synthesized from dolichol phosphate and GDP-Man by the enzyme Dol-P-Man synthetase. **G.** A second mannose is added in a (1,6) linkage, probably using Dol-P-Man as the source. **H.** A third mannose is added in a (1,2) linkage; again, the source is probably Dol-P-Man. **I.** An ethanolamine phosphate is added to the last mannose. In most cells, the acyl group is removed from the inositol; this does not occur readily in red cells. A second ethanolamine phosphate group is added to the first mannose residue, probably after the protein has been attached.

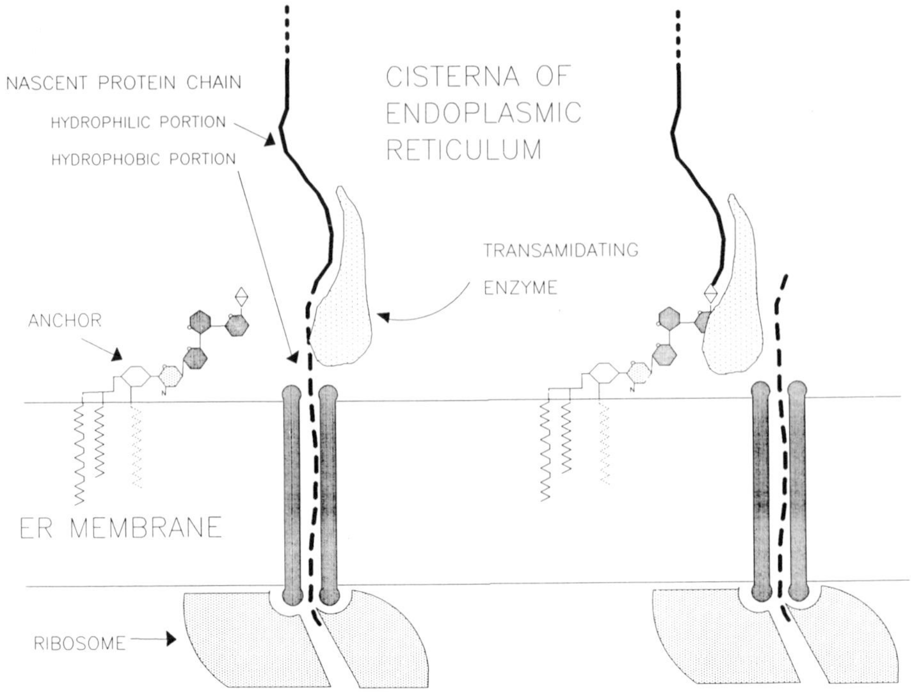

Figure 11.3. The translocation of the nascent protein chain to the preformed glycolipid anchor. The nascent protein is synthesized by ribosomes attached to the outer leaflet of the membrane of the endoplasmic reticulum. As the protein is extruded into the cisterna of the endoplasmic reticulum by the translocating mechanism, a putative transamidating enzyme binds to the signal sequence in the hydrophobic tail. This enzyme both cleaves the nascent protein and transfers it to the preformed phosphatidylinositol-glycan anchor.

stretch of hydrophobic amino acids, usually about 17 in number, near the carboxy terminus of the protein (Caras and Weddell 1989; Caras et al. 1987, 1989). In studies on placental alkaline phosphatase, the full length of this hydrophobic segment was found to be 29 residues; constructs with 17 residues were partially transferred to the anchor, but those of 13 residues were not appropriately formed and therefore remained inserted in the lipid bilayer (Berger et al. 1988). The substitution of one hydrophobic amino acid for another along much of the length of the hydrophobic segment does not alter processing (Caras and Weddell 1989). The preferred carboxy terminal amino acid on the nascent protein for attachment of the anchor is aspartate, although any of five others (glycine, alanine, cysteine, asparagine, or serine) can be substituted, with resultant lesser efficiency of enzymatic transfer (Micanovic et al. 1990). Processing of this segment of the protein occurs even though the anchor is not present to be attached (Bailey et al. 1989).

The normally anchored protein may be readily removed from the membrane by the actions of an enzyme able to cleave the phosphoinositol group from the diacyl- (or acylalkyl-) glycerol (Hereld et al. 1986). This is usually mediated by a phosphatidylinositol-specific phospholipase C, but can be mediated by a phosphatidylinositol-specific phospholipase D (Davitz et al. 1987b). The cellular enzyme is well described in trypanosomes; the equivalent enzyme is less well characterized in mammals.

The number of proteins known to be anchored in this way is continually increasing. These are usually identified by the fact that they may be removed from the cell surface by phosphatidylinositol-specific phospholipase C; the presence of the glycan anchor may then be determined biochemically. Table 11.1 lists such proteins.

As can be seen, proteins anchored in this way subserve a number of different functions for the cells. Many of the functions do not require transmembrane signaling, and it is difficult to see how any signal could be transmitted by a protein without a cytoplasmic portion. However, some of the functions do require transmembrane signaling, and the means by which this is effected is currently under investigation.

Some of the proteins contained in Table 11.1 are known to be normally present on human red cells. These are of particular importance because they bear antigens that may be recognized as blood group antigens and because, as outlined below, these proteins are missing to a greater or lesser degree from the abnormal cells in paroxysmal nocturnal hemoglobinuria.

PHOSPHATIDYLINOSITOL-GLYCAN LINKED PROTEINS IN PAROXYSMAL NOCTURNAL HEMOGLOBINURIA

Paroxysmal nocturnal hemoglobinuria (PNH) is a complex disorder of stem cells characterized by hemolytic anemia, unusual venous thrombosis, infections, and bone marrow hypoplasia (Rosse 1990b). In it, a population of abnormal stem cells arises that give rise to blood cells lacking in PI-glycan–linked surface proteins. These include membrane enzymes [acetylcholinesterase on red cells (Chow et al. 1985), alkaline phosphatase on granulocytes (Lewis and Dacie 1965), and 5′-ectonucleotidase on lymphocytes]; complement regulatory proteins [decay-accelerating factor, DAF, CD55) (Nicholson-Weller et al. 1983), "protectin" (membrane inhibitor of reactive lysis, MIRL, CD59) (Holguin et al. 1989), and C8 binding protein (C8 BP, homologous restriction factor) (Haensch et al. 1987)]; immunologic function proteins [lymphocyte function antigen-3 (LFA-3) (Selvaraj et al. 1988), Fc receptor III (Selvaraj et al. 1988), and CD14 (a protein of unknown function) (Simmons et al. 1989)]; and other proteins (folate receptor, etc.). Although the absence of some of these proteins has no deleterious effect on the function or survival of the cell, the absence of others is undoubtedly related to the pathogenesis of the disease.

Table 11.1. A Partial List of Proteins Known to Be Linked to the Membrane Through a Glycosyl-Phosphatidylinositol Anchor

Protozoan and helminthic surface proteins
Trypanosoma variable-surface glycoproteins
Leishmania surface glycoproteins
T. cruzi stage-specific antigens
Toxoplasma gondii surface antigen P30
Schistosoma mansoni surface antigens
Paramecium temperature-specific antigens
Plasmodium 195-kDa antigen
Cell adhesion proteins
Neural cell adhesion molecule (N-CAM)
Proteoheparin sulfate
Immunologic proteins or markers
Thy-1 (mouse)
Lymphocyte functional antigens-3 (LFA-3)
Blast-1
Fc receptor III (human)
CD14 (human)
Thymocyte surface proteins (2)
RT-6.2 (thymocyte differentiation antigen)
ThB and certain Qa antigens
Complement regulatory proteins
Decay-accelerating factor (DAF) (human)
Membrane inhibitor of reactive lysis (MIRL, CD59)
C8 binding protein
Membrane-bound enzymes
Alkaline phosphatase (human)
Acetylcholinesterase (human)
Acetylcholinesterase *(Drosophila)*
Alkaline phosphodiesterase I
Trehalase
Lymphocyte 5′-ectonucleotidase
Kidney microvillus ectoenzymes
Other
Folate binding protein
Neural-cell recognition protein
Carcinoembryonic antigen (CEA)
Scrapie prion protein
J11d (murine hematopoietic cell marker)
Placental p34 growth factor

Source: From Rosse 1990b.

The reason for the deficiency of these proteins is not clear. The mRNA for DAF (Stafford et al. 1988) and MIRL are present in the cells that do not express the surface protein; further, in some experiments, the protein is synthesized, apparently without the anchor (Carothers et al. 1990). It should be noted that multiple defects may underlie different forms of PNH. Indeed, an inherited complete deficiency of homologous restriction factor (MIRL) was found to result in PNH in the homozygote, who was apparently not deficient in other PI-glycan–linked surface proteins (Yamashima et al. 1990).

A model system for the deficiency of GPI-linked proteins has been developed from the cloning of mouse thymoma cell lines that lack the GPI-linked protein Thy-1 (Hyman and Cunningham 1986; Trowbridge et al. 1978; Teng et al. 1989). Several defects appear to result in the same phenotype, as shown by complementation studies. One of the defined defects is the deficiency of the enzyme mannosyl phosphoryldolichol synthetase, which is responsible for the biosynthesis of the mannose donor (DeGaspari et al. 1990); since the mannosyl residues are not available for the construction of the anchor, the protein is not expressed. Transfection of the gene for the enzyme from yeast corrected the defect in anchor synthesis and protein expression. Studies using similar techniques have demonstrated that, in PNH granulocytes, the complete anchor cannot be made or is made in undetectable amounts (Mahoney et al. 1991). These studies also suggest that, as with the Thy-1–deficient cell lines, any of several defects in anchor biosynthesis may result in the nonexpression of the protein.

THE COMPLEMENT REGULATORY PROTEINS

The direct relationship between the absence of surface proteins and the pathogenesis of the symptoms of PNH is best established for the complement regulatory proteins DAF and MIRL. Ham and associates first found that the red cells in PNH are sensitive to the hemolytic action of complement; this sensitivity is the basis for the tests diagnostic of PNH (the acidified serum lysis or Ham test, the sucrose lysis test, etc.) (Ham et al. 1937). This sensitivity is quantitated in the complement lysis sensitivity test of Rosse and Dacie (1966), in which cells sensitized with antibody are lysed by graded increases in complement. By this test, cells of marked sensitivity (PNH III cells) as well as cells of intermediate sensitivity (PNH II cells) may be defined. It was originally thought that most patients had PNH I (normal or nearly normal cells) and PNH III cells, but more detailed analysis has shown that cells of intermediate sensitivity are commonly found by special techniques (Rosse et al. 1974, 1991).

Nicholson-Weller and associates (1983) first demonstrated the absence of a complement regulatory protein, decay-accelerating factor (DAF, CD55), on the abnormal red cells in PNH. This protein has a molecular weight of about 69 kDa and is linked to the membrane by a PI-glycan anchor (Medof et al. 1986). It contains four so-called tandem repeats, each a sequence of about 66 amino acids (Medof et al. 1987b); these structures are common to proteins reacting with C3b and C4b of the complement sequence (Kristensen et al. 1986). The proposed structure of DAF is shown in Figure 11.4.

The function of DAF is to disrupt the enzymatic complexes responsible

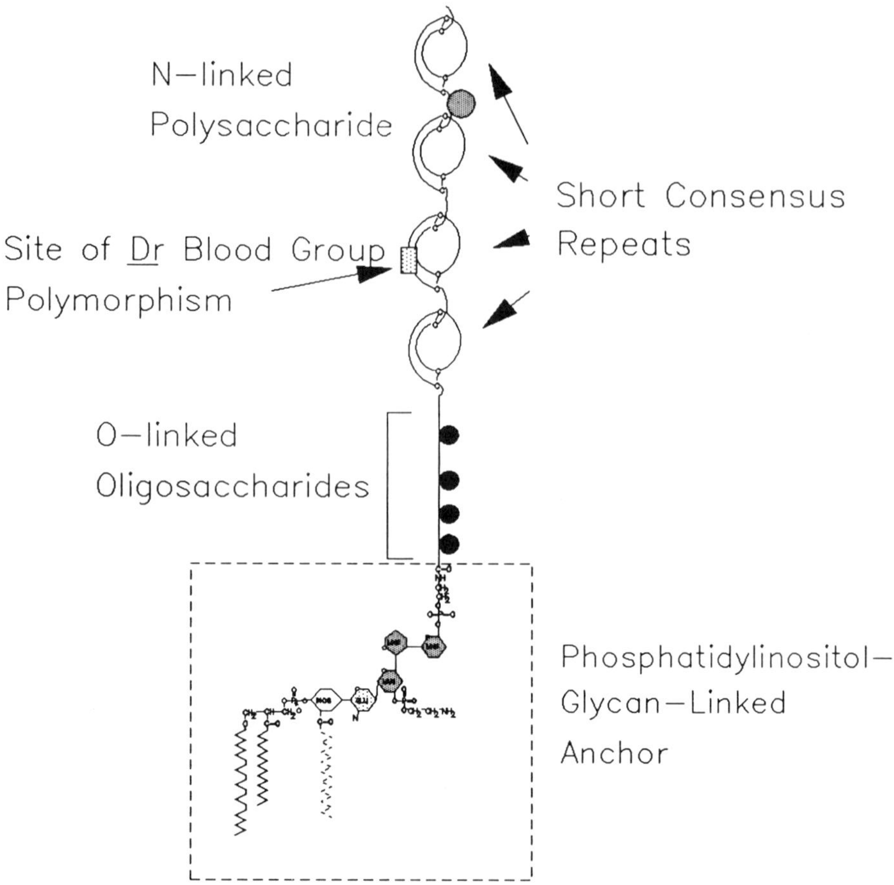

Figure 11.4. The structure of DAF. See text for explanation.

for the amplification of the activation of complement (Medof et al. 1984). In the classic pathway, this complex consists of C4b (bound to the membrane) and C2a (bound to C4b by Mg^{2+}); in the alternative pathway, the role of C4b is played by C3b and the role of C2a by factor Bb. These complexes act by binding substrate (C3) to C4b or C3b and cleaving from it the activation peptide by the enzyme C2a or Bb. These reactions provide an immense potential for the amplification of the reactions of complement.

The function of DAF is to disrupt these complexes, presumably by binding to C4b or C3b and dislocating the enzyme. If this down-regulation does not occur, then the enzymatic complex persists and the middle and final stages of complement activation are enhanced (Pangburn et al. 1983). Thus, much more C3b is activated and deposited on the membrane of defective PNH red cells than on normal cells (Parker et al. 1982).

During studies of the reactions of DAF, investigators realized that the lack of DAF could not alone account for the marked sensitivity to complement of the PNH III cells (Medof et al. 1987a). Inhibition of DAF activity on normal red cells by antibody resulted in cells that had the sensitivity of PNH II cells. It was thus suspected that a further defect was present in the PNH III cells that somehow increased the efficiency of the membrane attack complex, the group of proteins that is inserted into the membrane to bring about its disruption and the lysis of the cell.

Two further proteins, both PI-glycan linked, have been implicated in this respect. One, C8 binding protein, or homologous restriction factor, has a molecular weight of about 79 kDa and binds to C8, a property that is used in its purification (Hansch et al. 1987; Zalman et al. 1987). In the membrane, it presumably binds to C8 and interferes with the polymerization of C9, an important part of the formation of the complex. The protein is missing in abnormal PNH red cells.

A second protein, apparently not related, with similar functions is "protectin," also called membrane inhibitor of reactive lysis (MIRL), MEM 21, and CD59 (Holguin et al. 1990; Davies et al. 1989). This protein is about 18 kDa and is highly glycosylated. The sequence of the expressed protein is known and it has no homology with other proteins other than with certain murine lymphocyte signaling proteins. It also appears to interfere with the polymerization of C9, but the exact mechanism is not known.

The inhibition of this protein on normal red cells with specific antibody renders them as susceptible to lysis as PNH III cells. Further, the quantitative replacement of this protein in the membrane of PNH III cells renders them nearly as resistant to complement lysis as normal cells. Thus, MIRL appears to be the crucial protein in the defense of the membrane against the lytic action of complement.

It was originally thought that the cells of intermediate sensitivity (PNH II cells) lacked DAF but possessed MIRL. More careful studies have shown that the two proteins (and acetylcholinesterase) are equally expressed in decreased amounts on these cells and that the degree of complement sensitivity is directly related to the amount expressed (Rosse et al., unpublished data). This property, coupled with the finding that most patients have these cells of intermediate sensitivity, suggests that the defect in PNH is quantitative rather than purely qualitative.

One of the major complications of PNH is thrombosis of venous sites, particularly in the liver or splanchnic beds. It is known that the platelets are abnormal and lack both DAF (Devine et al. 1987) and MIRL (at least the 18-kDa variety), but it is not entirely clear that the tendency to thrombosis is related to the absence of these proteins. It has been known for some time that the platelets in PNH are more reactive in aggregation and release tests than are normal platelets (Dixon et al. 1977); only recently has it been shown that this increased reactivity is confined to the aggregation of the platelets by thrombin; PNH platelets require as little as one one-hundredth to one one-thousandth the concentration of thrombin for the aggregation as normal platelets. The inhibition of membrane DAF or MIRL of normal platelets does not seem to render them sensitive to this agonist, nor does the placement on the membrane of complexes of the complement sequence. Thus, there may be other, as yet undiscovered proteins that regulate thrombin activation of the platelet that are missing on the PNH platelet.

The absence of MIRL may have a role in the hypercoagulable state in PNH. When membrane attack complexes accumulate on the membrane surface of the normal platelet, they are gathered into a limited area and exocytosed by vesiculation (Sims et al. 1988). These vesicles also contain the binding site for the prothrombinase complex and are much more likely to activate clotting than is the membrane of the intact platelet. Since the platelets of PNH lack MIRL, many more membrane attack complexes may form on the cell membrane and more vesicles are produced (Sims et al. 1989). This may have a role in inducing the venous clotting characteristic of the disorder.

In the red cell, the lack of DAF and MIRL clearly results in the early destruction of the cell by complement; the life span of the most deficient cells is 16 to 20 days, as compared with 90 to 120 days for normal red cells (Rosse 1971). Hemolytic "crises" usually occur in the setting one would expect complement to be activated (infections, incompatible transfusions, etc.), and it is the complement-sensitive cells that are lysed. The nocturnal lysis experienced by some patients is thought to be due to the activation of complement by endotoxin absorbed during the night.

On the other hand, the defective platelets (Devine et al. 1987) and neutrophils (Brubaker et al. 1977) in PNH have a normal life span. This may be because the platelet is able to remove nascent membrane attack complexes by exocytosis. Further, these cells may have additional control proteins that are not PI-glycan linked and therefore are not missing.

IMMUNOLOGIC PROTEINS

Three proteins thought to be related to immune function are missing in the defective cells in PNH. The function of one, the Fc receptor III molecule on neutrophils, is well characterized (Selvaraj et al. 1988); it is the primary molecule mediating immune adherence for these cells. Its absence may explain why patients with PNH tolerate sepsis rather poorly, since the neutrophil is the main phagocytic cell of the blood.

The role of two other proteins known to be missing is less clear. LFA-3 is a signal-transducing protein that reacts with CD2 complex of the T cell (Krensky et al. 1983). One of its roles is signaling monocytes to produce IL-2; thus, PNH monocytes, which lack LFA-3, may not receive the signal and may not produce IL-2 in response to T-cell signaling.

CD14 is a molecule present on monocytes. Although it is a convenient marker, its function is not known. Therefore, the effect of its absence is also not clear.

It would be inviting to explain the relative or absolute marrow hypoplasia in PNH on the basis of the lack of PI-glycan–linked proteins. To date, that is not possible, but the area of the control of hematopoiesis in PNH clearly deserves investigation.

THE BLOOD GROUP ANTIGENS ON PHOSPHATIDYINOSITOL-GLYCAN LINKED PROTEINS

Human red cell blood group antigens often represent small differences in the structure of common expressed cell-surface proteins. Using a variety of methods, investigators identified a small number of human red cell blood group antigens as borne by phosphatidylinositol-linked membrane proteins (Telen et al. 1988, 1990). These antigens include those of the "Cromer-related" blood group, as well as the following smaller blood group antigen systems: John Milton Hagen (JMH), Holley-Gregory (Hy/Gy), Dombrock (Do^a/Do^b), and Cartwright (Yt^a/Yt^b). In the case of one Cromer-related antigen—Dr^a—the genetic basis of the antigen polymorphism has also been identified.

CROMER-RELATED BLOOD GROUP ANTIGENS ARE ON DECAY-ACCELERATING FACTOR

Cromer-related blood group antigens comprise a family of antigens expressed by all circulating hematopoietic cells (reviewed by Reid 1990). Many of the Cromer-related antigens defined to date are high-frequency antigens present on the cells of more than 99 percent of all donors. However, a few of the antigens produced by rare alleles have also been identified (Table 11.2). The many Cromer-related antigens were initially associated with one another because of the existence of two rare phenotypes, in which the expression of all these antigens is altered. One

Table 11.2. Cromer-Related Blood Group Antigens

High-Frequency Antigens	Low-Frequency Antigens
Cr^a	
Tc^a	Tc^b, Tc^c
Dr^a	
Es^a	
IFC	
WES^b	WES^a
UMC	

phenotype, termed Inab, expresses no detectable Cromer-related cell-surface antigens. Persons with this phenotype may produce an antibody (called anti-IFC) that reacts with all other red cells that express any Cromer-related antigens. The other, Dr(a−), lacks the Dr^a antigen but expresses all other Cromer-related antigens very weakly. Thus, antigens lacking from Inab cells and weakly expressed by Dr(a−) cells have been classified as Cromer-related.

The Cromer-related antigens comprise the first blood group antigen system shown to reside on a phosphatidylinositol-glycan–anchored protein. Initially, monoclonal antibodies with IFC-like reactivity, as well as human Cromer-related antisera, were found to identify a 70-kDa membrane protein in immunoblots of red cell membrane proteins (Spring et al. 1987). This protein was then proven to be DAF by a variety of methods (Telen et al. 1988). First, purified soluble DAF was able to completely inhibit the binding of human Cromer-related antibodies to human red cells. Second, human anti-Tc^a and anti-Cr^a identified DAF in immunoblots using purified DAF protein. Finally, DAF-deficient PNH cells also failed to express Cromer-related antigens, while DAF-positive cells from the same donors did express these antigens.

THE INAB (CROMER-NULL) PHENOTYPE

The identification of Cromer-related antigens on DAF allowed for the first time the recognition of a hereditary phenotype of cellular DAF deficiency. The Inab (Cromer-related antigen-negative) phenotype has now been found in six individuals. Study of cells from these persons has demonstrated that these cells express other PI-linked proteins—such as acetylcholinesterase, LFA-3, and CD59—normally (unlike PNH red cells) (Telen and Greene 1989b). However, neither murine monoclonal nor rabbit polyclonal antibodies to DAF bind to Inab red cells, lymphocytes, or platelets.

The finding of isolated DAF deficiency also allowed the determination of the importance of DAF in defense against autologous complement activation (Telen and Greene 1989b; Merry et al. 1989). Numerous in vitro tests of the regulation of complement activation demonstrated that Inab red cells were slightly more sensitive to lysis by complement than were normal red cells. In the complement lysis sensitivity assay of Rosse and Dacie, Inab cells were about 2.5 times more sensitive than normal cells. Furthermore, direct examination of C3 convertase decay demonstrated that C3 convertase decay was prolonged on Inab cells, to a degree comparable to that seen with PNH cells. However, no Inab donor has ever been reported to have a hemolytic syndrome, and the acidified serum lysis test was normal with Inab cells. Thus, a lack of DAF activity appeared associated with only modest in vitro defects and no significant in vivo hemolysis.

The existence of the Inab phenotype is also interesting because the mechanism whereby cell-surface DAF is lacking is not yet understood. Persons with this phenotype do not have a large deletion of chromosomal material, as other genes encoded by the regulation of complement activation locus on chromosome 1 are normally expressed. Such genes include the plasma proteins C4 binding protein and factor H (Telen and Rosse, unpublished observations). Furthermore, a reduced but detectable amount of DAF antigen activity can be found in the plasma of Inab donors (Telen and Greene, unpublished data). Direct investigation of the genetic basis of this phenotype in one person has further shown that the gene appears intact when restriction fragments are analyzed by Southern blotting (Tate et al. 1989). Moreover, a lymphoblastoid cell line made from the donor studied was found to contain normal-appearing DAF mRNA. Further investigation is under way to determine what type of mutation leads to the nonexpression of cell-surface DAF with concomitant expression of DAF in plasma. Also to be answered is the question of why Inab persons make the antibody whose specificity is designated anti-IFC. For, if they do produce DAF in at least the soluble form, then the antibody must be directed either against an epitope unique to the membrane-bound form or against an epitope present in normal DAF but not in the variant, which is expressed only in the soluble form.

THE DR(A−) PHENOTYPE

The Dr^a antigen is one of the high-incidence antigens of the Cromer-related system. Workers in Israel described rare persons who lack the Dr^a antigen (Levene et al. 1984, 1987). Interestingly, the cells from these persons also demonstrate only very weak expression of all other high-incidence Cromer-related antigens, such as Tc^a and Cr^a. Investigation of such cells using monoclonal and polyclonal antibodies to DAF has confirmed that these cells do indeed express markedly reduced amounts of DAF (Telen and Greene 1989a). The partial DAF deficiency is not, however, associated with in vitro enhancement of complement lysis sensitivity, as is the DAF defect of Inab cells, indicating that the DAF present is more or less functionally normal.

Biochemical and genetic analysis of the Dr(a−) phenotype has elucidated in part the nature of the defect of these cells (Lublin et al., 1991). Immunoblotting of DAF from Dr(a−) red cells demonstrated that Dr(a−) DAF appeared grossly normal but reduced in quantity in relationship to other membrane proteins. Analysis also showed that, although the molecular weight of the Dr(a−) DAF was grossly normal, variation of polyacrylamide concentration suggested that the Dr(a−) protein might have a slightly lower molecular weight. This was not due to lack of an N-linked oligosaccharide, as the expected decrease in molecular weight was obtained after treatment with endoglycosidase F.

Analysis of genomic DNA from donors with the Dr(a−) phenotype has demonstrated the molecular basis of the change in antigen expression.

When each of the nine exons of the DAF gene from Dr(a−) subjects was amplified by polymerase chain reaction (PCR) and sequenced, the Dr(a−) gene was found to contain a single point mutation compared with the wild-type Dr(a+) DAF gene. A C to T change in codon 165, in the exon encoding short consensus repeat IIIB, changes a serine to leucine. Thus, Leu165 DAF, or Dr(a−) DAF, constitutes the first reported polymorphism in the coding region of that gene.

Proof that the Ser to Leu alteration at codon 165 is the basis of the Dr(a−) phenotype was then provided by transfection experiments, in which CHO cells were transfected with either the wild-type or Dr(a−) DAF coding region DNA. Human anti-Dr^a sera reacted with wild-type transfectants but not with Leu165 transfectants. Demonstration that this point mutation was positively correlated with Dr phenotype has also allowed the correlation of phenotype with a restriction-fragment-length polymorphism (RFLP) using TaqI. This work has pioneered the application of RFLP analysis to confirm antigen phenotyping and the use of allele-specific transfectants to identify antibody specificity.

THE IDENTIFICATION OF THE PROTEIN BEARING JMH ANTIGENS

The John Milton Hagen (JMH) antigen was first identified by autoantibodies found, in general, in elderly patients whose own JMH antigen expression was weakened (Sabo et al. 1978). To date, only one family has been identified as illustrative of an inheritable JMH phenotype (Kollmar et al. 1981). Since the description of the original JMH antibodies, careful serologic investigation of JMH antibodies has also demonstrated that some alloantibodies recognize distinct epitopes within the JMH blood group (Moulds et al. 1982).

Studies using several such antisera, as well as a monoclonal antibody (Daniels and Knowles 1982, 1983), have now identified the protein that bears JMH antigens (Bobolis et al., unpublished data). This protein has an apparent molecular weight of 76 kDa and demonstrates a minimal increase in apparent molecular weight after exposure to disulfide-reducing agents, despite the fact that the epitopes recognized by all antibodies are destroyed by such reagents. This 76-kDa protein appears to be absent from JMH red cells. Numerous other PI-linked proteins—such as acetylcholinesterase, LFA-3, DAF, and MIRL (CD59)—are normally expressed by JMH red cells.

The linkage of JMH protein to the membrane by a PI anchor has now been confirmed directly using phosphatidylinositol-specific phospholipase C. Although phosphatidylinositol-specific phospholipase C cleaves only a small amount of JMH protein from red cells (most likely owing to a palmitoyl group, as in other PI-linked red cell proteins), JMH protein can be specifically detected in the supernate after the treatment of red cells with phosphatidylinositol-specific phospholipase C. Interestingly, however, incubation of red cells at 37°C without enzyme releases a protein of approximately 67 kDa, with JMH antigen activity. This protein appears likely to be a product of proteolysis, although the exact relationship of this spontaneously released protein to that released by phosphatidylinositol-specific phospholipase C has not been ascertained.

OTHER PI-LINKED ANTIGENS

The molecular bases of the other antigens thought to be PI-linked—that is, Hy/Gy, Do^a/Do^b, and Yt^a/Yt^b—have yet to be delineated. However, we can expect that investigation of these antigens should contribute new knowledge about already identified proteins or, like JMH, identify for us even more PI-linked proteins heretofore undiscovered.

ACKNOWLEDGMENTS

This work was performed during the tenure of the following grants from the National Institutes of Health: 5 R37 DK31379 (W.F.R.), and 1 RO1 HL44042 and K04 HL02233 (M.J.T.).

REFERENCES

Bailey, C. A., L. Gerber, A. D. Howard, and S. Udenfriend. 1989. Processing at the carboxyl terminus of nascent placental alkaline phosphatase in a cell-free system: Evidence for specific cleavage of a signal peptide. *Proc. Natl. Acad. Sci. U.S.A.* 86:22–26.

Berger, J., A. D. Howard, L. Brink, L. Gerber, J. Hauber, B. R. Cullen, and S. Udenfriend. 1988. COOH-terminal requirements for the correct processing of a phosphatidylinositol-glycan anchored protein. *J. Biol. Chem.* 263:10016–21.

Brubaker, L., L. J. Essig, and C. E. Mengel. 1977. Neutrophil life span in paroxysmal nocturnal hemoglobinuria. *Blood* 50:657–62.

Caras, I. W., and G. N. Weddell. 1989. Signal peptide for protein secretion directing glycophospholipid membrane anchor attachment. *Science* 243:1196–98.

Caras, I. W., G. N. Weddell, M. A. Davitz, V. Nussenzweig, and D. W. Martin, Jr. 1987. Signal for attachment of a phospholipid membrane anchor in decay accelerating factor. *Science* 238:1280–83.

Caras, I. W., G. N. Weddell, and S. R. Williams. 1989. Analysis of the signal for attachment of a glycophospholipid membrane anchor. *J. Cell Biol.* 108:1387–96.

Carothers, D. J., S. V. Hazra, S. W. Andreson, and M. E. Medof. 1990. Synthesis of aberrant decay-accelerating factor proteins by affected paroxysmal nocturnal hemoglobinuria leucocytes. *J. Clin. Invest.* 85:47–54.

Chow, F.-L., M. J. Telen, and W. F. Rosse. 1985. The acetylcholinesterase defect in paroxysmal nocturnal hemoglobinuria: Evidence that the enzyme is absent from the cell membrane. *Blood* 66:940–45.

Daniels, G. L., and R. W. Knowles. 1982. A monoclonal antibody to the high frequency red cell antigen JMH. *J. Immunogen.* 9:57-59.

———. 1983. Further analysis of the monoclonal antibody H8 demonstrating a JMH-related specificity. *J. Immunogenet.* 10:257–58.

Doering, T. I., W. J. Masterson, G. W. Hart, and P. T. Englund. 1990. Biosynthesis of glycosyl phosphatidylinositol membrane anchors. *J. Biol. Chem.* 265:611–14.

Davies, A., D. L. Simmons, G. Hale, R. A. Harrison, H. Tighe, P. J. Lachmann, and H. Waldmann. 1989. CD59, an LY-6-like protein expressed in human lymphoid cells, regulates the action of the complement membrane attack complex on homologous cells. *J. Exp. Med.* 170:637–54.

Davitz, M. A., A. M. Gurnett, M. G. Low, M. J. Turner, and V. Nussenzweig. 1987a. Decay-accelerating factor (DAF) shares a common carbohydrate determinant with the variant surface glycoprotein (VSG) of the African *Trypanosoma brucei. J. Immunol.* 138:520–23.

Davitz, M. A., D. Hereld, S. Shak, J. Krakow, P. T. Englund, and V. Nussenzweig. 1987b. A glycan-phosphatidylinositol–specific phospholipase D in human serum. *Science* 238:81–84.

DeGasperi R., L. J. Thomas, E. Sugiyama, H. M. Chang, P. J. Beck, P. Orlean, C. Albright, G. Waneck, J. F. Sambrook, C. D. Warren, and E. T. H. Yeh. 1990. Correction of a defect in mammalian GPI anchor biosynthesis by a transfected yeast gene. *Science* 250:988–90.

Devine, D. V., R. S. Siegel, and W. F. Rosse. 1987. Interactions of the platelets in paroxysmal nocturnal hemoglobinuria with complement. *J. Clin. Invest.* 79:131–37.

Dixon, R. H., and W. F. Rosse. 1977. Mechanism of complement activation on human blood platelets in vitro. *J. Clin. Invest.* 59:360–68.

Dustin, M. I., P. Selvaraj, R. J. Mattaliano, and T. A. Springer. 1987. Anchoring mechanisms for LFA-3 cell adhesion glycoprotein at membrane surface. *Nature* 329:846–48.

Ferguson, M. A. H., M. G. Low, and G. A. M. Cross. 1985. Glycosyl-sn-1,2-dimyristylphosphatidylinositol is covalently linked to *Trypanosoma brucei* variant surface glycoprotein. *J. Biol. Chem.* 260:14547–55.

Ham, T. H. 1937. Chronic hemolytic anemia with paroxysmal nocturnal hemoglobinuria: A study of the mechanism of hemolysis in relation to acid-base equilibrium. *N. Engl. J. Med.* 217:915–19.

Hansch, G. M., S. Schonermark, and D. Roelcke. 1987. Paroxysmal nocturnal hemoglobinuria type III: Lack of an erythrocyte membrane protein restricting the lysis of C5b-9. *J. Clin. Invest.* 80:7–12.

Hereld, D., J. L. Krakow, J. D. Bangs, G. W. Hart, and P. T. Englund. 1986. A phospholipase C from *Trypanosoma brucei* which selectively cleaves the glycolipid on the variant surface glycoprotein. *J. Biol. Chem.* 261:13813–19.

Holguin, M. H., L. R. Fredrick, N. J. Bernshaw, and C. J. Parker. 1989. Isolation and characterization of a membrane protein from normal human erythrocytes that inhibits reactive lysis of the erythrocytes of paroxysmal nocturnal hemoglobinuria. *J. Clin. Invest.* 84:7–17.

Hyman, R., and K. Cunningham. 1986. A Thy-1 mutant defining a gene acting in *trans* position to regulate cell surface Thy-1 glycoprotein expression and Thy-1 messenger RNA content. *Immunogenetics* 23:312–21.

Kollmar, M., S. F. South, and W. M. Tregallas. 1981. Evidence of genetic mechanism for the production of the JMH-negative phenotype. *Transfusion* 21:612.

Krensky, A. M., F. Sanchez-Madrid, E. Robbins, J. A. Nagy, T. A. Springer, and S. J. Burakoff. 1983. The functional significance, distribution, and structure of LFA-1, LFA-2, and LFA-3: Cell-surface antigens associated with CTL-target interactions. *J. Immunol.* 131:611–16.

Kristensen, T., R. A. Wetsel, and B. F. Tack. 1986. Structural analysis of human complement protein H: Homology with C4b-binding protein, a2-glycoprotein 1 and Ba fragment of B. *J. Immunol.* 136:3407–11.

Levene, C., N. Harel, G. Kende, S. Papo, M. F. Bradford, and G. L. Daniels. 1987. A second Dr(a−) proposita with anti-Dr[a] and a family with the Dr(a−) phenotype in two generations. *Transfusion* 27:64–65.
Levene, C., N. Harel, G. Lavie, S. Greenberg, B. Laird-Fryer, and G. L. Daniels. 1984. A "new" phenotype confirming a relationship between Cr[a] and Tc[a]. *Transfusion* 24:13–15.
Lewis, S. M., and J. V. Dacie. 1965. Neutrophil (leucocyte) alkaline phosphatase in paroxysmal nocturnal hemoglobinuria. *Br. J. Haematol.* 11:549–56.
Low, M. G. 1987. Biochemistry of the glycosyl-phosphatidylinositol membrane protein anchor. *Biochem. J.* 244:1–13.
———. 1989. Glycosyl-phosphatidylinositol: A versatile anchor for cell surface proteins. *FASEB J.* 3:1600–1608.
Lublin, D. M., E. S. Thompson, A. M. Green, C. Levene, and M. J. Telen. 1991. Dr(a−) polymorphism of decay accelerating factor. *J. Clin. Invest.* 87:1945-52.
Mahoney, J. F., M. Urakaze, S. Hall, R. DeGasperi, H.-M. Chang, C. D. Warren, A. Nicholson-Weller, W. F. Rosse, and E. T. H. Yeh. 1991. Defective glycosylphosphatidylinositol anchor synthesis in paroxysmal nocturnal hemoglobinuria. *Clin. Res.* 39:210a. (abstract).
Masterson, W. J., T. L. Doering, G. W. Hart, and P. T. Englund. 1989. A novel pathway for the glycan assembly: Biosynthesis of the glycosyl-phosphatidylinositol anchor of the trypanosome variant surface glycoprotein. *Cell* 56:793–800.
Medof, M. E., A. Gottleib, T. Kinoshita, S. Hall, R. Silber, V. Nussenzweig, and W. F. Rosse. 1987a. Relationship between decay-accelerating factor deficiency, diminished acetylcholinesterase activity, and defective terminal complement pathway restriction in paroxysmal nocturnal hemoglobinuria erythrocytes. *J. Clin. Invest.* 80:165–74.
Medof, M. E., T. Kinoshita, and V. Nussenzweig. 1984. Inhibition of complement activation on the surface of cells after incorporation of decay-accelerating factor (DAF) into their membranes. *J. Exp. Med.* 160:1558–78.
Medof, M. E., D. M. Lublin, V. M. Holers, D. J. Ayers, R. R. Getty, J. F. Leykam, J. P. Atkinson, and M. L. Tykocinski. 1987b. Cloning and characterization of cDNAs encoding the complete sequence of decay-accelerating factor of human complement. *Proc. Natl. Acad. Sci. U.S.A.* 84:2007–11.
Medof, M. E., E. I. Walter, W. L. Roberts, R. Haas, and T. L. Rosenberry. 1986. Decay accelerating factor of complement is anchored to cells by a C-terminal glycolipid. *Biochemistry* 25:6740–47.
Merry, A. H., V. I. Rawlinson, M. Uchikawa, M. R. Daha, and R. B. Sim. 1989. Studies on the sensitivity to complement-mediated lysis of erythrocytes (Inab phenotype) with a deficiency of DAF (decay-accelerating factor). *Br. J. Haematol.* 73:248–53.
Micanovic, R., L. D. Gerber, J. Berger, K. Kodukula, and S. Udenfriend. 1990. Selectivity of the cleavage/attachment site of phosphatidylinositol-glycan–anchored membrane proteins determined by site-specific mutagenesis at ASP-484 of placental alkaline phosphatase. *Proc. Natl. Acad. Sci. U.S.A.* 87:157–61.
Moulds, J. J., C. Levene, and S. Zimmerman. 1982. Serological evidence for heterogeneity among antibodies compatible with JMH-negative red cells. Proceedings of the Joint Meeting of the Nineteenth Congress of the International Society of Haematology and the Seventeenth Congress of the International Society of Blood Transfusion. p. 287.
Nicholson-Weller, A., J. P. March, S. I. Rosenfeld, and K. F. Austen. 1983. Affected erythrocytes of patients with paroxysmal nocturnal hemoglobinuria

are deficient in the complement regulatory protein, decay accelerating factor. *Proc. Natl. Acad. Sci. U.S.A.* 80:5066–70.

Pangburn, M. K., R. D. Schreiber, and H. J. Muller-Eberhard. 1983. Deficiency of an erythrocyte membrane protein with complement regulator activity in paroxysmal nocturnal hemoglobinuria. *Proc. Natl. Acad. Sci. U.S.A.* 80:5430–34.

Parker, C. J., P. J. Baker, and W. J. Rosse. 1982. Increased enzymatic activity in the alternative pathway convertase when bound to the erythrocytes of paroxysmal nocturnal hemoglobinuria. *J. Clin. Invest.* 69:337–46.

Reid, M. E. 1990. Cromer-related blood group antigens and the glycosyl-phosphatidylinositol–linked protein, decay-accelerating factor DAF (CD55). *Immunohematology* 6:27–29.

Roberts, W. L., B. H. Kim, and T. L. Rosenberry. 1987. Differences in the glycolipid membrane anchors of bovine and human erythcyte acetylcholinesterases. *Proc. Natl. Acad. Sci. U.S.A.* 84:7817–21.

Roberts, W. L., S. Santikarn, V. N. Reinhold, and T. L. Rosenberry. 1988. Structural characterization of the glycoinositol phospholipid membrane anchor of human erythrocyte acetylcholinesterase by fast atom bombardment mass spectrometry. *J. Biol. Chem.* 263:18776–84.

Rosse, W. F. 1971. The life-span of complement-sensitive and -insensitive red cells in paroxysmal nocturnal hemoglobinuria. *Blood* 37:556–62.

———. 1990a. Paroxysmal nocturnal hemoglobinuria. In *Clinical immunohematology: Basic concepts and clinical applications*. 593-648. Boston, Blackwell Scientific.

———. 1990b. Phosphatidylinositol-linked proteins and paroxysmal nocturnal hemoglobinuria. *Blood* 75:1595–1601.

Rosse, W. F., J. P. Adams, and A. M. Thorpe. 1974. The population of cells in paroxysmal nocturnal haemoglobinuria of intermediate sensitivity to complement lysis: Significance and mechanism of increased immune lysis. *Br. J. Haematol.* 28:181–90.

Rosse, W. F., and J. V. Dacie. 1966. Immune lysis of normal human and paroxysmal nocturnal hemoglobinuria red blood cells. I. The sensitivity of PNH red cells to lysis by complement and specific antibody. *J. Clin. Invest.* 45:736–48.

Rosse, W. F., S. Hoffman, M. Campbell, M. Borowitz, J. O. Moore, and C. J. Parker. 1991. The erythrocytes in paroxysmal nocturnal haemoglobinuria of intermediate sensitivity to complement lysis. *Br. J. Haematol.* 79:99–107.

Sabo, B., J. J. Moulds, and J. McCreary. 1978. Anti-JMH: Another high titer-low avidity antibody against a high frequency antigen. *Transfusion* 18:387. (abstract).

Selvaraj, P., W. F. Rosse, R. Silber, and T. A. Springer. 1988. The major Fc receptor in blood has a phosphotidylinositol anchor and is deficient in paroxysmal nocturnal hemoglobinuria. *Nature* 333:565–67.

Simmons D. L., S. Tan, D. G. Tenen, A. Nicholson-Weller, and B. Seed. 1989. Monocyte antigen CD14 is a phospholipid anchored membrane protein. *Blood* 3:284–89.

Sims, P. J., E. M. Faioni, T. Wiedmer, and S. J. Shattil. 1988. Complement proteins C5b-9 cause release of membrane vesicles from the platelet surface that are enriched in the membrane receptor for coagulation factor Va and express prothrombinase activity. *J. Biol. Chem.* 263:18205–12.

Sims, P. J., S. A. Rollins, and T. Wiedmer. 1989. Regulatory control of complement on blood platelets: Modulation of platelet procoagulant responses by a membrane inhibitor of the C5b-9 complex. *J. Biol. Chem.* 264:17049–57.

Spring, F. A., P. A. Judson, G. L. Daniels, S. F. Parsons, G. Mallinson, and D. J. Anstee. 1987. A human cell-surface glycoprotein that carries Cromer-related blood group antigens on erythrocytes and is also expressed on leucocytes and platelets. *Immunology* 62:307–13.

Stafford, H. A., M. L. Tykocinski, D. M. Lublin, V. M. Holers, W. F. Rosse, J. P. Atkinson, and M. E. Medof. 1988. Normal polymorphic variations and transcription of the decay-accelerating factor gene in paroxysmal nocturnal hemoglobinuria cells. *Proc. Natl. Acad. Sci. U.S.A.* 85:880–84.

Tate, C. G., M. Uchikawa, M. J. A. Tanner, P. A. Judson, S. F. Parsons, G. Mallinson, and D. J. Anstee. 1989. Studies on the defect which causes absence of decay-accelerating factor (DAF) from the peripheral blood cells of an individual with the Inab phenotype. *Biochem. J.* 261:489–93.

Telen, M. J., and A. M. Greene. 1989a. The Dr(a−) phenotype: Isolated partial deficiency of decay accelerating factor. *Blood* 74:147A. (abstract).

———. 1989b. The Inab phenotype: Characterization of the membrane protein and complement regulatory defect. *Blood* 74:437–41.

Telen, M. J., S. E. Hall, A. M. Green, J. J. Moulds, and W. F. Rosse. 1988. Identification of human erythrocyte blood group antigens on decay-accelerating factor (DAF) and identification of an erythrocyte phenotype negative for DAF. *J. Exp. Med.* 167:1993–98.

Telen, M. J., W. F. Rosse, C. J. Parker, M. K. Moulds, and J. J. Moulds. 1990. Evidence that several high-frequency human blood group antigens reside on phosphatidylinositol-linked erythrocyte membrane proteins. *Blood* 75:1404–7.

Teng, M.-H., S. Hedayati, A. A. Alexander, R. Barkin, R. S. Basch, and J. N. Busbaum. 1989. A Thy-1 negative lymphoma cell variant defective in the formation of glycosyl-phosphatidylinositol membrane protein anchors. *Mol. Immunol.* 26:391–402.

Trowbridge, I. S., R. Hyman, and C. Mazauskas. 1978. The synthesis and properties of T25 glycoprotein in Thy-1 negative mutant lymphoma cells. *Cell* 14:21–32.

Yamashima, M., E. Ueda, T. Kinoshita, T. Takami, A. Ojima, H. Ono, H. Tanaka, N. Kondo, T. Orii, N. Okada, H. Okada, K. Inoue, and T. Kitani. 1990. Inherited complete deficiency of 20-kilodalton homologous restriction factor (CD59) as a cause of paroxysmal nocturnal hemoglobinuria. *N. Engl. J. Med.* 323:1184–89.

Zalman, L. S., L. M. Wood, M. M. Frank, and H. J. Muller-Eberhard. 1987. Deficiency of the homologous restriction factor in paroxysmal nocturnal hemoglobinuria. *J. Exp. Med.* 165:572–77.

12

RED CELL ANTIGENS AS RECEPTORS FOR MALARIA PARASITES

Terence J. Hadley, M.D.
and Louis H. Miller, M.D.

Malaria is caused by protozoa of the genus *Plasmodium,* which are transmitted to humans by the bite of the female anopheline mosquito. Four species of human malaria are known: *P. falciparum, P. vivax, P. ovale,* and *P. malariae.* Of these, *P. falciparum* and *P. vivax* are responsible for most human disease. *Plasmodium falciparum* invades red cells of all ages, resulting in high levels of parasitemia, often killing the person. *Plasmodium vivax* invades reticulocytes, resulting in lower levels of parasitemia and considerable morbidity, although death is less frequent. In vitro culture systems and animal models exist for both *P. falciparum* and *P. vivax,* but not for *P. ovale* or *P. malariae.*

When the mosquito takes a blood meal, parasites enter the bloodstream and invade hepatocytes, where they divide into thousands of merozoites. The hepatic stage of the infection is asymptomatic. After 1 to 2 weeks, merozoites emerge from the liver and invade red cells. The asexual red cell stage of the infection is the symptomatic stage, characterized by fever, myalgias, malaise, and anemia; in the case of *P. falciparum,* the infection may result in renal failure, pulmonary edema, cerebral malaria, and death. The malaria parasite is an obligate intracellular parasite; it must invade red cells to survive and multiply. Once inside a red cell, a malarial parasite develops sequentially into a ring form (which has the appearance of a ring when blood films are stained with Giemsa), a more mature form, termed a *trophozoite,* and finally a dividing form, termed a *schizont.* Schizont-infected red cells rupture and release approximately six to twenty new parasites (merozoites), which invade other red cells. The cycle of invasion, division, rupture, and reinvasion leads to an increasing parasitemia, with its resultant morbidity and mortality. Inhibition of the invasion would break this cycle and prevent the disease. Numerous studies indicate that malaria parasites possess ligands that bind to receptors on the red cell membrane and that receptor-ligand interactions are required for invasion (Miller et al. 1975, 1977; Pasvol et al. 1982; Perkins 1984; Hadley et al. 1986; Hadley and Miller 1988). Understanding the molecular basis of the invasion may lead to strategies for controlling the disease.

THE MORPHOLOGY OF INVASION

The invasion of a red cell by a merozoite is a multistep process, summarized in Figure 12.1 (Dvorak et al. 1975; Aikawa et al. 1978). The ability of a merozoite to attach to a red cell depends on the species of malaria and the species of the host from which the red cell is derived (McGhee 1953; Butcher et al. 1973; Mason et al. 1977; Miller et al. 1977). The specificity of the initial attachment indicates that receptors are involved at this step. Following the initial attachment, the merozoite reorients so that its apical end is in apposition to the red cell membrane. The molecular mechanism of the reorientation is unknown. When apical attachment occurs, the red cell undergoes a wave of deformation that appears to coincide with the release of the contents of a pair of apical organelles. A junction forms in a caplike distribution between the apical end of the merozoite and the red cell. The junction is an area of close apposition and molecular interaction between the red cell membrane and the surface of the merozoite. It is characterized by an electron-dense layer beneath the red cell membrane in the area where the red cell membrane is in apposition with the merozoite. As the invasion proceeds, the junction forms a circumferential band around the merozoite and moves from the apical end of the merozoite to the caudal end, bringing the merozoite into the red cell. Following the entry of the parasite into the red cell, a resealing of the red cell membrane occurs.

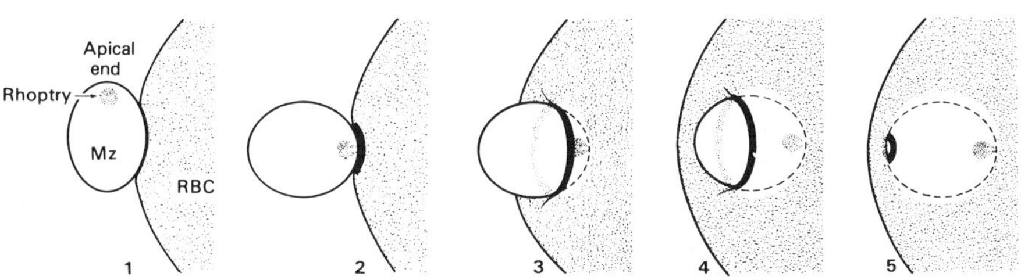

Figure 12.1. A schematic representation of a merozoite (Mz) invading a red cell (RBC). Following initial attachment (1), the merozoite reorients itself such that its apical end is in apposition to the red cell (2). The apical end is defined by organelles involved in invasion, which include the rhoptry. A junction forms between merozoite and red cell and is characterized by a region of electron density (on electron microscopy) beneath the red cell membrane (2). As the invasion proceeds, the junction moves as a circumferential band from the apical end to the posterior end of the merozoite, bringing the merozoite into the vacuole (3–5).

DUFFY ANTIGENS AND INVASION

A laboratory model that has proven useful in studying invasion is the monkey malaria, *P. knowlesi,* which infects Old World monkeys such as the Rhesus monkey and the kra monkey. *Plasmodium knowlesi* can also invade the red cells of humans and New World monkeys (except *Cebus appella*). Molecular analysis indicates that *P. knowlesi* is more closely related to the human malaria *P. vivax* than to the human malaria *P. falciparum* (McCutchan et al. 1984). *Plasmodium knowlesi* parasites can invade all human red cells tested except those that lack Duffy blood group antigens Fy^a and Fy^b (Miller et al. 1975). The resistance of $Fy(a-b-)$ red cells to invasion by *P. knowlesi* suggested that Fy^a and Fy^b are associated with a ligand used by this parasite. The finding that anti-Fy^a and anti-Fy^b block the invasion of *P. knowlesi* into $Fy\ (a+b-)$ and $Fy(a-b+)$ red cells, respectively, further supports this conclusion. Other studies demonstrated that *P. knowlesi* merozoites can attach to Duffy-negative red cells and undergo apical reorientation (Miller et al. 1979). Thus the initial attachment and apical reorientation are independent of Duffy blood group antigens; however, electron microscopic studies demonstrated that the morphology of apical attachment of *P. knowlesi* to Duffy-negative red cells is different from that of apical attachment to Duffy-positive red cells. Specifically, apical attachment to Duffy-negative red cells is characterized by a fine fibrillar material extending between the parasite and red cell, whereas apical attachment to Duffy-positive red cells is characterized by the formation of the junction. The data indicate that the formation of the junction between *P. knowlesi* and the red cell requires the presence of Duffy Fy^a- or Fy^b-related structures on the red cell membrane. The failure of *P. knowlesi* to invade Duffy-negative red cells appears to be related not to the failure of attachment but to the failure of junction formation. A concept implicit in these data is that at least two receptor-ligand interactions (and probably more) are required for invasion: one for the initial attachment, which is present on both Duffy-positive and Duffy-negative red cells, and another for junction formation, which is present only on Duffy-positive red cells.

Observations regarding Duffy blood group antigens and *P. knowlesi* have been extended to the human malaria *P. vivax*. When neurosyphilis was treated in the 1930s by infecting patients with malaria, it was noted that many black people are resistant to infection with *P. vivax* (Boyd and Stratman-Thomas 1933; Young et al. 1955). A study on blood group antigens of black people in New York City indicated that about 70 percent are Duffy negative (Sanger et al. 1955). A survey of blood group antigens among West Africans indicated that more than 95 percent are Duffy negative (Mourant and Kopec 1976). These observations, coupled with the data obtained with *P. knowlesi,* led to the hypothesis that *P. vivax* parasites also require the presence of Duffy antigen Fy^a or Fy^b for invasion. This hypothesis was borne out in several studies, which demonstrated that individuals who are Duffy negative are indeed resistant to infection with *P. vivax* (Miller et al. 1976, 1978; Spencer et al. 1978). Methods have been developed to study invasion by *P. vivax* in vitro, and it has been shown that this parasite cannot invade Duffy-negative red cells (Barnwell et al. 1989). Thus, *P. vivax,* as well as *P. knowlesi,* requires that presence of an Fy^a- or Fy^b-related red cell membrane receptor to invade human red cells.

Plasmodium vivax can also invade the red cells of the New World monkeys *Aotus trivirgatus* (owl monkey) and *Saimiri sciureus* (squirrel monkey). The red cells of the owl monkey possess Fy^b and Fy^{ab} [a Duffy antigen common to both Fy(a+b−) and Fy(a−b+) red cells] when typed with human antisera; the red cells of the squirrel monkey possess Fy^{ab}. *Plasmodium vivax* cannot invade the red cells of the New World monkey *Cebus apella,* which also possess Fy^{ab}, or the red cells of Old World monkeys such as *Macaca mulatta,* which possess both Fy^b and Fy^{ab} (Barnwell et al. 1989). The only murine monoclonal antibody to the human Duffy blood group system is anti-Fy6 (Nichols et al. 1987). Anti-Fy6 reacts with human Fy(a+b−), Fy(a−b+), and Fy(a+b+) red cells, but not with human Fy(a−b−) red cells. The Fy6 epitope has been shown to be separate from other Duffy epitopes such as Fy^{ab}. Anti-Fy6 reacts with the red cells of New World monkeys except *Cebus apella* and does not react with the red cells of Old World monkeys. Thus the distribution of the Fy6 antigenic epitope among primates correlates with the susceptibility of red cells to invasion by *P. vivax* (Table 12.1). This correlation suggests that the Fy6 may be the epitope recognized by *P. vivax* merozoites. *Plasmodium knowlesi,* which invades the red cells of Old World monkeys, must recognize a site on the Duffy blood group antigen other than Fy6, as Fy6 is not present on Old World monkey (Rhesus and kra) red cells.

Plasmodium vivax, unlike *P. knowlesi,* preferentially invades human reticulocytes. Thus, *P. vivax* parasites possess a ligand that binds to a reticulocyte-specific receptor in addition to a ligand that binds to a Duffy-related receptor. The reticulocyte-specific receptor has not been identified. Studies on the biology and cell biology of *P. knowlesi* and *P. vivax* provided convincing evidence that malaria parasites possess ligands for red cell receptors. These same studies suggested the concept that more than one receptor-ligand interaction is involved in invasion. Data from studies on *P. falciparum* further confirmed and extended the concept that more than one receptor-ligand interaction is involved in invasion.

SIALIC ACID AND PLASMODIUM FALCIPARUM

Plasmodium falciparum is the human malaria that causes most malaria-related mortalities. Unlike *P. vivax,* which has a preference for reticulocytes, *P. falciparum* invades red cells of all ages. *Plasmodium falciparum*

Table 12.1. The Correlation Between Duffy Blood Group Antigens on Red Cells and Susceptibility to *Plasmodium* Invasion*

	Fy^a	Fy^b	Fy3	Fy6	*P. vivax* Invasion	*P. knowlesi* Invasion
Human						
Fy (a+b−)	+	−	+	+	+	+
Fy (a−b+)	−	+	+	+	+	+
Fy (a−b−)	−	−	−	−	−	−
Old World Monkeys						
Rhesus	−	+	+	−	−	+
Kra	−	+	+	−	−	+
New World Monkeys						
Aotus	−	+	+	+	+	+
Squirrel	−	−	+	+	+	+
Marmoset	−	−	+	+	+	+
Cebus	−	−	+	−	−	−
Subprimate	−	−	−	−	−	−

*Note the association of the presence of the Fy6 antigen with invasion by *P. vivax*. The domains recognized by *P. knowlesi* have not been identified.

Key: + = positive correlation; − = negative correlation.

infections can therefore result in very high parasitemias and life-threatening complications, such as fulminant hemolysis, renal failure, pulmonary edema, and cerebral malaria. Studies on the red cell receptors for *P. falciparum* demonstrated differences from the requirements for *P. vivax* and *P. knowlesi*. *Plasmodium falciparum* does not require the presence of Fy^a or Fy^b for invasion. Duffy-negative red cells are invaded as efficiently as Duffy-positive red cells. It was observed, however, that neuraminidase treatment of human red cells results in decreased invasion by *P. falciparum* (Miller et al. 1977; Perkins 1981; Breuer et al. 1983). Furthermore, En(a−) red cells that lack glycophorin A (GPA) show a reduced susceptibility to invasion (Miller et al. 1977; Pasvol et al. 1982).

The first study on En(a−) red cells showed only a 50 percent reduction in invasion, which was similar to the reduction seen with neuraminidase-treated red cells in the same study (Miller et al. 1977). Since the reduction in invasion of En(a−) red cells was only 50 percent, it was concluded that other receptors on the red cell membrane, in addition to GPA, must be important for invasion. Interestingly, a subsequent study demonstrated a 90 percent reduction in the invasion by *P. falciparum* into En(a−) red cells (Pasvol et al. 1982). Other investigators also obtained 90 percent reductions in the invasion into neuraminidase-treated red cells. Different results obtained in different laboratories with En(a−) red cells and neuraminidase-treated red cells suggested the possibility that the structure or expression of ligands may vary among different strains of *P. falciparum*. This possibility was investigated by examining the invasion of different strains into sialic acid–deficient red cells under identical experimental conditions (Mitchell et al. 1986; Hadley et al. 1987; Perkins and Holt 1988). These experiments demonstrated that different strains of *P. falciparum* do vary in the ability to invade sialic acid–deficient red cells. Some strains invade neuraminidase-treated red cells with 50 percent efficiency compared with normal red cells; other strains invade neuraminidase-treated red cells with only 5 percent efficiency compared with normal red cells.

Studies indicating heterogeneity among *P. falciparum* parasites in terms of their invasion requirement for sialic acid also provided information on the role of GPA and GPB. Strains that showed a marked reduction of invasion into neuraminidase-treated red cells also showed a marked reduction into En(a−) red cells that lack GPA and into M^kM^k red cells that lack both GPA and GPB (Hadley et al. 1987, 1990). Strains that showed only a 50 percent reduction of invasion into neuraminidase-treated red cells showed only a 50 percent reduction into En(a−) or M^kM^k red cells. When these latter strains were tested with neuraminidase-treated M^kM^k red cells, the invasion remained around 50 percent. Thus, the absence of GPA and GPB did not impede the invasion to any degree greater than neuraminidase treatment. This finding suggests that GPA and, possibly, GPB, are important for invasion because they carry most of the sialic acid on the red cell membrane. The data suggest that sialic acid, rather than a peptide domain, constitutes one receptor for the parasite on GPA and GPB.

Recent data indicate that cloned parasites can change their phenotypic requirement for sialic acid from one of being totally dependent on sialic acid for invasion to one of being totally independent of sialic acid (Dolan et al. 1990). Cloned parasites from a single strain of *P. falciparum* were cultured in neuraminidase-treated red cells. Under these conditions, most clones do not grow and are soon lost from culture; however, it was noted that one clone, which initially disappeared from culture in neuraminidase-treated red cells (as detected by blood films stained with Giemsa and examined by light microscopy), reappeared after 10 to 12 days. This parasite, selected for its ability to grow and multiply in neuraminidase-treated red cells, was then tested for its ability to invade neuraminidase-treated red cells. Invasion studies demonstrated that this parasite could invade neuraminidase-treated red cells as efficiently as it could invade normal red cells. The parent clone, from which this parasite was derived, continued to demonstrate marked reductions in invasion into neuraminidase-treated red cells. The new sialic acid–independent parasite was shown by molecular fingerprinting to be the same as the sialic acid–dependent parent clone. The switch in invasion capability from sialic acid dependence to sialic acid independence probably results from the expression of a sialic acid–independent ligand on the new parasite.

The above data indicate that there are at least two pathways for invasion by *P. falciparum:* a sialic acid–dependent pathway and a sialic acid–independent pathway. Furthermore, *P. falciparum* parasites, adapted to culture, appear heterogeneous in their ability to use these pathways. Some parasites are almost totally dependent on the presence of red cell sialic acid for invasion, whereas other parasites are almost totally independent of red cell membrane sialic acid. This heterogeneity probably depends on the relative presence or absence of ligands on the parasite for sialic acid or for a sialic acid–independent receptor. The sialic acid–independent receptor for invasion has not yet been identified.

An important question related to sialic acid is does the parasite recognize a structural conformation of sialic acid, or does the sialic acid provide a negative charge to which the parasite binds by a charge-charge interaction? Studies using Cad red cells suggested that parasites recognize a structural conformation rather than a negative charge per se (Cartron et al. 1983). Cad red cells have an additional neutral sugar (N-acetylgalactosamine) linked to the penultimate sugar (galactose) on O-linked oligosaccharides, including those present on the glycophorins. This additional sugar does not change the charge of the red cell, but may alter the conformation or accessibility of adjacent sialic-acid residues. *Plasmodium falciparum* parasites that depend on sialic acid for optimal invasion show reduced invasion into Cad red cells.

Another line of evidence indicating that the structural conformation of sialic acid is important is based on the invasion of *P. falciparum* into murine red cells (Klotz et al. 1987). Genetic analysis has shown that *P. falciparum* is more closely related to rodent and avian malarias than to other primate malarias (McCutchan et al. 1984). Although *P. falciparum* cannot produce an in vivo infection in mice, it can invade murine red cells in vitro. Unlike human red cells, which possess N-acetylneuraminic acid as the only form of sialic acid, murine red cells contain N-acetylneuraminic acid, N-glycolylneuraminic acid, and 9-O-acetyl-N-acetylneuraminic acid. Treatment of murine red cells with influenza C esterase cleaves the 9-O-acetyl group from 9-O-acetyl-N-acetylneuraminic acid, converting it to N-acetylneuraminic acid, the human form of sialic acid. This treatment enhances invasion by *P. falciparum,* suggesting that the acetyl group on the 9 carbon sterically interferes with reception (Klotz et al., unpublished data). The fact that parasites can distinguish between N-acetylneuraminic acid and 9-O-acetyl-N-acetylneuraminic acid supports the concept that the parasite receptor recognizes a structural conformation of sialic acid rather than only negative charge.

GLYCOPHORIN AND PLASMODIUM FALCIPARUM

There is a controversy regarding whether or not a peptide portion of GPA also constitutes a binding site for the parasite. A peptide of GPA, consisting of amino acids 65 to 69 (peptide 65-69), has been shown to inhibit invasion in vitro (Tounkara et al. 1986). Peptides flanking peptide 65-69 were inhibitory, thereby exluding toxicity introduced by the peptide-purification procedure. Nevertheless, interpretation of inhibition studies can be problematic because it is difficult to exclude the toxicity of the peptide per se (Hermentin et al. 1986, 1987). Subtle toxicity or nonspecific inhibition through hydrophobic interactions may not be apparent by the morphologic appearance of the parasite or even by its ability to incorporate radiolabeled metabolites. Also, inhibition of invasion can potentially occur by mechanisms other than receptor blockade. For example, a peptide may inhibit a proteolytic enzyme that is necessary for rupture or invasion. It would be of interest to test the effect of peptide 65-69 on invasion by *P. knowlesi,* a parasite that does not require GPA for invasion. If peptide 65-69 were to inhibit *P. knowlesi,* mechanisms other than receptor blockade would have to be considered. The chymotryptic peptide containing amino acids 1 to 64 of GPA has also been shown to inhibit invasion; however, this peptide contains O-linked oligosaccharides, and the inhibition may be due to specific receptor blockade by N-acetylneuraminic acid on the O-linked oligosaccharides (Hermentin et al. 1987).

The amino acid sequence of the GPA may be important because it determines the density or clustering of O-linked oligosaccharides containing N-acetylneuraminic acid. The chymotryptic peptide of GPA, peptide 1-64, contains densely clustered O-linked oligosaccharides and inhibits invasion, whereas fetuin, which contains similar O-linked oligosaccharides and N-acetylneuraminic acid, does not inhibit invasion (Hermentin et al. 1986). However, the O-linked oligosaccharides on fetuin are not as densely clustered as those on GPA. The concept that the distribution of N-acetylneuraminic acid is important for parasite recognition requires further investigation.

Initially, it was hoped that the identification and purification of red cell receptors for parasite binding would enable investigators to use these receptors as affinity substrates for the identification and purification of parasite receptors. This approach has been taken using GPA in an attempt to purify a *P. falciparum* ligand. Extracts of radiolabeled *P. falciparum* parasites were incubated with GPA immobilized on acrylamide beads (Perkins 1984). A 130-kDa *P. falciparum* protein that binds to GPA on acrylamide beads was purified. However, a subsequent study demonstrated that the 130-kDa protein binds to positively charged acrylamide beads alone, thus calling into question the specificity of binding (van Schravendijk et al. 1987).

THE DUFFY BLOOD GROUP ANTIGEN

Theoretically, immobilized Duffy antigen could be used to affinity-purify ligands from *P. knowlesi* or *P. vivax.* Experiments using this approach have not yet been reported because, until recently, the Duffy antigen had not been purified. The Duffy antigen was identified by immunoblotting with anti-Fy^a (Hadley et al. 1984). The Duffy protein migrates as a broad band between 35 and 43 kDa when whole red cell membranes are analyzed by sodium dodecyl sulfate–polyacrylamide gel electrophoresis (SDS-PAGE) followed by immunoblotting with anti-Fy^a. Its susceptibility to proteases indicates that it is a protein. Purification of the Duffy protein has been complicated by the fact that it is a minor red cell membrane protein with an estimated number of 5000 to 20,000 copies per red cell (in contrast to GPA, which is present in around 300,000 copies per red cell) and by the fact that it appears to interact with other membrane proteins (possibly through hydrophobic interactions) during purification.

A monoclonal antibody (anti-Fy6) has been produced against an epitope on the Duffy protein, designated Fy6 (Nichols et al. 1987). Anti-Fy6 was used to purify the Duffy protein (Chaudhuri et al. 1989). The purification scheme involved binding the monoclonal antibody to intact red cells, lysing the red cells in hypotonic buffer, solubilizing the membranes (with bound antibody) in Triton X-100, and precipitating Duffy–anti-Duffy immune complexes with anti-mouse IgG-sepharose. Precipitated proteins were analyzed for Duffy reactivity by SDS-PAGE followed by immunoblotting with anti-Fy6. Three Duffy-reactive bands were identified, designated pD, pB, and pA. pD has an apparent molecular weight of 36 to 46 kDa, which is consistent with the Fy^a reactive protein previously identified. pB has an apparent molecular weight of around 100 kDa, and pA has an apparent molecular weight of more than 200 kDa. When pD was electroeluted from the 36- to 46-kDa region of the gel, stored at −20°C or 4°C, and reanalyzed by SDS-PAGE followed by immunoblotting, pD, pB, and pA were again noted. This finding suggests that pB is probably a dimer and pA is probably an oligomer of pD. pD from Fy(a+b−) red cells was shown by two-dimensional peptide mapping to differ from pD from Fy(a−b+) red cells. The apparent molecular weight of pD as detected with anti-Fy6 did not change after treatment with glycosidases. In contrast, we and others have observed a shift in the apparent molecular weight of the Duffy protein (as recognized by anti-Fy^a) after treatment of intact membranes and partially purified protein with neuraminidase and endoglycosidase F (Hadley et al. 1984; Tanner et al. 1988). The shift observed with neuraminidase appeared to affect a subset of Duffy-reactive molecules as analyzed by immunoblotting with anti-Fy^a. After neuraminidase treatment of membranes, Duffy reactivity was seen at a slightly lower molecular weight, in addition to Duffy reactivity at the original molecular weight (35 to 43 kDa). It is possible that the Duffy blood group protein is heterogeneous in terms of its glycosylation and in terms of its reactivity with neuraminidase, endoglycosidase F, and anti-Fy6. Alternatively, it is possible that the shift in molecular weight observed after treatment with endoglycosidase F is due to proteolysis by trace amounts of proteases contaminating these enzymes. Although the experiments were done in the presence of several protease inhibitors, it is difficult to formally exclude proteolysis. The shift in molecular weight seen after neuraminidase treatment is unlikely to be due to proteolysis, as *Vibrio cholerae* neuraminidase was used and this enzyme is not known to be contaminated with proteases. Further experiments are required to resolve the question of whether the Duffy protein is variably glycosylated.

RED CELL BINDING PROTEINS

THE IDENTIFICATION OF PARASITE LIGANDS

The use of immobilized receptors as affinity substrates offers a potentially useful approach to the identification and purification of parasite ligands. Thus far, however, this approach has yielded inconclusive results in the case of *P. falciparum* and, until recently, has not been possible with *P. knowlesi* or *P. vivax*. An alternative approach to identifying parasite ligands uses intact red cells as an affinity substrate (Camus and Hadley 1986). This approach was taken for several reasons. First, other approaches to the identification of parasite ligands had been inconclusive. Second, it was reasoned that parasite ligands should bind to red cells and that intact red cells might provide optimal binding because the receptor would be in its native configuration in the intact membrane. Third, the specificity of binding could be tested by using different red cells to test for binding, some of which were susceptible to invasion and others of which were resistant to invasion. Parasite ligands that bind to intact red cells were sought in culture supernatants for the following reasons. First, culture supernatants were known to contain many malarial proteins, and working with culture supernatants avoided the use of detergents that would lyse intact red cells. Second, it had shown by immunofluorescence that malarial antigens from culture were associated with the surface of uninfected red cells (Mendis et al. 1983). Third, membrane receptor proteins, such as the Tac protein of the interleukin-2 receptor, had been reported to be present in culture supernatants in other biologic systems (Waldman 1986-87).

Experiments on red cell binding proteins were carried out in the following manner. Purified trophozoite- and schizont-infected red cells were cultured in the presence of ^{3}H-isoleucine so that parasite proteins were radiolabeled. Cultured parasites were permitted to mature and rupture from infected red cells. Culture supernatants containing radiolabeled parasite proteins were incubated with intact, uninfected red cells. The red cells were washed, lysed with nonionic detergent, and radiolabeled. Parasite proteins that had bound to the surface of the red cell were immunoprecipitated with polyclonal hyperimmune sera from monkeys that had been repeatedly infected with *P. falciparum.* The technique of identifying red cell binding proteins was subsequently modified to avoid the immunoprecipitaton step (Haynes et al. 1988).

The initial experiments were done with *P. falciparum* culture supernatants and red cells from various humans, nonhuman primates, and subprimates and with red cells after treatment with neuraminidase, trypsin, and chymotrypsin (Camus and Hadley 1986; Orlandi et al. 1990). A protein with an apparent molecular weight of 175 kDa on SDS-PAGE was identified which bound to red cells that could be invaded by *P. falciparum* but not to red cells that could not be invaded. For example, the 175-kDa protein bound to *Aotus* red cells (which were invaded), but not to guinea pig red cells (which were not invaded). It bound to chymotrypsin-treated red cells (which were invaded) but not to trypsin-treated red cells (which showed markedly reduced invasion). The binding of the 175-kDa protein to red cells was dependent on red cell sialic acid, as the protein did not bind to neuraminidase-treated red cells (which showed markedly reduced invasion). Because of the specificity of binding, it was postulated that the 175-kDa red cell binding protein is the sialic acid–dependent ligand of *P. falciparum.*

Using similar techniques for the identification of ligands, Perkins and Rocco (1988) identified a soluble protein of *P. falciparum* that binds to human red cells in a sialic acid–dependent fashion. This protein was reported to have a slightly higher apparent molecular weight (200 kDa as determined by SDS-PAGE) than the 175-kDa red cell binding protein described by Camus and Hadley (1985). The apparent molecular weight of the 175-kDa protein can be shifted upward, depending on the percentage of polyacrylamide used. The 200-kDa red cell binding protein was immunoprecipitated by antisera to the major surface glycoprotein on merozoites, MSA 1, a protein that has been characterized in a number of laboratories. In the study by Camus and Hadley, monoclonal antibodies against MSA 1 did not immunoprecipitate the 175-kDa red cell binding protein. It is possible that there are two different red cell binding proteins, both of which bind in a sialic acid–dependent fashion. An important question remains, however: if there are indeed two different red cell binding proteins that are sialic acid–dependent, why did each laboratory not find both proteins, as they were using similar assay methods? Red cell binding proteins have been examined from a number of different strains of *P. falciparum.* Both the MSA 1 and the sialic acid binding protein, originally designated as 175 kDa, have variable molecular weights with different strains. Thus, each laboratory studying red cell binding proteins should have observed both proteins. Two possibilities remain to be resolved: (1) both laboratories are studying the same molecule and, for technical reasons, claiming that it is different; or (2) there are two different sialic acid–dependent red cell binding proteins and each laboratory is not identifying one because of undefined differences in their reagents.

The results obtained with *P. falciparum* prompted similar experiments with *P. knowlesi,* the parasite that had been used to define many aspects of malarial invasion. It was postulated that if the 175-kDa red cell binding protein of *P. falciparum* is indeed a ligand, then an analogous protein might be present in *P. knowlesi* and *P. vivax. Plasmodium knowlesi,* unlike most cultured strains of *P. falciparum,* does not depend on red cell sialic acid for invasion. Therefore, it was postulated that a red cell binding protein of *P. knowlesi* should bind independently of red cell sialic acid. It was further postulated that *P. knowlesi* might produce a protein that binds to red cells in a Duffy-dependent fashion. This would comprise additional evidence that red cell binding proteins of both *P. knowlesi* and *P. falciparum* bind with specificity and therefore are probably ligands. Experiments using *P. knowlesi* identified a 135-kDa red cell binding antigen that did indeed bind to human red cells in a Duffy-dependent fashion (i.e., it bound to Duffy-positive human red cells but not to Duffy-negative human red cells) (Haynes et al. 1988; Miller et al. 1989). Binding of the 135-kDa red cell binding protein of *P. knowlesi* was not dependent on red cell membrane sialic acid, as was the binding of the 175-kDa protein of *P. falciparum.* Furthermore, when the 135-kDa protein was eluted from Duffy-positive red cells and used to probe a blot of red cell membrane proteins separated by SDS-PAGE, it bound to the 35 to 43 kDa region of the blot, the precise area where the Duffy protein migrates. Binding of the 135-kDa red cell binding protein of *P. knowlesi* to human Fy(a+b−) and Fy(a−b+) red cells was blocked by anti-Fy^a and anti-Fy6 monoclonal antibody, respectively. These data indicate that the 135-kDa red cell binding protein of *P. knowlesi* binds to the Duffy protein per se and is probably the parasite ligand for the Duffy receptor.

A red cell binding protein (135 to 140 kDa) similar to that of *P. knowlesi* has been identified from *P. vivax* (Wertheimer and Barnwell 1989). The red cell binding protein of *P. vivax* binds to Duffy-positive human red cells but not to Duffy-negative human red cells. In contrast to the 135-kDa protein of *P. knowlesi,* the 135- to 140-kDa protein of *P. vivax* does not bind to Rhesus red cells. This supports the specificity of binding, because Rhesus red cells cannot be invaded by *P. vivax* parasites.

Rhesus red cells type as Fy(a−b+) and also express the Fy^{ab} antigen. However, they do not react with the monoclonal anti-Fy6, as do human red cells, indicating that differences exist between the Duffy protein of humans and that of Rhesus monkeys. Such differences may underlie the inability of *P. vivax* to invade Rhesus red cells.

Another important feature of the invasion of *P. knowlesi* into Rhesus red cells is that invasion can occur even after the Duffy antigen (Fy^b) has been removed by chymotrypsin. Thus, whereas invasion of *P. knowlesi* into human red cells is dependent on the presence of Duffy antigens, invasion into Rhesus red cells can occur independent of Duffy antigens. The nature of the Duffy-independent pathway or receptor is unknown. The picture that is emerging from studies on *P. knowlesi* and *P. falciparum* is that invasion by these parasites may not be limited by the absence of a single receptor; alternative pathways are present. It is not clear if there are alternative receptors at each step of the multistep invasion process or if alternative receptors exist at only one step. Since it is crucial to the parasite's survival to invade red cells, it is not surprising that alternative pathways for invasion have evolved. What is surprising is that *P. vivax* has not evolved an alternative pathway that would circumvent its requirement for Duffy antigens. This requirement has virtually excluded *P. vivax* from West Africa, where more than 95 percent of the population is Duffy negative.

Another important feature of the invasion of *P. vivax* into human red cells is that the parasite has a preference for reticulocytes. A 250-kDa red cell binding protein that binds preferentially to reticulocytes has been identified and is probably the reticulocyte-specific ligand. The receptor on reticulocytes for this protein has not yet been identified.

THE CLONING OF PARASITE LIGANDS

The method used to clone parasite ligands for binding to the Duffy blood group antigen (the Duffy ligands of *P. knowlesi* and *P. vivax*) and sialic acid on glycophorin (the glycophorin ligand of *P. falciparum*) was based on the method used for identifying the parasite ligands. Soluble proteins were affinity-purified on red cells, eluted from the red cells, separated by PAGE, and electroblotted to nitrocellulose. Antibodies from hyperimmune serum were reacted with the strip of nitrocellulose that contained the ligand. Eluted antibody was used to screen λgtll expression libraries. Cloned genes were then shown to encode receptors by the production of antibodies to multiple regions of the proteins. Definitive proof that these are indeed receptor molecules will require the binding of red cells to receptor gene products expressed in eukaryotic expression systems.

Plasmodium knowlesi has a gene family consisting of three genes on three different chromosomes (Adams et al. 1990). Antisera to a fusion protein expressing a peptide sequence shared by all three gene products was used to identify a set of three proteins translated in vitro from parasite mRNA. These proteins, 180 kDa, 170 kDa, and 165 kDa, were also precipitated by an antibody produced against a shared C-terminal peptide sequence. Experiments indicate that these three proteins do not arise from alternate splicing but are transcribed separately from three different genes. Immunoprecipitations from detergent-extracted parasites identified a 148/145-kDa doublet. Pulse-chase experiments indicate that the 145-kDa protein does not arise from the 148-kDa protein. During the chase period, a 138/135-kDa doublet appears in culture supernatants, indicating that these proteins are probably proteolytic products of the higher-molecular-weight precursors. There is no evidence from pulse-chase experiments that the 135-kDa protein is derived from the 138-kDa protein. The 135-kDa protein is the Duffy-dependent red cell binding protein that binds to human, Rhesus, and New World monkey red cells. The 138-kDa protein is an erythrocyte-binding protein that binds only to Rhesus red cells.

Antibodies to homologous regions of these proteins were also used to determine their location within the parasite by immunoelectronmicroscopy. These proteins are located within the micronemes at the apical end of the parasite. This location is also consistent with their function as ligands, as these proteins could be transported to the merozoite surface at or near the time of invasion. Alternatively, soluble ligands may function as a bridge between another parasite molecule and the red cell surface.

The cloned portion of the *P. knowlesi* gene was used to identify and clone the gene encoding the 135- to 140-kDa red cell binding protein of *P. vivax* (Fang et al. 1991). In contrast to *P. knowlesi,* a single gene, rather than a gene family, was identified. In the sequences of *P. vivax* and *P. knowlesi* on the N-terminal side of the transmembrane region, two areas of high homology are separated by an area of no homology. In the two homologous regions, 65.4 percent and 61 percent of the amino acids of *P. vivax* are identical to those found in the α *P. knowlesi* gene. The cysteines in both of these homologous regions are in identified positions in *P. vivax* and *P. knowlesi,* indicating a similar tertiary structure of the protein in each species. It is predicted that the cysteine-rich homologous regions of *P. knowlesi* and *P. vivax* will be found to contain the binding site for the Duffy protein. The nonhomologous region between the homologous regions is proline-rich and hydrophilic, suggestive of a hinge region.

The gene that codes for the 175-kDa red cell binding protein of *P. falciparum* (Sim et al. 1990) is not homologous to the genes of *P. knowlesi* and *P. vivax* described above. Antibodies against a peptide corresponding to amino acid residues 1062 to 1103 of the *P. falciparum* gene blocked the invasion of the parasite into red cells and also blocked the binding of the 175-kDa red cell binding protein to red cells (Sim et al. 1990). The anti–175-kDa antibodies also reacted by immunofluorescence in a dotlike pattern at the apical region of merozoites, consistent with the location of the protein in an apical organelle. It is not known whether this protein (or the Duffy-dependent ligands of *P. knowlesi* and *P. vivax*) is expressed constitutively on the surface of the merozoite or whether it is transported there at or near the time of rupture and invasion.

FUTURE RESEARCH

The cell biology of invasion at the molecular level is little understood. The sequence of receptor-ligand interactions from initial recognition to internalization has yet to be defined. For example, the molecules involved in initial recognition between merozoite and red cell are unknown. Is there a significance to the choice of red cell molecules used for attachment—that is, are these important for signals to the cytoskeleton or reorganization at the membrane? Why do *P. knowlesi* and *P. vivax* bind to the Duffy blood group antigen and *P. falciparum* to sialic acid on GPA? The biochemistry of the Duffy blood group system is at a rudimentary stage and may amplify our understanding of the cell biology of invasion. The reticulocyte receptor has presumably been selected for by a parasite requirement for growth in young red cells, but the molecule involved has not been defined. It is expected that basic research in this area will lead to novel approaches to vaccines and chemotherapy.

REFERENCES

Adams, J. H., D. E. Hudson, M. Torii, G. E. Ward, T. E. Wellems, M. Aikawa, and L. H. Miller. 1990. The Duffy receptor family of *Plasmodium knowlesi* is located within the micronemes of invasive malaria merozoites. *Cell* 63:141–53.

Aikawa, M., L. H. Miller, J. Johnson, and J. Rabbege. 1978. Erythrocyte entry by malaria parasites: A moving junction between erythrocyte and parasite. *J. Cell Biol.* 77:72–82.

Barnwell, J. W., M. E. Nichols, and P. Rubinstein. 1989. *In vitro* evaluation of the role of the Duffy blood group in erythrocyte invasion by *Plasmodium vivax*. *J. Exp. Med.* 169:1795–1802.

Boyd, M. F., and W. K. Stratman-Thomas. 1933. Studies on benign tertian malaria: On the refractoriness of Negroes to inoculation with *Plasmodium vivax*. *Am. J. Hyg.* 18:485–89.

Breuer, W. V., H. Ginsburg, and Z. I. Cabantchik. 1983. An assay of malaria parasite invasion into human erythrocytes: The effects of chemical and enzymatic modification of erythrocyte membrane components. *Biochim. Biophys. Acta* 755:263–71.

Butcher, G. A., G. H. Mitchell, and S. Cohen. 1973. Mechanism of host specificity in malarial infection. *Nature* 244:40–42.

Camus, D., and T. J. Hadley. 1985. A *Plasmodium falciparum* antigen that binds to host erythrocytes and merozoites. *Science* 230:553–56.

Cartron, J. P., O. Prou, M. Luiller, and J. P. Soulier. 1983. Susceptibility to invasion by *Plasmodium falciparum* of some human erythrocytes carrying rare blood group antigens. *Br. J. Haematol.* 55:639–47.

Chaudhuri, A., V. Zbrezna, C. Johnson, M. Nichols, P. Rubinstein, W. L. Marsh, and A. O. Pogo. 1989. Purification and characterization of an erythrocyte membrane protein complex carrying Duffy blood group antigenicity: Possible receptor for *Plasmodium vivax* and *Plasmodium knowlesi* malaria parasite. *J. Biol. Chem.* 264:13770–74.

Dolan, S. A., L. H. Miller, and T. E. Wellems. 1990. Evidence for a switching mechanism in the invasion of erythrocytes by *Plasmodium falciparum*. *J. Clin. Invest.* 86:618–24.

Dvorak, J. A., L. H. Miller, W. C. Whitehouse, and T. Shiroishi. 1975. Invasion of erythrocytes by malaria merozoites. *Science* 187:748–49.

Fang, X., D. C. Kaslow, J. H. Adams, and L. H. Miller. 1991. Cloning of the *Plasmodium vivax* Duffy receptor. *Mol. Biochem. Parasitol.* 44:125–32.

Hadley, T. J., P. H. David, M. H. McGinniss, and L. H. Miller. 1984. Identification of an erythrocyte component carrying the Duffy blood group Fy^a antigen. *Science* 223:597–99.

Hadley, T. J., F. W. Klotz, D. J. Anstee, J. D. Haynes, and L. H. Miller. 1990. Invasion of erythrocytes deficient in glycophorin C by *Plasmodium falciparum* malaria parasites. In *Cellular and molecular biology of normal and abnormal erythroid membranes.* UCLA Symposia on Molecular and Cellular Biology 118:301–14.

Hadley, T. J., F. W. Klotz, and L. H. Miller. 1986. Invasion of erythrocytes by malaria parasites: A cellular and molecular overview. *Ann. Rev. Microbiol.* 40:451–77.

Hadley, T. J., and L. H. Miller. 1988. Invasion of erythrocytes by malaria parasites: Erythrocyte ligands and parasite receptors. *Prog. Allergy* 41:49–71.

Hadley, T. J., F. W. Klotz, G. Pasvol, J. D. Haynes, M. H. McGinniss, Y. Okubo, and L. H. Miller. 1987. *Falciparum* malaria parasites invade erythrocytes that lack glycophorin A and B (M^kM^k): Strain differences indicate receptor heterogeneity and two pathways for invasion. *J. Clin. Invest.* 80:1190–93.

Haynes, J. D., J. P. Dalton, F. W. Klotz, M. H. McGinniss, T. J. Hadley, D. E. Hudson, and L. H. Miller. 1988. Receptor-like specificity of a *Plasmodium knowlesi* malarial protein that binds to Duffy antigen ligands on erythrocytes. *J. Exp. Med.* 167:1873–81.

Hermentin, P., G. Neunziger, B. Enders, and W. Dahr. 1987. Toxic effect of isolated glycophorin A on the *in vitro* growth of *Plasmodium falciparum. Blut* 54:115–22.

Hermentin, P., G. Neunziger, H. Paulsen, F. R. Kolar, R. Seiler, W. Dahr, and B. Enders. 1986. Toxicity of hydrophobic groupings and the role of carbohydrates in *Plasmodium falciparum* infection. *Behring Inst. Mitt.* 80:64–73.

Klotz, F. W., J. D. Chulay, W. Daniel, and L. H. Miller. 1987. Invasion of mouse erythrocytes by human malaria parasite, *Plasmodium falciparum. J. Exp. Med.* 165:359–67.

Mason, S. J., L. H. Miller, T. Shiroishi, J. A. Dvorak, and M. H. McGinniss. 1977. The Duffy blood group determinants: Their role in the susceptibility of human and animal erythrocytes to *Plasmodium knowlesi* malaria. *Br. J. Haematol.* 36:327–35.

McCutchan, T. F., J. B. Dame, L. H. Miller, and J. Barnwell. 1984. Evolutionary relatedness of *Plasmodium* species as determined by the structure of DNA. *Science* 225:808–11.

McGhee, R. B. 1953. The infection by *Plasmodium lophurae* of duck erythrocytes in the chicken embryo. *J. Exp. Med.* 97:773–82.

Mendis, K. N., P. H. David, M. Hommel, R. Carter, and L. Miller. 1983. Immunity to malarial antigens on the surface of *Plasmodium falciparum*–infected erythrocytes. *Am. J. Trop. Med. Hyg.* 32:926–30.

Miller, L. H., M. Aikawa, J. G. Johnson, and T. Shiroishi. 1979. Interaction between cytochalasin B–treated malarial parasites and erythrocytes: Attachment and junction formation. *J. Exp. Med.* 149:172–85.

Miller, L. H., J. D. Haynes, F. M. McAuliffe, T. Shiroishi, J. Durocher, and M. H. McGinniss. 1977. Evidence for differences in erythrocyte surface receptors for the malaria parasites *Plasmodium falciparum* and *Plasmodium knowlesi. J. Exp. Med.* 146:277–81.

Miller, L. H., D. Hudson, and J. D. Haynes. 1989. Identification of *Plasmodium knowlesi* erythrocyte binding proteins. *Mol. Biochem. Parasitol.* 36:177–86.

Miller, L. H., S. J. Mason, D. F. Clyde, and M. H. McGinniss. 1976. The resistance factor to *Plasmodium vivax* in blacks: The Duffy-blood-group genotype, *FyFy*. *N. Engl. J. Med.* 295:302–4.

Miller, L. H., S. J. Mason, J. A. Dvorak, M. G. McGinniss, and I. K. Rothman. 1975. Erythrocyte receptors for (*Plasmodium knowlesi*) malaria: Duffy blood group determinants. *Science* 189:561–63.

Miller, L. H., M. H. McGinniss, P. V. Holland, and P. Sigmon. 1978. The Duffy blood group phenotype in American blacks with *Plasmodium vivax* in Vietnam. *Am. J. Trop. Med. Hyg.* 27:1069–72.

Mitchell, G. H., T. J. Hadley, F. W. Klotz, M. H. McGinniss, and L. H. Miller. 1986. Invasion of erythrocytes by *Plasmodium falciparum* malaria parasites: Evidence for receptor heterogeneity and two receptors. *Blood* 67:1519–21.

Mourant, A. E., and A. C. Kopec. 1976. *The distribution of human blood groups and other polymorphisms.* 2nd ed. London, Oxford University Press.

Nichols, M. E., P. Rubinstein, J. Barnwell, S. Rodriquez de Cordoba, and R. Rosenfield. 1987. A new human Duffy blood group specificity defined by a murine monoclonal antibody: Immunogenetics and association with susceptibility to *Plasmodium vivax*. *J. Exp. Med.* 166:776–85.

Orlandi, P. A., B. K. L. Sim, J. D. Chulay, and J. D. Haynes. 1990. Characterization of the 175-kilodalton erythrocyte binding antigen of *Plasmodium falciparum*. *Mol. Biochem. Parasitol.* 40:285–94.

Pasvol, G., J. S. Wainscoat, and D. J. Weatherall. 1982. Erythrocytes deficient in glycophorin resist invasion by the malarial parasite, *Plasmodium falciparum*. *Nature* 297:64–66.

Perkins, M. E. 1981. Inhibitory effects of erythrocyte membrane proteins on the *in vitro* invasion of the human malarial parasite (*Plasmodium falciparum*) into its host cell. *J. Cell Biol.* 90:563–67.

———. 1984. Surface proteins of *Plasmodium falciparum* merozoites binding to the erythrocyte receptor, glycophorin. *J. Exp. Med.* 160:788–98.

Perkins, M. E., and E. H. Holt. 1988. Erythrocyte receptor recognition varies in *Plasmodium falciparum* isolates. *Mol. Biochem. Parasitol.* 27:23–34.

Perkins, M. E., and L. J. Rocco. 1988. Sialic acid–dependent binding of *Plasmodium falciparum* merozoite surface antigen, Pf 200, to human erythrocytes. *J. Immunol.* 141:3190–96.

Sanger, R., R. R. Race, and J. Jack. 1955. The Duffy blood groups of New York Negroes: The phenotype Fy(a − b −). *Br. J. Haematol.* 1:370–74.

Sim, B. K. L., P. A. Orlandi, J. D. Haynes, F. W. Klotz, J. M. Carter, D. Camus, H. E. Zegens, and J. D. Chulay. 1990. Primary structure of the 175-K *Plasmodium falciparum* binding antigen and identification of a peptide which elicits antibodies that inhibit malaria merozoite invasion. *J. Cell Biol.* 111:1877–84.

Spencer, H. C., L. H. Miller, W. E. Collins, C. Knud-Hansen, M. McGinniss, R. A. Lobos, and R. A. Feldman. 1978. The Duffy blood group and resistance to *Plasmodium vivax* in Honduras. *Am. J. Trop. Med. Hyg.* 27:664–70.

Tanner, M. J. A., D. J. Anstee, G. Mallinson, K. Ridgwell, P. G. Martin, N. D. Avent, and S. F. Parsons. 1988. Effect of endoglycosidase F-peptidyl N-glycosidase F preparations on the surface components of the human erythrocyte. *Carbohydr. Res.* 178:203–12.

Tounkara, A., F. Piller, D. Blanchard, J. P. Cartron, B. Ferrari, and A. Pavia. 1986. Evaluation of receptor sites for *Plasmodium falciparum* on human erythrocytes. In *Peptides: A chemical synthesis of peptides relevant to glycophorin.* D. Theodoropoulas, ed. 619–22. Amsterdam, Walter D. Gruyter.

van Schravendijk, M. R., R. J. M. Wilson, and C. Newbold. 1987. Possible pitfalls in the identification of glycophorin-binding proteins of *Plasmodium falciparum*. *J. Exp. Med.* 166:376–90.

Waldman, T. A. 1986–87. The multichain interleukin-2 receptor from gene to bedside. *Harvey Lect.* 82:1–17.

Wertheimer, S. P., and J. W. Barnwell. 1989. *Plasmodium vivax* interaction with the human Duffy blood group glycoprotein: Identification of a parasite receptor-like protein. *Exp. Parasitol.* 69:340–50.

Young, M. D., D. E. Eyles, R. W. Burgess, and G. M. Jeffrey. 1955. Experimental testing of the immunity of Negroes to *Plasmodium vivax*. *J. Parasitol.* 41:315–28.

13

HEMPAS AND OTHER CONGENITAL DYSERYTHROPOIETIC ANEMIAS

Michiko N. Fukuda, Ph.D.

Congenital dyserythropoietic anemias (CDAs) are a group of relatively rare but well-defined genetic diseases. They result from several distinct cellular abnormalities; the most common type is the result of abnormal glycosylation of red cell integral membrane polypeptides. Congenital dyserythropoietic anemias are characterized by ineffective erythropoiesis and morphologic abnormalities of the erythroblasts (Wolff and Von Hofe 1951).

In 1968, Heimpel and Wendt classified CDAs into three types. Later, variants and unclassified CDAs were described (Boogaerts and Verwilghen 1982), but the original classification has not only retained its validity but also has received strong support from ultrastructural, serologic, and biochemical findings. Although numerous observations have shown fundamental difference among the three types of CDA, common manifestations appear as gross abnormalities in membrane structures and multinuclearity in erythroblasts. The most recent study indicated that the primary gene defect of CDA type II (HEMPAS) occurs in the gene encoding a glycosylation enzyme (Fukuda et al. 1990). This defect brings changes in physical properties of plasma membrane glycoproteins and further disturbs membrane organization in erythroid cells (Fukuda et al. 1986b). Both CDA type I and CDA type III show morphologic abnormalities in nuclei and nuclear membranes (Lewis et al. 1972; Björksten et al. 1978). The breakdown of the membrane envelope is more severe in CDA type I than in CDA type III erythroblasts. This chapter summarizes observations and findings of CDAs. In particular, CDA type II (HEMPAS) will be described in detail, based on the recent studies on the primary gene defect.

CONGENITAL DYSERYTHROPOIETIC ANEMIA TYPE I

Type I CDA is quite rare: only about 30 cases have been reported in the literature. The patients are mildly or severely anemic. The onset was seen in early childhood, as early as two months in one case (Mori et al. 1986), or was not recognized until the patient was older than 30 years in other cases (Lewis et al. 1972). Inheritance of CDA type I is autosomal recessive.

The anemia is due to ineffective erythropoiesis in the patient's bone marrow, which clearly demonstrates erythroid hyperplasia. The majority of the red cell precursors beyond the stage of the proerythroblast and early basophilic erythroblasts show striking morphologic abnormalities in nuclei (Heimpel et al. 1971; Lewis et al. 1972). These abnormalities include uneven condensation and spongy appearance of chromatin, incomplete separation of nuclei, and spindles bridging the nuclei of two cells. Binucleated cells that appear to have resulted from incomplete nuclear division can be seen clearly under a light microscope. Close examination by electron microscopy shows the presence of cytoplasmic organelles such as mitochondria in the nucleus, indicating cytoplasmic invagination into the nucleus. In the late erythroblasts, polyribosomes appear to be less frequent than normal. Mature red cells do not show significant ultrastructural abnormalities (Lewis et al. 1972).

The disappearance of the nuclear envelope, appearance of similar membrane structures in the cytoplasm, and appearance of the widening nuclear pores strongly suggest that the anomaly of CDA type I is closely related to the nuclear envelope. Hiraoka and colleagues (1983) suggested that the primary abnormality is in the nuclear membrane itself, a conclusion based on their observations with thin-section and freeze-fracture electron microscopy of CDA type I erythroblasts. The nuclear envelopes of erythroblasts frequently lacked heterochromatin in wide areas and often showed a marked nuclear invagination and/or evagination. This was associated with the invasion of cytoplasmic organelles into the nuclear space and occasionally with extrusion of the nuclear contents into the cytoplasm. There were no nuclear pores on the invaginated or the evaginated portions of the nuclear envelope where the perinuclear cisternae were compressed to lose the cisternal space or widened to contain membrane debris.

Heimpel and colleagues (1971) suggested that an aberrant interaction exists between hemoglobin and nuclear membrane components. From their observation they stated that the nuclear changes are absent in early basophilic stages and present at the time of hemoglobinization. Wickramasinghe and Pippard (1986) reported an unbalanced globin-chain synthesis with increased α:β globin-chain synthesis ratios in two CDA type I patients. Occasionally, intracytoplasmic inclusions are seen in erythroblasts, and they are indistinguishable from precipitated α-chains. Electron microscopic autoradiography studies showed that a high proportion of the erythroblasts contain morphologically abnormal nuclei and suffered from impairment or arrest of DNA, RNA, and protein synthesis. The failure of macromolecule synthesis follows rather than precedes the development of the Swiss cheese–like nuclear morphology, which suggests that the primary biochemical lesion may be in the nuclear proteins of the cells

(Wickramasinghe and Pippard 1986). The abnormality in nucleoprotein synthesis may lead to various secondary effects, including the impairment of erythroblast proliferation. It is therefore possible that the ultrastructural abnormalities affecting the nuclear envelope may also arise as a consequence of an abnormality in nuclear protein, possibly leading to a change in the normal interaction between nuclear proteins and the nuclear membrane. Cytokinetic studies (Queisser et al. 1971) as well as spectrophotometric analysis (Meuret et al. 1972) have also suggested an underlying disturbance in nuclear protein synthesis, which leads to abnormal mitotic divisions.

The biochemical analysis of CDA type I erythroblasts and erythrocytes has been limited to date. Gel electrophoretic analysis of red cell membrane proteins detected no anomalies to CDA type I (Anselstetter et al. 1977; Alloisio et al. 1982), which is in contrast to CDA type II. In summary, presently existing data on CDA type I suggest that this disease is caused by a defect in the nuclear membrane or nuclear protein.

CONGENITAL DYSERYTHROPOIETIC ANEMIA TYPE II (HEMPAS)

Congenital dyserythropoietic anemia type II is also an autosomal-recessive disorder and is the most common CDA. Patients with CDA type II suffer from a lifelong but in most cases mild anemia (Crookston et al. 1969; Verwilghen et al. 1973). They show various other symptoms, such as hemosiderosis, secondary tissue cirrhosis, and gallstones. Although hemosiderosis is also seen in other anemias, the magnitude of iron overload and frequency of liver cirrosis in CDA type II are remarkable (Faruqui et al. 1982; Halpern et al. 1985; Bird et al. 1987). In severe cases, widening of the diploe of the skull, consequent abnormal facies, and mental and sensory abnormalities have been recorded (Verwilghen et al. 1973).

MORPHOLOGIC OBSERVATIONS

The bone marrow of patients with CDA type II shows erythroid hyperplasia. Up to one third of the late erythroblasts are bi- or multinucleated, while early erythroblasts are relatively normal (Fresco 1981). Karyotype and chromosomal banding from CDA type II did not show chromosomal inversions, deletions, or translocations (Roodman et al. 1982). Multinuclearity is believed to have resulted from the failure of cell division. Electron microscopic examinations demonstrated nuclear changes similar to some of those found in CDA type I. There is uneven condensation of chromatin, with extensive contact of the noncondensed chromatin to the nuclear envelope. In contrast to CDA type I, there is no penetration of the cytoplasmic components into the nuclear region. Therefore, the nuclear envelope and nuclear pores appear to be normal.

One feature that was considered unique to CDA type II is the so-called double membrane effect, which is a linear structure running parallel to and beneath the plasma membranes of erythroblasts and erythrocytes (Hug et al. 1972). The second kind of membrane is clearly not a duplication of plasma membrane (Fukuda et al. 1987b) and can also be seen in erythroblasts from patients with other congenital and acquired anemias (Frisch et al. 1974). Therefore, this morphologic feature is not necessarily specific to the CDA type II condition.

SEROLOGIC CHARACTERISTICS

Congenital dyserythropoietic anemia type II has also been called HEMPAS, since this disease was characterized as *h*ereditary *e*rythroblastic *m*ultinuclearity *a*ssociated with a *p*ositive *a*cidified *s*erum lysis test (Crookston et al. 1969). HEMPAS red cells give a positive acidified serum lysis test when cells are mixed with sera from about 30 percent of normal individuals, while the patient's own serum does not have such activity. Presumably, HEMPAS red cells have a HEMPAS antigen, and some normal sera contain anti-HEMPAS IgM alloantibody. There are, however, CDA type II cases that are negative in the acidified serum lysis test (Boogaerts and Verwilghen 1982). The biochemical nature of the HEMPAS antigen is not known.

Red cells from patients with HEMPAS are agglutinated strongly by anti-i antibodies as well as anti-I antibodies (Verwilghen et al. 1973). I/i antigens are carbohydrate antigens determined by branched (I antigen) and linear (i antigen) N-acetyllactosamine repeating structures (Hakomori 1981). The I/i-antigen carbohydrates attach to band 3 and band 4.5 glycoproteins as well as to ceramide on the red cell surface. Red cells from normal adults express I antigen, and red cells from fetuses express i antigen (Marsh 1961). The developmental change of I/i antigens correlates to the structural change from linear to branched polylactosamines of red cell glycoproteins and glycolipids. Red cells from patients with HEMPAS are, however, strongly positive for both I and i antigens. It is known that the red cells from severe anemias such as thalassemia contain fetal-type (i-active) red cells owing to the bone marrow stress (Giblett and Crookston 1964). However, i-active red cells appearing in patients with thalassemia account for a subpopulation of the red cells, in contrast to HEMPAS. The elevation of the I/i antigens is universally seen in all HEMPAS red cells. The i antigen is also increased in red cells from HEMPAS heterozygotes (parents or children of patients with HEMPAS); otherwise, they cannot be distinguished from normal red cells. The appearance of i antigen is a useful diagnostic marker for identifying a HEMPAS heterozygote (Verwilghen et al. 1973).

BIOCHEMICAL ANALYSIS

In 1977, Anselstetter and associates found that band 3 glycoproteins from CDA type II (HEMPAS) red cells migrate faster than those from normal controls upon sodium dodecyl sulfate–polyacrylamide gel electrophoresis

(SDS-PAGE). This characteristic of HEMPAS band 3 has been well documented since then (Alloisio et al. 1982; Baines et al. 1982; Fukuda et al. 1984c, see Fig. 13.1). Such a shift in the molecular weight of membrane proteins is not detected in red cells from normal individuals or from patients with other hematologic disorders. Proteolytic cleavage study of HEMPAS band 3 showed no sign of deletion of the peptide segment; thus, the decrease of molecular weight appeared to be the result of an underglycosylation of this protein (Baines et al. 1982). Decreased glycosylation of band 3 and band 4.5 glycoproteins was demonstrated by cell-surface labeling and chemical carbohydrate analysis (Scartezzini et al. 1982; Fukuda et al. 1984c; Mawby et al. 1983; Zdebska et al. 1987).

In normal red cells, band 3 and band 4.5 glycoproteins are glycosylated by polylactosaminoglycans, whereas in HEMPAS red cells these glycoproteins are glycosylated by truncated short oligosaccharides (Fukuda et

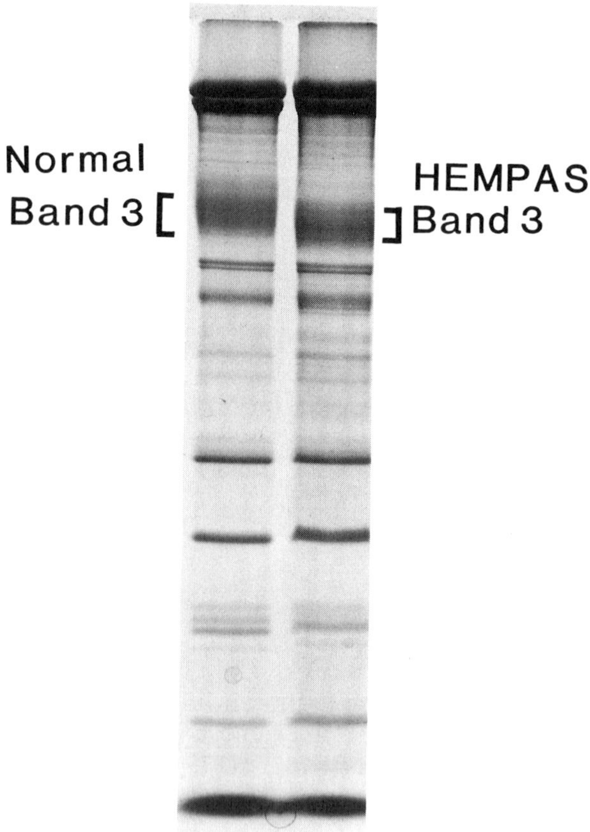

Figure 13.1. SDS-PAGE of red cell membrane proteins. Note that band 3 glycoprotein from CDA type II HEMPAS migrates slightly faster than that from normal red cell membranes.

al. 1987a, 1990). Furthermore, the polylactosamines appear in a 30- to 40-kDa region as new molecular species (Fukuda et al. 1984c). These polylactosamine components, characteristic for HEMPAS red cells, have been identified as polylactosaminyl-ceramides (Fukuda et al. 1986a; Zdebska et al. 1987). Increases in the amounts of lactosylceramide, lacto-N-triaosylceramide, and lacto-N-*neo*tetraosylceramide in HEMPAS red cells were noticed earlier (Joseph and Gockerman 1975), which is consistent with an increase of polyglycosylceramides in HEMPAS. Thus it appears that a genetic factor of HEMPAS blocks the polylactosamine formation on proteins and shifts the polylactosamines to the lipid acceptors (Fig. 13.2).

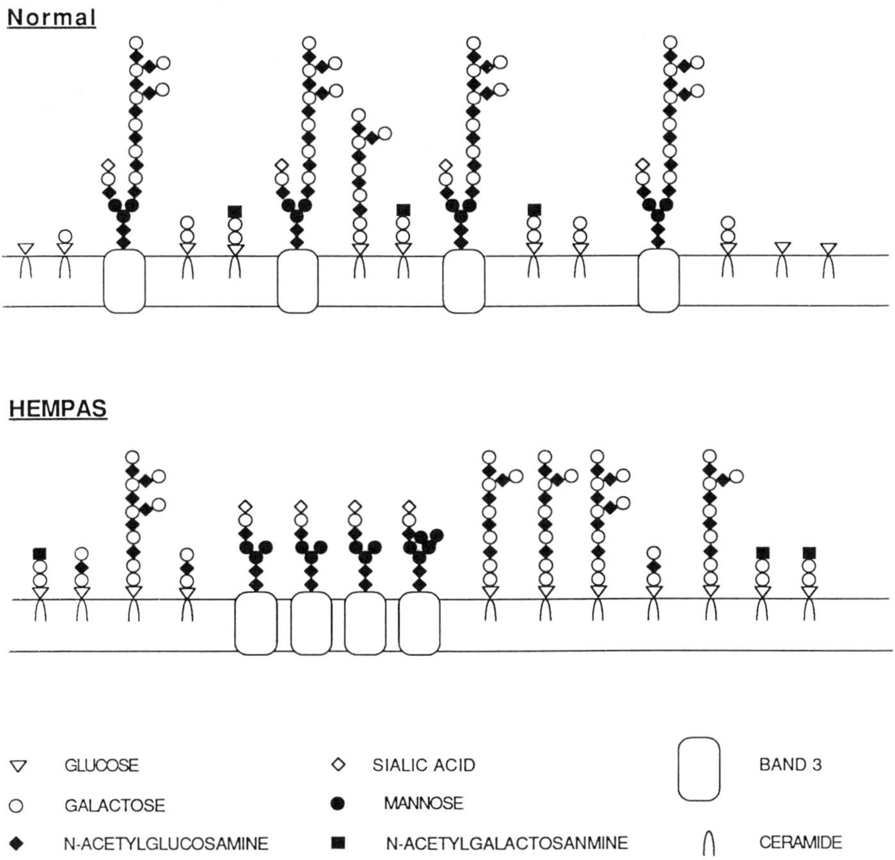

Figure 13.2. Glycoproteins and glycolipids in normal and HEMPAS red cell membranes. In normal red cells, band 3 is glycosylated by a large carbohydrate, polylactosaminoglycan. However, in HEMPAS red cells, polylactosamines attach to lipid acceptor, and band 3 contains truncated oligosaccharides. Underglycosylated band 3's cluster in HEMPAS red cell membranes, resulting in macroscopic membrane disorganization. (*Source:* Adapted from Fukuda et al. 1989.)

THE PRIMARY GENE DEFECT OF HEMPAS

A clue to the primary defect of HEMPAS was obtained by structural analysis of band 3 carbohydrates isolated from HEMPAS red cells (Fukuda et al. 1987a). Before this analysis, carbohydrate structures of normal adult and fetal band 3 glycoproteins had been extensively analyzed (Fukuda et al. 1984a, 1984b), which enabled us to compare the band 3 carbohydrate structures between normal and HEMPAS red cells. Band 3 from normal red cells has a large carbohydrate chain, composed of a biantennary trimannosyl core with polylactosamine side chains. In contrast, band 3 from HEMPAS red cells revealed truncated hybrid type structures (see Fig. 13.2). This evidence, together with the lowered activity of N-acetylglucosaminyltransferase II (GnT II) in some HEMPAS cases (Fukuda et al. 1987a) and low activity of α-mannosidase II (α-MII) in another HEMPAS case (Fukuda et al. 1990), suggests that the primary enzyme deficiency of HEMPAS is in GnT II or α-MII (Fig. 13.3).

A HEMPAS case (G.C.) has been identified as being defective in the α-MII gene (Fukuda et al. 1990). HEMPAS G.C. cells demonstrated a

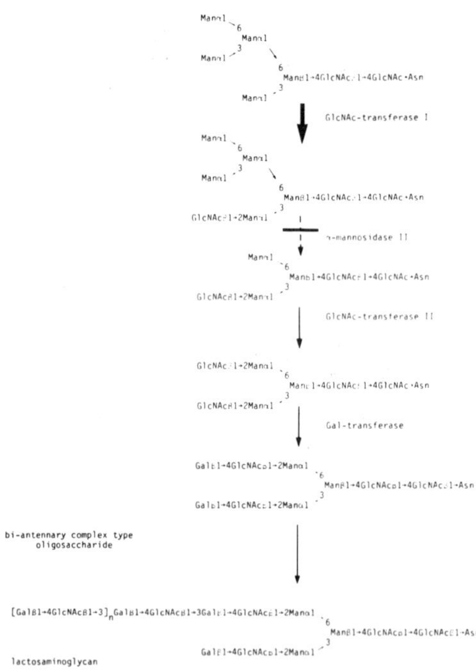

Figure 13.3. Biosynthesis steps of Asn-linked oligosaccharides. Nascent proteins receive high-mannose oligosaccharide en bloc in the endoplasmic reticulum. The high-mannose oligosaccharides are processed to trimannosyl core oligosaccharide in *cis* and medial Golgi, and then matured to complex-type and further to polylactosaminoglycans in *trans* Golgi. The genetic defect of α-MII (or GnT II) blocks the processing of Asn-linked oligosaccharides, resulting in incomplete synthesis of polylactosaminoglycans on proteins.

normal level of GnT I, GnT II, and galactosyltransferase (GT) activities but a low α-MII activity. Low expression of α-MII mRNA was then demonstrated by Northern RNA blot. Poly(A)+mRNA from HEMPAS G.C. cells shows less than 10 percent of normal level of α-MII mRNA (Fig. 13.4). Since no abnormal RNA species are detected in poly(A)+mRNA as well as in total RNA, the most likely defect of G.C.'s α-MII gene is a mutation in its promoter region, resulting in inefficient transcription. Isolation and nucleotide sequencing of the α-MII gene from HEMPAS G.C. may define the genetic defect of α-MII that occurred in this patient. Presently it is not clear whether HEMPAS is a genetically heterogeneous collection of glycosylation deficiencies or a genetically homogeneous defect with heterogeneous expression. The cDNA for GnT II has not yet been isolated, so it remains uncertain whether HEMPAS cases with low GnT II activity truly are defective in GnT II gene.

VARIANTS

Besides typical patients with HEMPAS, variants have been reported (Boogaerts and Verwilghen 1982). Several HEMPAS variants are negative in the acidified serum lysis test, and thus apparently lack the HEMPAS

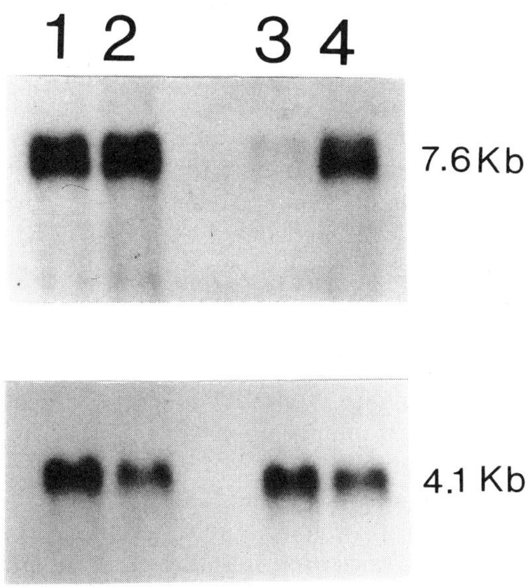

Figure 13.4. A Northern blot of poly(A)+mRNA from normal controls and patients with HEMPAS. Upper panel: poly(A)+mRNA was hydridized with a cDNA probe for α-MII. Lower panel: the same filter was rehybridized with a cDNA probe for GT. HEMPAS patient B.S. (lane 1), B.R. (lane 2), G.C. (lane 3), and normal control (lane 4). (*Source:* Adapted from Fukuda et al. 1990.)

antigen (Vermylen et al. 1986; Dvilansky et al. 1974). Some variants showed ultrastructural abnormalities not only in erythroid cells but also in granulocytes and/or platelets (Vermylen et al. 1986; Lowenthal et al. 1980). Variants with nuclear abnormalities, an anomaly known to be characteristic to CDA type I, have also been reported (Seip et al. 1975; Weiss et al. 1975; Bethlenfalvay et al. 1985). Some of the variants may be merely a reflection of the extreme manifestation of HEMPAS defect. The magnitude of illness and variation of phenotype probably depend on the mutation, such as a specific point mutation or deletion. Patients with HEMPAS associated with other genetic and nongenetic factors may result in phenotypes unusual to HEMPAS. HEMPAS cases have been reported with defective glucose-6-phosphate dehydrogenase (Ventura et al. 1984), transient autoantibody to Rh D antigen (Krikler et al. 1984), and a rare Kell phenotype (Lowenthal et al. 1980).

HEMPAS variant G.K. was analyzed extensively (Lowenthal et al. 1980; Harlow and Lowenthal 1982; Fukuda et al. 1989). The red cells of variant G.K. were negative in the acidified serum lysis test. The I/i antigens were positive, but were not as strong as typical HEMPAS red cells. The patient suffered from anemia and hemosiderosis. Atypical to HEMPAS, patient G.K. had severe gout and showed deformation of his joints. Although independent to the HEMPAS gene defect, G.K.'s red cells belong to the rare phenotype Kp^b. His bone marrow showed a high incidence of multinucleated erythroblasts. The examination by electron microscopy showed membrane duplication not only in erythroblasts but also in granulocytes and platelets. Cell-surface labeling showed a striking difference from other HEMPAS red cells: G.K.'s red cells virtually lack polylactosamines either on proteins or on lipids. Enzyme activity assay then showed only 24 percent of the normal galactosyltransferase (GT) activity in his microsome membranes, while his serum exhibited concomitantly high GT activity. It was speculated then that G.K. has a defective GT. The keratansulfate level in G.K. was unusually low, which is consistent with the low GT activity in his cells.

Cloning of cDNAs encoding human GT shows that human GT is a type II membrane protein made of 400 amino acids (Masri et al. 1988). Only one hydrophobic domain is present near the NH_2 terminus, which functions as both signal and membrane-anchoring domain. The GT gene from variant G.K. was amplified by polymerase chain reaction (PCR) using his genomic DNA as a template. The nucleotide sequence of the amplified DNA, however, revealed no mutation in exon 1 of G.K.'s GT gene, which contains the translation initiation site, membrane-anchoring domain, and proteolytic cleavage site (Fukuda and Masri, unpublished data). The reduced level of membrane-bound form GT in G.K. therefore cannot be explained by the mutation in the membrane-anchoring domain or proteolytic cleavage site of GT gene. Since G.K.'s red cells contain high mannose-type oligosaccharides, possible gene defects in Golgi α-MII and other glycosylation enzymes remain to be investigated.

THE LINK BETWEEN THE PRIMARY GENE DEFECT AND DISEASED PHENOTYPES

Band 3 is the major intrinsic protein of red cell membranes, constituting up to 30 percent of the total membrane proteins. The lack of the large carbohydrate moiety from HEMPAS band 3 increases the hydrophobicity of this protein. Immunoelectron microscopy and freeze-fracture electron microscopy demonstrated clustering of band 3 molecules in HEMPAS red cell membranes (Fukuda et al. 1986b). In HEMPAS reticulocytes, band 3 molecules are seen as single gold particles, while the clustering pattern of band 3 was demonstrated in both immature and mature red cells. These observations suggest that the clustering process takes place inside the young red cells at the time that the intracellular membrane systems disappear.

The cytoplasmic domain of band 3 provides a binding site for several other proteins. The clustering of band 3 may result in the abnormal localization of associated proteins and lipids. For example, the association to spectrin through ankyrin should be considered one of the factors for the irregularly contracted shape of HEMPAS red cells. It is likely that the clustering of band 3 molecules results in an irregular network of membrane skeletons. If so, such red cells would easily be deformed.

Multinuclearity seen in HEMPAS erythroblasts may be a consequence of defective glycosylation of membrane proteins. During the maturation of erythroblasts, I/i antigens (polylactosamines) increase in the late erythroblast stage (Fukuda et al. 1981). In the erythroblasts, the membrane glycoprotein(s) may be abnormally distributed if polylactosamine formation on proteins is blocked, which may result in the disturbance of their normal functions, such as cell division.

Red cell polylactosaminoglycans are unique because they have a biantennary core structure (Fukuda et al. 1984a, 1984b). Polylactosamines are preferentially attached to one of the arms (see Figs. 13.2 and 13.3). A lowered activity of α-MII (or GnT II) may result in the drastic failure of polylactosaminoglycan formation in red cell glycoproteins.

In many cells other than red cells, polylactosamines have tri- and tetraantennary core structures. For example, the majority of polylactosaminoglycans from granulocytes, teratocarcinoma cells, and lymphoma cells attach to tetraantennary cores. In these cells, low α-MII (or GnT II) activity does not necessarily inhibit polylactosamine formation on proteins. Such differences in core structures must be responsible for the apparently erythroid-specific manifestation of the HEMPAS defect.

Besides anemia, HEMPAS is associated with liver cirrhosis and secondary tissue siderosis (Crookston et al. 1969; Faruqui et al. 1982; Halpern et al. 1985; Bird et al 1987). It is likely that the primary gene defect of the glycosylation enzyme affects liver cells. In fact, incompletely processed Asn-linked glycans have been detected in HEMPAS patients' serum glycoproteins (Fukuda et al., unpublished data), of which the majority are synthesized in the hepatocytes and secreted into the circulation. The serum glycoproteins with truncated oligosaccharides would be recognized by lectin-like receptors on the surface of hepatocytes and the Kupffer cells, and also by the macrophages in the reticuloendothelial system. The quantity of serum glycoproteins to be cleared from circulation through these systems is enormous and could eventually cause cirrhosis and siderosis in patients with HEMPAS.

A high incidence of diabetes and gallstones may be linked to the primary gene defect of glycosylation enzymes. Further study is necessary to define whether abnormal glycosylation induces autoimmunity of pancreas cells and triggers diabetes, or whether abnormal glycosylation increases the risk of gallstones.

On the other hand, many tissues and organs apparently are unaffected by the HEMPAS condition. In many tissues and organs, altered carbohydrates may not necessarily cause ill effects. In baby hamster kidney mutant cell lines that are defective in α-MII and GnT II, no noticeable cellular anomaly is detected (Gleeson et al. 1985; Hughes and Feeney 1986). Since patients with HEMPAS apparently develop normally throughout the embryonic stages, the presence of developmental stage-specific isozymes should be considered. The GT isozyme, GT-2, is known to be expressed in the human fetus (Nozawa et al. 1990). Interestingly, the anemia of two siblings with HEMPAS improved after they developed large mediastinal masses contiguous with the vertebral bodies (Lugassy et al. 1986). In these paravertebral extramedullary masses (presumably a benign tumor), normal red cells are produced and correct HEMPAS anemia. It seems possible that an embryonic isozyme is expressed in the paravertebral mass.

CONGENITAL DYSERYTHROPOIETIC ANEMIA TYPE III

Congenital dyserythropoietic anemia type III is the rarest of the three types of CDA. It is characterized by (1) a macrocytic anemia that is detected during infancy or childhood; (2) an abnormality of erythroblast proliferation that results in the formation of many binucleated and multinucleated erythroblasts and giant mono- or multinucleated erythroblasts; and (3) a marked erythroid hyperplasia in bone marrow due to an ineffective erythropoiesis (Wolff and Von Hofe 1951; Bergströn and Jacobson 1962; Goudsmit et al. 1972). Family studies on CDA type III established autosomal-dominant inheritance of this disease (Goudsmit et al. 1977; Bergströn and Jacobson 1962). Lymphocytes from patients with CDA type III were found not to have abnormal chromosomal banding patterns (Björksten et al. 1978). The ultrastructure of bone marrow granulocytes and megakaryocytes appeared normal. Erythropoietic cells in the early stages of differentiation also appeared normal. In late erythroblasts, giant and multinucleated erythroblasts are seen with incomplete separation of nuclei between two erythroblasts. The nuclear membranes are disrupted. Clefts and blebs were detected in nuclear membranes.

Nuclear envelope anomalies in CDA type III erythroblasts are distinct from those of the CDA type I. In CDA type I there is loss of the nuclear envelope, "spongy" appearance of the chromatin, cytoplasmic connections between cells, and cytoplasm and/or cytoplasmic organelles within nuclear regions. None of these features is detected in CDA type III. Clefts and blebs within the nuclear region are more frequent in CDA type III than in CDA type I. Clefts and blebs are detected in CDA type I, but only in early erythroblasts or pre-erythroblasts. Common to CDA type I and III erythroblasts, they contain myelin figures, mitochondria filled with electron-dense material (presumably deposits of iron), and autolytic areas within the cytoplasm. Autophagic vacuoles and siderosomes were more often found in CDA type III than in type I.

The nucleus of CDA type III erythroblasts showed hyperdiploid DNA content (Wickramasinghe and Goudsmit 1979). Quantitation of DNA by ^{3}H-thymidine incorporation and Feulgen microspectrophotometry revealed that some mono- and multinucleated erythroblasts had a total DNA content two to 20 times higher than normal. In multinucleated erythroblasts, only some of the nuclei within the same cell incorporated ^{3}H-thymidine. Individual nuclei within the same cell had differences in diameter, shape, and DNA content. The nuclei that failed to synthesize DNA always showed abnormal morphology in the electron micrographs, such as abnormally dense heterochromatin or euchromatin, or degenerating nuclei with a Swiss cheese appearance.

Incorporation of ^{3}H-uridine and ^{3}H-leucine visualized by autoradiography demonstrated that cells with ultrastructurally abnormal nuclei failed to synthesize RNA or protein. Such erythroblasts are usually surrounded by bone marrow macrophages and are undergoing phagocytosis.

UNCLASSIFIED CONGENITAL DYSERYTHROPOIETIC ANEMIAS

Several reported cases do not fit into the three types of CDA (Boogaerts and Verwilghen 1982; Sansone 1978). Ohisalo and colleagues (1988) described a new CDA patient whose inheritance was apparently dominant. Further, this female patient showed numerous anomalies and at the age of 37 died of hemolysis and hemochromatosis. She had shown jaundice since the age of 8 months but was otherwise healthy. Her serum ferritin level and iron turnover rate were higher than normal, her liver showed no sign of cirrhosis, and her red cells showed no anomaly in glycosylation. The acidified serum test was positive, but the sera, which showed positive lysis to HEMPAS red cells, did not lyse this patient's red cells. Agglutination by anti-i was negative. These observations excluded CDA type II (HEMPAS). The nuclei of her erythroblasts showed morphologic anomalies, such as nuclear membrane budding, and numerous punched-out areas of heterochromatin. The reported case is apparently a heterozygote of CDA that may be related to CDA type III, judging by the dominant inheritance and nuclear abnormality.

Pothier and colleagues (1987) analyzed unclassified CDA red cells. The patient's blood showed macrocytes and red cells with basophilic stippling. Acidified serum test and i antigen were negative; thus, CDA type II (HEMPAS) was excluded. SDS-PAGE analysis of the red cell membrane proteins demonstrated 96, 82, 68, and 67 kDa bands. These bands also exist in normal membranes and cytosol in very low quantities. Identification of the aberrant peptides was attempted by proteolytic digestion of membrane proteins and by immunoblotting using antibodies to spectrin, band 3, band 4.1, band 4.5, and serum albumin. However, the analysis did not identify the origin of the peptides. The reason for the increased abundance of these peptides remains unknown, but similar biochemical analyses may be productively used in future cases of CDA.

Bird and associates (1986) described CDA type IV showing a morphology very similar to HEMPAS but without the double membranes. The acidified serum lysis test was negative and nuclear chromatin changes typical of CDA type I were not detected in this case. The patient developed a marked peripheral erythroblastosis after splenectomy and her anemia improved.

Carter and associates (1989) reported a CDA variant who was born from first-cousin parents. The mother's seven pregnancies had either ended in spontaneous abortion or were uneventful. The mother gave birth to two infants who were hydropic and died in infancy. A female child described in the report was noted to be pale and hydropic at birth, with hepatosplenomegaly. She has been dependent on transfusions. Her bone marrow shows multinucleated erythroblasts. Electron microscopy showed various ultrastructure abnormalities, including large autophagic vacuoles, irregular nuclear outlines, intranuclear clefts, and karyorrhexis.

An unusual type of CDA with thalassemia features of Kurdish Jewish origin was reported (Berrebi and Nir 1978). A male patient's red cells showed a positive acidified serum lysis test, but the i antigen was negative. Ultrastructural studies showed irregular nuclear envelopes, perinuclear cisternae, and the intrusion of cytoplasmic material into the nucleus. Thus this patient shows features of both CDA type I and CDA type II (HEMPAS). Similarly, CDA cases that show features of both CDA types I and II have been reported by Vermylen (1986) and Weiss (1975) and their associates.

FUTURE RESEARCH

The most important objective of research on CDA is to identify the primary gene defects. We obtained a clue for CDA type II HEMPAS, in which the α-MII gene is probably defective (Fukuda et al. 1990). Determination of the gene defects is needed at the nucleotide sequence level in each CDA type II cases. Information on the gene defect will allow us to test heterozygotes in each HEMPAS family. Future development of gene therapy may also be applied to the HEMPAS disease.

Biochemical analysis of nuclear proteins and nuclear membranes from CDA types I and III should be carried out in the near future. Basic information about nuclear proteins and nuclear membranes is still limited. However, analysis of CDA types I and III should contribute to the understanding of the normal and pathogenic roles of nuclear proteins. Also, as the red cell has proved to be an excellent model for biochemical and cell biologic investigation, with particular relevance in human genetic diseases, the investigation of abnormal membrane polypeptides in CDA red cells may provide significant insight.

REFERENCES

Alloisio, N., P. Jaccoud, E. Dorleac, L. Morle, N. Philippe, G. Margueritte, P. A. Bryon, and J. Delaunay. 1982. Alteration of globin chain synthesis and of red cell membrane proteins in congenital dyserythropoietic anemia I and II. *Pediatr. Res.* 16:1016–21.

Anselstetter, V., H.-J. Horstmann, and H. Heimpel. 1977. Congenital dyserythropoietic anaemia, type I and II: Aberrant pattern of erythrocyte membrane proteins in CDAII, as revealed by two-dimensional polyacrylamide gel electrophoresis. *Br. J. Haematol.* 35:209–15.

Baines, A. J., J. P. S. Banga, W. B. Gratzer, D. C. Linchi, and E. R. Huehns. 1982. Red cell membrane protein anomalies in congenital dyserythropoietic anemia, type II (HEMPAS). *Br. J. Haematol.* 50:563–74.

Bergströn, I., and L. Jacobson. 1962. Hereditary benign erythroreticulosis. *Blood* 19:296–303.

Berrebi, A., and E. Nir. 1978. An unusual type of congenital dyserythropoietic anemia with thalassemia features. *Isr. J. Med. Sci.* 14:1135–37.

Bethlenfalvay, N. C., C. S. Hadnagy, and H. Heimpel. 1985. Unclassified type of congenital dyserythropoietic anaemia (CDA) with prominent peripheral erythroblastosis. *Br. J. Haematol.* 60:541–50.

Bird, A. R., P. Jacobs, and P. Moores. 1987. Congenital dyserythropoietic anemia (type II) presenting with haemosiderosis. *Acta Haematol.* 78:33–36.

Bird, A. R., C. D. Karabus, and P. S. Hartley. 1986. Unclassified type of congenital dyserythropoietic anemia (CDA) with prominent peripheral erythroblasts. *Br. J. Haematol.* 63:797–98.

Björksten, B., G. Holmgren, R. Roos, and R. Stenling. 1978. Congenital dyserythropoietic anaemia type III: An electron microscopic study. *Br. J. Haematol.* 38:37–42.

Boogaerts, M. A., and R. L. Verwilghen. 1982. Variants of congenital dyserythropoietic anemia: An update. *Haematologia* 15:211–19.

Carter, C., P. J. Darbyshire, and S. N. Wickramashinghe. 1989. A congenital dyserythropoietic anaemia variant presenting as hydrops fetalis. *Br. J. Haematol.* 72:289–90.

Crookston, J. H., M. C. Crookston, K. L. Burnie, W. H. Francombe, J. V. Dacie, J. A. Davis, and S. M. Lewis. 1969. Hereditary erythroblastic multinuclearity associated with a positive acidified-serum test: A typical congenital dyserythropoietic anaemia. *Br. J. Haematol.* 17:11–26.

Dvilansky, A., S. Sukenik, J. Stern, and M. Djaldetti. 1974. Congenital dyserythropoietic anemia with ultrastructure findings compatible with both types I and II. *Acta Haematol.* 53:161–68.

Faruqui, S., A. Abraham, M. R. Berenfeld, and T. G. Gabuzda. 1982. Normal serum ferritin level in a patient with HEMPAS syndrome and iron overload. *Am. J. Clin. Pathol.* 78:97–101.

Fresco, R. 1981. Electron microscopy in the diagnosis of the bone marrow disorders of the erythroid series. *Semin. Hematol.* 18:279–92.

Frisch, B., S. M. Lewis, and D. Sherman. 1974. The ultrastructure of dyserythropoiesis in aplastic anemia. *Br. J. Haematol.* 29:545–52.

Fukuda, M. N., B. Bothner, P. Scartezzini, and A. Dell. 1986a. Isolation and characterization of poly-N-acetyllactosaminylceramides accumulated in the erythrocytes of congenital dyserythropoietic anemia type II patients. *Chem. Phys. Lipids* 42:185–97.

Fukuda, M., A. Dell, and M. N. Fukuda. 1984a. Structure of fetal lactosaminoglycan: The carbohydrate moiety of band 3 isolated from human umbilical cord erythrocytes. *J. Biol. Chem.* 259:4782–91.

Fukuda, M., A. Dell, J. E. Oates, and M. N. Fukuda. 1984b. Structure of branched lactosaminoglycans, the carbohydrate moiety of band 3 isolated from adult human erythrocytes. *J. Biol. Chem.* 259:8260–73.

Fukuda, M. N., A. Dell, and P. Scartezzini. 1987a. Primary defect of congenital dyserythropoietic anemia type II: Failure in glycosylation of erythrocyte lactosaminoglycan proteins caused by lowered N-acetylglucosaminyltransferase II. *J. Biol. Chem.* 262:7195–7206.

Fukuda, M., M. N. Fukuda, T. Papayannopoulou, and S. Hakomori. 1981. Membrane differentiation in human erythroid cells: Unique profiles of cell surface glycoproteins expressed in erythroblasts in culture and K562 human leukemic cells. In *Hemoglobins in development and differentiation.* G. Stamatoyannopoulos and A. W. Nienhuis, eds. 433–41. New York, Alan R Liss.

Fukuda, M. N., G. Klier, and P. Scartezzini. 1986b. Anomalous clustering of underglycosylated band 3 in erythrocytes and their precursor cells in congenital dyserythropoietic anemia type II. *Blood* 68:521–29.

———. 1987b. Congenital dyserythropoietic anaemia type II (HEMPAS): Characterization of aberrant intracellular organelles by immunogold electron microscopy. *Br. J. Haematol.* 67:95–101.

Fukuda, M. N., K. A. Masri, A. Dell, L. Luzzatto, and K. W. Moremen. 1990. Incomplete synthesis of N-glycans in congenital dyserythropoietic anemia type II (HEMPAS) caused by a defect in the gene encoding α-mannosidase II. *Proc. Natl. Acad. Sci. U.S.A.* 87:7443–47.

Fukuda, M. N., K. A. Masri, A. Dell, E. J.-M. Thonar, G. Klier, and R. M. Lowenthal. 1989. Defective glycosylation of erythrocyte membrane glycoconjugates in a variant of congenital dyserythropoietic anemia type II. *Blood* 73:1331–39.

Fukuda, M. N., T. Papayannopoulou, E. C. Gordon-Smith, H. Rochant, and U. Testa. 1984c. Defect in glycosylation of erythrocyte membrane proteins in congenital dyserythropoietic anaemia type II (HEMPAS). *Br. J. Haematol.* 56:55–68.

Giblett, E. R., and M. C. Crookston. 1964. Agglutinability of red cells by anti-i in patients with thalassemia major and other haematological disorders. *Nature* 201:1138–39.

Gleeson, P. A., J. Feeney, and R. C. Hughes. 1985. Structures of N-glycans of a Ricin-resistant mutant of baby hamster kidney cells: Synthesis of high-mannose and hybrid N-glycans. *Biochemistry* 24:493–503.

Goudsmit, R. 1977. Congenital dyserythropoietic anemia type III. In *Dyserythropoiesis.* S. M. Lewis and R. L. Verwilghen, eds 83. New York, Academic Press.

Hakomori, S. 1981. Blood group ABH and Ii antigens of human erythrocytes: Chemistry polymorphism and their developmental change. *Semin. Hematol.* 18:39–62.

Halpern, Z., R. Rahmani, and Y. Levo. 1985. Severe hemochromatosis: The predominant clinical manifestation of congenital dyserythropoietic anemia type II. *Acta Haematol.* 74:178–80.

Harlow, R. W. H., and R. M. Lowenthal. 1982. Erythrocyte membrane proteins in an usual case of congenital dyserythropoietic anaemia type II (CDA II). *Br. J. Haematol.* 50:35–41.

Heimpel, H., J. Forteza-Vila, W. Queisser, and E. Spiertz. 1971. Electron and light microscopic study of the erythroblasts of patients with congenital dyserythropoietic anemia. *Blood* 37:299–310.

Heimpel, H., and F. Wendt. 1968. Congenital dyserythropoietic anaemia with karyorrhexis and multinuclearity of erythroblasts. *Helv. Med. Acta* 34:103–15.

Hiraoka, A., Y. Kanayama, T. Yonezawa, T. Kitani, S. Tarui, and P. H. Hashimoto. 1983. Congenital dyserythropoietic anemia type I: A freeze-fracture and thin section electron microscopic study. *Blut* 46:329–38.

Hug, C., K. Y. Wong, and B. C. Lampkin. 1972. Congenital dyserythropoietic anemia type II: Ultrastructure of erythroid cells and hepatocytes. *Lab. Invest.* 26;11–21.

Hughes, R. C., and J. Feeney. 1986. Ricin-resistant mutants of baby-hamster-kidney cells deficient in α-mannosidase II–catalyzed processing of asparagine-linked oligosaccharides *Eur. J. Biochem.* 158:227–37.

Joseph, K. C., and J. P. Gockerman. 1975. Accumulation of glycolipids containing N-acetylglucosamine in erythrocyte stroma of patients with congenital dyserythropoietic anemia type II (HEMPAS). *Biochem. Biophys. Res. Commun.* 65:146–51.

Krikler, S. H., D. J. Ferguson, J. J. Akabutu, and C. G. Lomas. 1984. Transient anti-D in an Rh-positive patient with congenital dyserythropoietic anemia type II. *Transfusion* 24:169–70.

Lewis, S. M., D. A. Nelson, and C. S. Pitcher. 1972. Clinical and ultrastructural aspects of congenital dyserythropoietic anemia type I. *Br. J. Haematol.* 23:113–19.

Lowenthal, R. M., K. A. Marsden, C. L. Dewar, and G. R. Thompson. 1980. Congenital dyserythropoietic anaemia (CDA) with severe gout, rare Kell phenotype and erythrocyte, granulocyte and platelet reduplication: A new variant of CDA type II. *Br. J. Haematol.* 44:211–20.

Lugassy, G., J. Michaeli, N. Harats, E. Libson, and E. A. Rachmilewitz. 1986. Paravertebral extramedullary hematopoiesis associated with improvement of anemia in congenital dyserythropoietic anemia type II. *Am. J. Hematol.* 22:295–300.

Marsh, W. L. 1961. Anti-i: Cold antibody defining Ii relationship in human red cells. *Br. J. Haematol.* 7:200–209.

Masri, K. A., H. E. Appert, and M. N. Fukuda. 1988. Identification of the full-length coding sequence for human galactosyltransferase (β-N-acetylglucosamine: B1,4-galactosyltransferase). *Biochem. Biophys. Res. Commun.* 157:657–63.

Mawby, W. J., M. J. A. Tanner, D. J. Anstee, and J. R. Clamp. 1983. Incomplete glycosylation of erythrocyte membrane proteins in congenital dyserythropoietic anaemia type II (CDAII). *Br. J. Haematol.* 55:357–68.

Meuret, G., P. Tschan, G. Schlüter, D. G. Keyserlinck, and I. Boll. 1972. DNA-, histone-, RNA-, hemoglobin- content and DNA synthesis in erythroblasts in a case of congenital dyserythropoietic anemia type I. *Blut* 24:32–41.

Mori, P. G., F. Favareto, A. Achenone, A. C. Molinari, E. Boeri, L. Massimo, R. Bandelloni, and G. Sansone. 1986. Congenital dyserythropoietic anemia type I. *Acta Haematol.* 75:219–23.

Nozawa, S., M. Yajima, T. Sakuma, Y. Udagawa, K. Kiguchi, M. Sakayori, S. Narisawa, R. Iizuka, and M. Uemura. 1990. Cancer-associated galactosyltransferase as a new tumor marker for ovarian clear cell carcinoma. *Cancer Res.* 50:754–59.

Ohisalo, J. J., J. Viitala, R. Lintula, and T. Ruutn. 1988. A new congenital dyserthropoietic anemia. *Br. J. Haematol.* 68:111–14.

Pothier, B., L. Morle, N. Alloisio, M. T. Ducluzeau, C. Feo, D. Blanchard, J.-P. Cartron, M. Garbarz, I. Chaveroche, P. Boivin, J. Favre-Gilly, and J. Delaunay. 1987. Aberrant pattern of red cell membrane and cytosolic proteins in a case of congenital dyserythropoietic anemia. *Br. J. Haematol.* 66:393–400.

Queisser, W., E. Spiertz, E. Jost, and H. Heimpel. 1971. Proliferation disturbances of erythroblasts in congenital dyserythropoietic anemia type I and II. *Acta Haematol.* 45:65–76.

Roodman, G. D., C. N. Clare, and G. Mills. 1982. Congenital dyserythropoietic anaemia type II (CDA-II): Chromosomal banding studies and adherent cell effects on erythroid colony (CFU-E) and burst (P.FU-E) formation. *Br. J. Haematol.* 50:499–507.

Sansone, G. 1978. A new type of congenital dyserythropoietic anemia. *Br. J. Haematol.* 39:537–43.

Scartezzini, P., G. L. Forni, M. Baldi, C. Izzo, and G. Sansone. 1982. Decreased glycosylation of band 3 and band 4.5 glycoproteins of erythrocyte membrane in congenital dyserythropoietic anaemia type II. *Br. J. Haematol.* 51:569–76.

Seip, M., S. Skrede, K. S. Bjerve, T. Novig, and P. I. Gaarder. 1975. Congenital dyserythropoietic anaemia with features of both type I and type II. *Scand. J. Haematol.* 15:272–86.

Ventura, A., F. Panizon, M. R. Soranzo, G. Veneziano, G. Sansone, U. Testa, and L. Luzzatto. 1984. Congenital dyserythropoietic anemia type II associated with a new type of G6PD deficiency (G6PD Gabrovizza). *Acta Haematol.* 71:227–34.

Vermylen, C., J. M. Scheiff, J. Rodhain, J. Ninane, and G. Cornu. 1986. A variant of the congenital dyserythropoietic anemia type II with structural abnormalities in the granulocytic series. *Eur. J. Pediatr.* 145:232–35.

Verwilghen, R. L., S. M. Lewis, J. V. Dacie, and M. C. Crookston. 1973. HEMPAS: Congenital dyserythropoietic anaemia (type II). *Q. J. Med.* 42:257–78.

Weiss, S., U. Grafter, E. Van der Lijn, and M. Djaldetti. 1975. Congenital dyserythropoietic anemia with peculiar nuclear abnormality. *Scand. J. Haematol.* 15:261–71.

Wickramashinghe, S. N., and R. Goudsmit. 1979. Some aspects of the biology of multinucleate and giant mononucleate erythroblasts in a patient with CDA, type III. *Br. J. Haematol.* 41:485–95.

Wickramasinghe, S. N., and M. J. Pippard. 1986. Studies of erythroblast function in congenital dyserythropoietic anemia. type I: Evidence of impaired DNA, RNA, and protein synthesis and unbalanced globin chain synthesis in ultrastructurally abnormal cells. *J. Clin. Pathol.* 39:881–90.

Wolff, J. A., and F. H. Van Hofe. 1951. Familial erythroid multinuclearity. *Blood* 6:1274–83.

Zdebska, E., V. Anselstetter, T. Pacuszka, R. Krauze, A. Chelstowska, H. Heimpel, and J. Koscielak. 1987. Glycolipids and glycopeptides of red cell membranes in congenital dyserythropoietic anemia type II (CDAII). *Br. J. Haematol.* 66:385–91.

INDEX